Quantum pharmacology

Second edition

W. G. Richards, MA, DPhil (Oxon), CChem, FRSC
Lecturer in Physical Chemistry, Oxford University, and Fellow of Brasenose College

Butterworths
London . Boston . Singapore . Sydney . Wellington . Durban . Toronto

First published 1977
Second edition, 1983

© **Butterworth & Co (Publishers) Ltd. 1983**

British Library Cataloguing in Publication Data

Richards, W. G.
  Quantum pharmacology.—2nd ed.
  1. Pharmacology   2. Quantum theory
  I. Title
  615′.19′00153012   RM103

  ISBN 0–408–70950–2

Filmset in Monophoto Times by Northumberland Press Ltd, Gateshead
Printed and Bound in Great Britain by Mackays of Chatham, Kent.

Preface to second edition

The guarded optimism of the first edition of this book has proved to be well justified. In the intervening five years many of the hopes and speculations have become reality. Many pharmaceutical companies now employ specialists using theoretical methods; graduate students with experience in this area are much in demand.

Sceptics used to ask the small body of practitioners to name the drug discovered by theory. Still there is no simple answer to that question, but there are many instances where theoretical calculations have made a significant contribution towards the development of novel active compounds. Evidence for this includes the naming of computational chemists on patents.

The process is accelerating, above all due to developments in the computing world. The day of the minicomputer is being followed by the era of the micro. The most recent microcomputers have the sort of computing power previously associated with expensive mainframe machines. The use of mini- and microcomputers obviates the need for professional operators and has removed the cost restriction which meant that only generously funded academic institutions could explore the field. In addition, the new generation of computer graphics devices, especially those incorporating colour, permit the results of theoretical calculation to be displayed in a readily assimilable form.

The range of problems being studied has expanded so that now one of the more active areas is the field of agrochemicals: herbicides, fungicides and pesticides. Improvements in theoretical methods as well as computers have permitted the study of larger and larger molecules and systems of molecules, to the extent that perhaps the most exciting current work is in the realm of enzyme binding sites. If ever a drug is found using almost solely theoretical methods, it is likely to be by the design of completely novel enzyme blockers.

The new edition follows the pattern of the original. Part I, a summary of molecular pharmacology, has been extensively rewritten. Part II, the summary of molecular quantum mechanics, has relatively minor changes. The third section, on applications, is almost entirely new. The bibliography which constitutes Part IV has been brought up to date to December 1981.

Many colleagues and former students have been of significant help in the revision but I must thank in particular Keith Davies, Graham Durant, Keith Heritage, George Jaroskiewicz and above all Hilary Little. Joy Johnson again typed the manuscript and drawings were done by David Kozlow, save for those produced using computer graphics by Keith Davies.

Preface to first edition

It is tempting to add a question mark to the title of this book. Even the generous-spirited may feel that it is premature to start applying the methods of molecular quantum mechanics to the problems of medicinal chemistry, while sceptics will certainly feel that pharmacology is far too complex to be clarified by purely theoretical calculations.

These doubtful views are not in line with the current state of either molecular pharmacology or molecular quantum mechanics. Both subjects have advanced to the point where the problems of one are susceptible to the methods of the other. A major factor which has prevented widespread application of quantum chemistry to medicinal chemistry has been the fact that very few people are experts in both disciplines. In general, medicinal chemists are trained as organic chemists, while quantum mechanicians are more at home with computers and algebra than with dose–response curves or nerve impulses.

The aim of this book is to enable the medicinal chemist and pharmacologist to appreciate enough of the methods and uses of molecular quantum mechanics to apply the techniques, and to show the theoretician who has the techniques available, what problems may be clarified by these methods.

The field is one of great complications with many major questions unanswered, so that it is important to proceed with caution. Unfortunately, merely running a molecular orbital calculation for a given molecule is so simple once one is shown how to use a standard computer program that some over-facile work has been published. This should not, however, compromise the whole subject. With care the contribution of theoretical methods can be illuminating and should stand alongside and complement the experimental structural methods such as X-ray diffraction and nuclear magnetic resonance.

The intention is that this book should serve as an introduction for two sets of experts into the field of the other, or a newcomer into both. The work is divided into four parts so that readers familiar with the content of one particular section can avoid it and find the rest of the topic complete. After giving a brief selective account of molecular pharmacology and molecular quantum mechanics, the applications of one to the other are treated in Part III. Finally, Part IV is a complete bibliography of the subject up to the end of 1976. In this way researchers new to the topic and stimulated to try out the techniques, which can be done with no previous background using generally available computer programs, will have available a complete account of all previous work.

In writing a book which crosses the boundaries between scientific disciplines one is dependent on help from friends and colleagues. The following people, listed alphabetically, gave me assistance either by discussion or by reading parts of the manuscript, but I must single out Dr Barrie Hesp of ICI Pharmaceuticals Division whose help and patience have been invaluable. I should like to express my appreciation to John Barltrop, David Beveridge, Alison Brading, Robin Ganellin, Keith Heritage, Stephen Moore and John Northup. I am also indebted to David Kozlow and Maria Weil who did the drawings and to Joy Johnson who typed the original manuscript.

Finally I should like to thank Butterworths whose generous fellowship enabled me to write this book in three of the world's loveliest and most stimulating locations.

Berkeley, Oxford, Stanford   W.G.R.

Contents

Introduction

The men of genius who developed quantum mechanics in the 1920s and 1930s predicted an end to experimental chemistry, suggesting that it would become merely a branch of applied mathematics. Those early hopes or fears have proved groundless. Despite the fact that, in principle, the solution of the Schrödinger wave equation contains all the answers, in practice experimental chemistry still thrives.

For a period of over thirty years the theoretical chemist had to be content with perfect solutions of equations for the hydrogen atom and approximate solutions for a narrow range of very small chemical entities such as the helium atom, the hydrogen molecular ion and daringly enough, the hydrogen molecule. If one reads some theoretical chemical journals, one could be forgiven for believing that these small systems remain the obsession of theoreticians. However, since about 1960 there has been a rapid qualitative and quantitative change; a change brought about not by theoretical advances but by the advent of increasingly powerful computers.

Using what are only crude brute-force mathematical techniques, the computer has enabled the theoretical chemist to solve an approximate form of the Schrödinger equation to an arbitrary level of accuracy for larger and larger molecular systems. There are now numerous examples where these theoretical calculations can produce more precise details of molecular properties than can experiment. Such calculations may be expensive in terms of computer time and one may question the intrinsic value of some of the calculations which are performed, but it is not open to question that at the present time the methods of molecular quantum mechanics are sufficiently sophisticated to answer questions of molecular physics. For example, the water molecule, H_2O, has a bond angle between the two OH bonds which may be computed to an accuracy beyond the measuring capacity of spectroscopy. The barrier to inversion of the ammonia molecule, NH_3, can be calculated to any desired accuracy if one takes enough care with the computation. Even a tiny energy difference such as that between the energy levels responsible for the radio-astronomical detection of CH has been calculated more accurately than laboratory experiment allows.

In many ways the problems of molecular physics in which one considers an *isolated molecular species* are solved. It may be preferable or cheaper to measure a molecular property, such as a bond length or dipole movement, than it is to calculate the value, but the calculation can be done. In this realm the calculation will be more useful when the experiment cannot be performed, perhaps because the molecular species cannot be synthesized or is unstable and short-lived under experimental conditions. The calculations treat the molecule as totally isolated in space. This is a reasonable approximation to the experimental situation pertaining in gas-phase spectroscopic studies or in interstellar space.

The molecules which are within the scope of the most accurate theoretical methods are only slightly smaller in terms of the number of atoms they contain than many of the molecules which are of key importance to molecular pharmacologists, such as neuro-transmitters or drugs. It is tempting then to use the same type of theoretical calculation to probe the questions to which the pharmacologist would like an answer.

Before yielding to this temptation, however, several very important extra qualifications and safeguards must be discussed. There are many aspects of pharmacology which must be stressed if the theoretical calculations are not to be so naive as to be ludicrous.

An obvious theoretical restriction is imposed by the fact that the interesting molecules are large by comparison with those handled confidently by theoretical chemists. This means that even if the more rigorous methods of calculating molecular wave functions are employed, then large amounts of computer time may be required. As an alternative, one of the more rapid but less reliable approximate methods may be used. It will become clear later when we discuss the problems in more detail that the substitution of approximate for more rigorous theoretical methods is even more likely to be necessary because we will be interested not in one single molecular entity, but in a series of compounds and furthermore a range of geometries, conformations and tautomeric or ionic forms of each. The necessity of doing a large number of calculations may force us to use the approximate or semi-empirical molecular orbital methods for the immediate future.

None of the semi-empirical or *ab initio* molecular orbital methods is sufficiently reliable for its predictions to be accepted without question. Thus a primary qualification on any theoretical calculation is that the results and predictions should be in accord with some measured physical property. The obvious experimental results which can be used to test the reasonableness of calculations are X-ray crystallographic data, n.m.r. solution conformation or dipole moments for charge distributions with, in some cases where the data are available, nuclear quadrupole resonance studies or neutron scattering results.

The theoretical calculations should be consistent with these experimental findings; not necessarily in perfect agreement, since it must be stressed yet again that the calculations refer in general to the isolated gas-phase molecule, while crystallography is performed on a solid form and n.m.r. most frequently on rather concentrated solutions.

Not one of these three environments is exactly appropriate to the situation where the molecule of interest is involved in a biological process in a living system. In such surroundings it may be in a lipid or aqueous phase with a protein surface and a variety of ions in the vicinity, and in an ionic form different from the most abundant species which is found in solution at so-called 'physiological' pH.

Much effort is being expended by theoreticians on the fascinating problem of just how water as a solvent affects the gas-phase molecule. This difficult and worthwhile problem will not, if solved, provide all the answers which would make the results of gas-phase calculations transferable to the biological situation.

The nature of the appropriate biological environment of a pharmacologically interesting molecule at the active moment is unknown. Consequently, the only way to make any progress in understanding is to do what is normally done in biological experiments when there are many variables, some of which are unknown, and one wishes to isolate the effect of a particular parameter. The normal practice is to do a lot of experiments and then to use statistics to highlight important and significant relationships between activities and parameters. This is quite different from the manner in which a physicist uses statistics. He tends to measure one thing knowing that all other variables are constant and statistics are only employed as a means of estimating the accuracy with which a single property has been measured as the result of a series of repetitive experiments.

The problem of the exact nature of the appropriate environment puts the theoretical chemists in exactly the same quandary as any medicinal chemist seeking a relationship between molecular structure and biological activity. We will of necessity have to consider a series of chemically similar molecules with a range of biological activities and seek a consistent theory which will explain the biological variation. The choice of such a series will be arbitrary within certain limits and only statistical support will be satisfactory if a convincing theory emerges.

Many calculations on single molecular species have been published as separate articles. These are not without interest and have proved helpful to experimentalists, but on their own they cannot logically provide a theoretical explanation of any form of activity. A set of calculations on a single molecule, which may supply, for example, a potential energy surface for the changing conformation of a flexible molecular species, ought to be considered as a sophisticated form of molecular model building rather than an end in itself.

Any medicinal chemist who has sought to understand the relationship between structure and activity will have found molecular models such as Dreiding models or the approximate space-filling CPK (Corey, Pauling, Kolthun) models profoundly illuminating. The models give a good indication of which molecular shapes of the small biological molecule are ruled out on atom–atom repulsion grounds. Whereas space-filling models represent atoms as shapes with hard edges, calculations provide 'soft-edges' in the form of a varying potential energy as one group of a molecule approaches another, rather than an 'on-off' indication at the point where hard edges touch.

At least in the field of small molecules no one has the effrontery to publish the results of playing around with molecular models, but the same cannot be said of those who perform calculations. Conformational calculations on single species are interesting but they must be insufficient to provide a theory of activity. A precise description of the molecular shape and charge distribution which is essential for activity can only come from the study of a series of compounds, preferably with each member of the series considered in a wide range of conformations of all possible ionic and tautomeric forms. The reliability of the theory can then be judged objectively by the number of compounds fitting the theory; confidence can be increased by adding test examples and the theory is capable of refutation or modification by means of further experiment.

For the theoretician, working in his own form of isolated environment, the desirability of working with a series of compounds and their activities presents a further problem. From where can he obtain the data? This may appear to be a ridiculous question when the pharmacological literature is full of lists of similar compounds with varying activities of one sort or another. However, as we will discuss later, the pharmacologist has many problems in producing data on biological activities because of the number of possible variables. Much published work refers to experiments on live animals (*in vivo* experiments) where such variables as the weight, age or sex of the animal may be significant, as may factors such as absorption and metabolism. Even experiments on tissues or parts of living systems (*in vitro* experiments) may be crucially dependent on the precise way in which the experiment has been performed. It is a great trap for a theoretician with a background in physical science to treat published biological data as he would published physical measurements. Data on the same problem from different sources may not be comparable. In the experience of the author the safest and most satisfactory way of dealing with this problem is to work directly with the organic chemists who are making the molecules and in collaboration with the pharmacologists who are making the biological measurements. This may mean that the ideal collaboration is with the research group of a pharmaceutical company and in the experience of the author few collaborations have ever proved so stimulating or scientifically beneficial.

With so many cautionary words it is perhaps necessary to state clearly why, if there are so many hazards, it still seems timely to apply the methods of theoretical chemistry to pharmacology, apart from the desire of scientists in a pure and relatively esoteric field to tackle problems of obvious importance and, dare one say it, relevance. There are a number of reasons ranging from the pure to the practical and even commercial.

Firstly, there may be factors of importance which cannot be discovered in any other way than by calculation. Structures measured by crystallographers or n.m.r. spectroscopists are used in considerations of structure and activity but, apart from the obvious fact of the environmental effect, there is no logical reason to suppose that a small molecule performs its functions in the biological context while in the stable shape adopted in the solid state or in bulk solution. Indeed in many areas of physical biochemistry, induced changes of conformation on binding of one molecular species to another are an essential feature. Satisfactory calculations should indicate not only which forms of a molecule are likely to be possible crystal structures or solution structures (and these are frequently not identical even for simple molecules) but also the whole range of possible shapes within any given energy above the most stable form. Detailed use of calculations may indicate a precise non-equilibrium form which is a prerequisite for activity, or the barriers to interconversion of one metastable form to another and approximate rate constants for the transition. In this way, the theoretical calculations are a complementary and possibly essential addition to experimental structural studies. If we consider the conformational potential energy of a molecule as represented on a map with energy contours, then, if we neglect environmental perturbations, the X-ray data will provide a single point on the surface probably corresponding to the lowest point; n.m.r. will provide details of areas of the map surrounding any minimum deep enough to provide a sizeable population of conformers in an equilibrium situation, while theoretical calculations can, with care, provide full details of the whole map, the peaks and slopes as well as the valleys.

Another advantage of calculations is that they are capable of producing not only the energy of the molecule for a given configuration of the constituent atoms, but also any molecular property either of the entire molecule or more importantly at localized points within the molecule. Much effort in the realm of structure–activity work consists of correlating activity with measured bulk-molecular properties. Theoretical calculations offer the possibility of correlating not just a property of the whole molecule, such as dipole moment, but rather the charge on particular atoms or any other sub-molecular property.

Of all the many properties of a molecule which may be computed from a quantum mechanical calculation perhaps the most widely useful is the electronic distribution or the potential field which electrons and nuclei generate. The chemistry and biological activity of molecules must ultimately be explicable in terms of the behaviour of electrons. Until very recently the only drawback to the use of this fundamental information has been the difficulty of displaying the information in a comprehensible manner. The growth of sophisticated computer graphics systems has removed the dilemma and promises to provide a major stimulus to the use of quantum mechanical methods.

Once calculations have proved that they can yield a satisfactory explanation of activity, then a third potential advantage becomes apparent. The calculations may be performed without first synthesizing the molecule. Thus, if there is confidence in the calculations, they can then be run before the organic chemist does his synthetic work and the pharmacologist his testing. Ideally, this would greatly reduce the number of molecules synthesized and screened by removing the ones which are unlikely to be interesting. This state of affairs is only dawning, but if achieved would make the work of the organic chemist more stimulating as he would have to design specific properties into the smaller number of molecules he was making. It would also have the commercial attraction of reducing the number of compounds synthesized and screened in the search for more effective drugs.

Although the problems involved are far from simple, it does seem that there is every advantage in applying quantum mechanics to pharmacological problems. Quantum mechanics is particularly appropriate as it can tell us in a fairly direct way about the density of electrons in molecules. It must be remembered that atomic nuclei just provide a framework on which to hang varying electron densities. When a small molecule approaches the active site of a receptor molecule it is the varying charge density of the two species which will interact. If loose terminology may be applied, the receptor 'sees' a structured cloud of electron density, not a set of point atoms.

It is perhaps presumptuous but illuminating to try to define the question to which the pharmacologist and medicinal chemist would like an answer. They would like to know 'what is the precise three-dimensional electron density adopted by an active molecule at the instant it performs its essential role?' Molecular quantum mechanics may be the best means of providing an answer.

Part I

Molecular pharmacology

Chapter 1

Small molecules in biology

The success of molecular biology has convinced almost everyone that biology is in principle ultimately explicable in molecular terms. It is obvious that biological structures are based on proteins, nucleic acids, polysaccharides, lipids and other polymeric organic molecules. Strangely enough, in many respects these huge molecular species involving many thousands of atoms are better understood than the small molecules with only perhaps about twenty atoms which are also of great importance in biology, even if present in tiny quantities.

The chief role of the small molecule is in control systems. Even with plants the use of small molecules in control is obvious and demonstrable. Hormones are frequently small molecules. Very small quantities may dramatically affect growth or behaviour, not only in plants but also in human beings. The reproductive cycle in women, for example, is controlled by steroid hormones released into the blood stream. Hormones provide slow response and long-lasting control since the 'message' in the form of a molecular substance is carried in the blood and takes some time to reach all areas of the living system. Its effect lasts for as long as there are hormone molecules present. For the higher organisms rapid response and control are provided by the nervous system. The body is far more than a set of functioning structures. It can detect changes affecting it and reacts by readjusting itself. Nerve cells are not indefinitely long conductors like wires, but have discrete lengths. The connection between nerve cells and between nerves and the muscles they control is of a chemical nature. These chemicals, or *neuro-transmitters*, are small molecules which again are highly potent in the sense that injection of very small amounts into a living system can have a dramatic effect.

Much of pharmacology is concerned with the study of the mode of action of these various neuro-transmitters, and molecular pharmacology attempts to define the role of the transmitter in molecular terms.

Some molecules synthesized by the organic chemist and usually similar to the naturally occurring active molecule but not found in the living system will, when injected, produce a similar effect to the natural compound possibly by acting in its place. Such molecules, along with the naturally occurring molecules, are referred to as *agonists*.

The theory of the mode of action of small molecules in biological control

3

which we will discuss in more detail later involves the interaction between the small molecule and a macromolecule with a specific active site. That is, the small molecule, perhaps a neuro-transmitter or synthetic agonist, interacts with a *receptor*. Some synthetic non-natural molecules may bind to the same receptor as a naturally active molecule in such a way that the receptor is blocked and the natural transmitter is rendered ineffective. Such blocking molecules are called *antagonists*. Antagonists may bind in exactly the same or similar manner as the molecule which they are preventing from acting or may have their effect as a result of some other interference with the natural process. In the next chapter we will consider this in more detail.

Drugs include both agonists and antagonists which produce a result which is clinically desirable in a given instance, such as the lowering of blood pressure or increase of heart-rate.

Molecular pharmacology is at its most advanced state when consideration is focused on the role of a particular molecule in a biological mechanism in which the nature of the small molecule is highly specific: minute changes in chemical structure give enormous changes in biological activity. Other active molecules have low specificity or seem to have an effect based on physical properties, such as colligative properties, rather than chemical structure.

For the latter case, the explanation of activity is not as precisely molecular as in the cases where binding between the small molecule and the receptor produces the ultimate observed reaction. For this reason we will discuss mostly the cases where receptor ideas seem to be most well-founded, considering first of all the nervous system.

Nerves

The nervous system consists of a network of *nerves*. Some can transmit messages about the detection of stimuli to the brain and are called *sensory nerves*; others working in the opposite direction, carrying the message which leads to some reaction, are called *motor nerves*. The message is in the form of an electrical impulse. A nerve is a collection of *nerve fibres* gathered together like the strands of an electric cable (*Figure 1.1*). Each nerve fibre

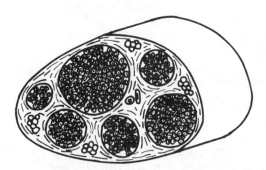

Figure 1.1. Cross section of a nerve trunk with individual nerve fibres grouped into six separate groups

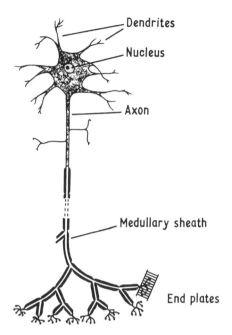

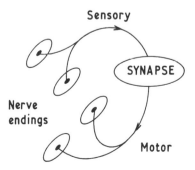

Figure 1.2. A nerve cell or neuron

or neuron is a single cell, with a cell body, and an elongated process, the *axon* (*Figure 1.2*).

The sensory nerves are stimulated to transmit an electrical impulse by some change in the environment of the peripheral nerve endings such as temperature, or a mechanical disturbance. The motor nerves carry the electrical impulse which initiates the mechanical response in the form of a muscle movement or change in the activity of an organ.

In more primitive forms of life a sensory nerve is connected directly with the corresponding motor nerve at a so-called *synapse* or junction (*Figure 1.3*). These synapses are also found in the nervous systems of higher creatures and above all in the brain. They are the site of action of many drugs.

If the sensory impulse is strong enough, the motor nerve is stimulated and the part of the animal disturbed is provoked into appropriate action.

In the vertebrates the sensory and motor impulses are coordinated within the *central nervous system* or CNS. This involves the brain and spinal cord.

Figure 1.3. Sensory and motor nerves connected via a synapse

The latter, which lies in the hollow parts of the vertebrae forming the spine, is continuous with the brain. The sensory and motor nerves join the cord at points between the spinal vertebrae, sensory nerves at the back and motor fibres at the front. The two types of nerve are often connected by short nerve cells which lie in the *grey matter* of the cord giving a *reflex arc* which permits an automatic reflex response similar to that of lower life although this may be overruled by higher control. The nerve cells are also connected with the brain via cells whose axons are in the *white matter* (*Figure 1.4*).

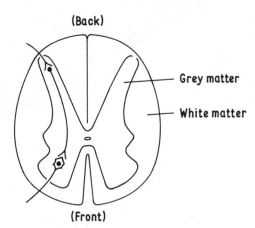

Figure 1.4. Nerve connections in the spinal cord

Cell Membranes

The cell membrane is not just a boundary but plays a vital part in the functioning of the cell. It is responsible for maintaining the chemical and structural integrity of the cell. It controls the movement of ions, nutrients, drugs and other molecules into and out of the cell. In addition it must be the membrane which first responds to external stimuli such as in the recognition of foreign substances or circulating hormones, and indeed during nerve transmission.

A schematic view of a cell membrane is given in *Figure 1.5*. As can be seen it is composed of a bilayer of phospholipid, containing a percentage of cholesterol surrounded on each side by protein molecules. Some proteins lie within the bilayer and some pass right through. Immediately on the outer surface of the cell are mucopolysaccharides which provide the recognition sites and which furnish a transition between the fatty lipid layers and the bulk aqueous phase outside the cell. In plants and bacteria the carbohydrate also has structural significance.

The proteins compose over half the membrane and are responsible for its functions. They are closely bound to the other molecules in the membrane and this binding is important in preserving the finer functions. The protein molecules control the movement of ions, which would not pass through the hydrophobic areas of the bilayer, by providing areas of polar environment.

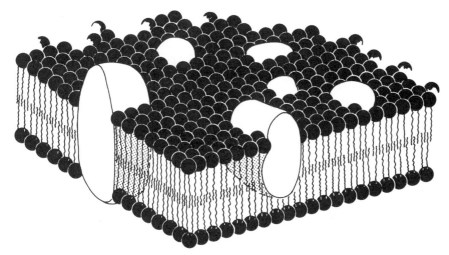

Figure 1.5. Schematic view of a cell membrane showing a lipid bilayer with protein molecules embedded in the matrix

These areas have been described as 'pores' or 'channels'. Alternatively they could take the form of 'carriers' but their exact form is uncertain. The active transport of ions, involving the use of energy is also carried out by the proteins.

Changes in ionic permeability form the basis of neuronal transmission, both in the conduction of action potentials along axons and at synapses. These changes are thought to be brought about by changes in protein conformation.

Action Potentials

When a nerve cell is at rest there is a potential difference between the inside and the outside of the cell amounting to about -90 mV owing to the fact that the concentration of sodium and potassium ions differs in the two environments. The resting nerve has a much higher permeability to K^+ than Na^+. There is a higher concentration of Na^+ than of K^+ outside the nerve cell and the converse is true inside. When a nerve impulse passes the cell

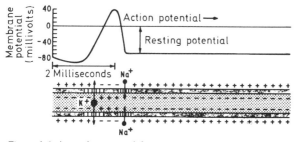

Figure 1.6. An action potential

becomes more permeable to Na^+ than K^+ and the sign of the concentration potential changes as illustrated in *Figure 1.6*. The so-called action potential is thus a propagation of the change in permeability of the cell membrane. It is an 'all or none' effect. A nerve either transmits the action potential or it does not. The response is not graded. The passing of the nervous message along a nerve cell thus corresponds to the movement of this action potential down the cell from one end to the other. When the message reaches a synapse at the end of the nerve the chemical neuro-transmitter is emitted.

The classification of nerves

We have so far distinguished sensory and motor nerves. Motor nerves, however, can be further classified. There are *voluntary* motor nerves which control limbs, for example, and which are operated at will. Frequently voluntary nerves are merely called motor nerves. The muscles used are of the *striated* or *skeletal* muscle type such as those in the arm.

At this level the other major motor nerves are the *autonomic* vegetative or involuntary nerves. These autonomic nerves primarily control organs such as the heart and uterus or blood vessels which are not operated at will, but maintain a stable internal environment or *homeostasis*.

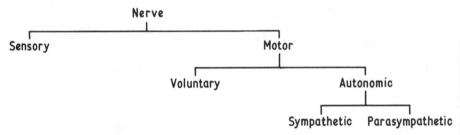

Figure 1.7. The classification of nerves

The organs of the body are doubly served by nerves giving a further subdivision of autonomic nerves into *sympathetic* and *parasympathetic* types. The divisions are summarized in *Figure 1.7* and *Table 1.1* shows the effect of sympathetic and parasympathetic stimulation on a few organs. The standard summary of this subdivision is to say that sympathetic stimulation prepares an animal for flight or fight and thus the expenditure of energy, while parasympathetic stimulation allows the body to undergo activity resulting in the conservation and restoration of energy.

Neuron structure and junctions

Like almost all living cells, the nerve cell consists of a membrane surrounding cellular material in which there is a nucleus. The nerve cell is differentiated from other types of cell by virtue of the fact that it is shaped like a long fibre and the nucleus only occupies a small percentage of the cell volume.

TABLE 1.1. Effects of stimulation of sympathetic and parasympathetic nerves on organs of the body

Organ	Sympathetic	Parasympathetic
Blood vessels	Constriction, except coronary vessels which are dilated	Usually nil
Heart	Acceleration and augmentation	Inhibition
Eye:		
Iris	Contraction of radial muscle	Contraction of circular muscle
Ciliary muscle	Nil	Contraction
Skin:		
Sweat secretion	Augmentation	Nil
Erection of hairs	Increased	Nil
Salivary glands	Slight secretion	Free secretion and vasodilatation
Stomach:		
Contractions	Inhibition	Augmentation
Secretions	—	Increase
Sphincters	Contraction or relaxation	Relaxation or contraction
Intestinal movements	Inhibition	Augmentation
Gall bladder	Relaxation	Contraction
Liver	Glycogenolysis	Nil
Spleen	Contraction	Nil
Pancreatic secretion	—	Increase
Bronchial muscles	Relaxation	Contraction
Bronchial secretion	Nil	Increase
Ureter	Relaxation	Contraction
Bladder:		
Fundus	Relaxation	Contraction
Sphincter	Contraction	Relaxation
Uterus	Contraction and relaxation	

The part surrounding the nucleus has many appendages called dendrites but only one fibre, the axon, which carries the impulses.

The nerve fibre is surrounded by a membrane and there may in addition be a sheath of the protein myelin which acts as an electrical insulator. Such nerves are said to be myelinated, or medullated.

Gaps between nerve cells are called synapses. Clusters of synapses which act as a sort of relay system in the peripheral nervous system are called *ganglia*. Ganglia are however more than mere gaps. At a synapse there is a specific structure where chemical transmission takes place.

The disposition of the ganglion with respect to the spinal cord and innervated organ or muscle depends on the type of nerve.

The structure of a sensory nerve is summarized in *Figure 1.8*. Such nerves

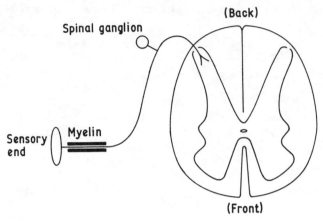

Figure 1.8. Structure of a sensory nerve

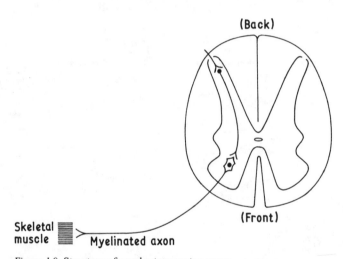

Figure 1.9. Structure of a voluntary motor nerve

are frequently myelinated. Voluntary nerves, which are also myelinated, run from their dendrites and nuclei in the anterior part of the cord to their peripheral termination (*Figure 1.9*).

There are distinct anatomical differences between the subdivisions of the autonomic nerves. The sympathetic nerves have a ganglion just outside the spinal cord (*Figure 1.10*).

The parasympathetic nerves have their ganglia very close to or even in the organ (*Figure 1.11*).

The two types of autonomic nerves leave the spinal cord at different and distinct points (*Figure 1.12*).

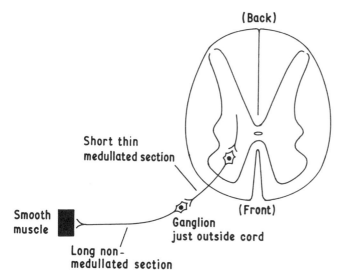

Figure 1.10 Structure of a sympathetic nerve

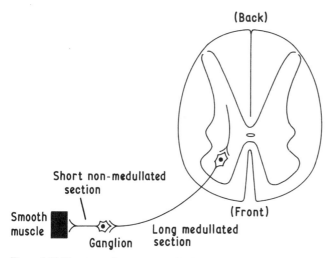

Figure 1.11 Structure of a parasympathetic nerve

Nerve transmitters

A point of key importance in this very complex topic is the manner in which the nerve impulse is passed across the synapses between the ends of nerves and the muscles they control and across synaptic gaps in ganglia. There is much variation in the size of synaptic gaps, particularly in the central nervous system. They may be of the order 200 to 500Å wide although in some cases they are thought to be as wide as 10000Å. These are extremely wide gaps if thought of in molecular terms.

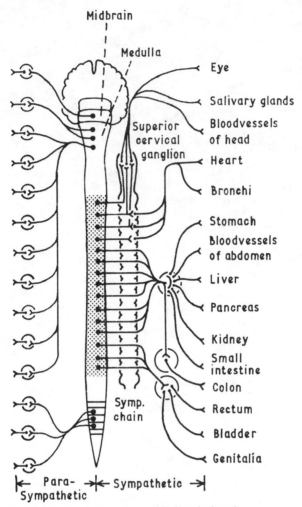

Midbrain

Medulla

Eye

Salivary glands

Superior
cervical
ganglion

Bloodvessels
of head

Heart

Bronchi

Stomach

Bloodvessels
of abdomen

Liver

Pancreas

Kidney

Small
intestine

Colon

Symp.
chain

Rectum

Bladder

Genitalia

|← Para- →|←— Sympathetic —→|
Sympathetic

Figure 1.12. Nerve connections with the spinal cord

After years of controversy it is now accepted that the transmission is chemical. That is, a chemical neuro-transmitter is released from one side of the gap, diffuses to the other side and causes some change in the second cell which propagates the impulse.

Combination of transmitter with sites on the post-synaptic membrane results in specific changes in the ionic conductance of the membrane in the post-synaptic region leading to local membrane potential changes. These changes lead to the next stage which may be triggering of action potentials, muscle contraction or glandular secretion, depending on the particular post-synaptic structure. The conductance changes which occur are different at each type of synapse and may involve various ions, for example, Na^+, K^+ or Cl^-. At the skeletal neuromuscular junctions and at the so-called nicotinic sites in ganglia the combination of acetylcholine results in an increase in the permeability of the membrane to Na^+ and K^+. The result is a depolarization as the ions move down their concentration gradients so that there is a reduction in the resting membrane potential. In other instances the binding of a transmitter produces an increase in Cl^- permeability or a decrease in K^+ conductance. The latter, which is thought to occur at some so-called muscarinic sites, also results in depolarization.

At other sites the action of the transmitter causes a hyperpolarization of the post-synaptic membrane and this decreases the excitability of the post-synaptic cell. Synapses where this takes place are known as inhibitory synapses. An example of a conductance change which can bring this about is the increase in K^+ permeability produced by noradrenaline in the intestine.

It is the existence of these chemical neuro-transmitters or neural hormones and the fact that they are small molecules which makes pharmacology a chemical subject in principle open to investigation based on quantum mechanics.

It is interesting to ponder as to why nature uses chemical transmitters. The reason probably arises from the fact that nervous conduction is an 'all or none' effect; the nerve passes a message or it does not do so and there is no variation in the strength of the message. An obvious method to convert from this digital response to a graded or analogue effect is to allow the nerves to emit a chemical at the ends; several nerves will produce chemicals whose total concentration can be summed at the receptors in the spinal cord. A finite number of receptors will ensure that there is a maximum possible effect of nervous stimulation and the system cannot be overloaded. Chemical transmission also provides the potential for interactions between various junctions and the possibility of feedback.

The actual identification of the transmitter substances is far from simple and not all those suggested have been proved convincingly to be such. The sort of evidence necessary to settle such an issue can be summarized as follows:

(1) If a substance is postulated as a transmitter, it should be liberated when a nerve is stimulated and not when it is not.
(2) There should be enzymes present capable of the synthesis of the molecule and some mechanism for its rapid removal.
(3) Injection at the appropriate site (neuromuscular junction or synapse) of the postulated transmitter should reproduce stimulation, especially in terms of conductance changes.
(4) If a blocking agent is available, then it should stop both natural stimulation and that provoked by injection of the putative transmitter.

The results of investigations along these lines for the gaps in the motor nerve system are summarized in *Figure 1.13*.

The voluntary motor nerve ending emits acetylcholine across the neuromuscular junction with skeletal muscle. Curare is an antagonist of this action and nicotine an agonist.

In the autonomic system all ganglia employ acetylcholine as the main transmitter both in parasympathetic and sympathetic nerves. Antagonists show slightly different action potential profiles from those at the skeletal muscle junction so that although receptors in the autonomic system are frequently called nicotinic receptors they are not identical to those involving voluntary muscles.

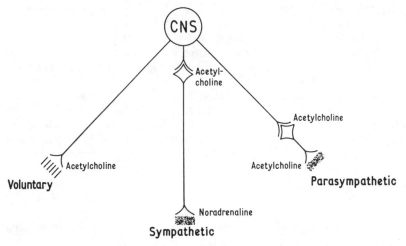

Figure 1.13. Chemical transmitters in the peripheral motor nervous system

An example of an antagonist of ganglionic transmission is hexamethonium. At the parasympathetic neuroeffector junction the transmitter is again acetylcholine although in this case the receptors are called 'muscarinic' as muscarine was found to act as an agonist at these sites. Antagonist action here is illustrated by atropine.

Sympathetic neuroeffector junctions use noradrenaline as the transmitter (norepinephrine in US terminology). Adrenaline will also have agonist actions at these sites. They are divided, on the basis of the actions of agonist and antagonist drugs into alpha- and beta-receptors. Examples of drugs with antagonist actions at these sites are phentolamine which acts at alpha-receptors and propranolol for the beta-receptors. All these details will be amplified in later chapters.

Synaptic actions of neuro-transmitters

It is in the synaptic gap between neurons or at the gap between nerve and muscle that transmission is by chemical agent so that it is on this process that the attention of molecular pharmacology must be directed. It is here that molecular interference with control systems is possible.

A crude outline of the essentials of transmission by acetylcholine is illustrated in *Figure 1.14*. Vesicles containing acetylcholine are present in the axon terminal. Stimulation of the nerve causes the release of the transmitter which diffuses across the gap causing a change in the post-junctional membrane permeability to Na^+ and K^-. The release requires the presence of Ca^{2+} and can be inhibited by Mg^{2+}. To ensure that the effect of acetylcholine release is only of brief duration the enzyme acetylcholinesterase is present to destroy the transmitter.

The binding of transmitter to the receptor causes the change in membrane ion permeability. The precise manner in which this is achieved is not yet

(a)

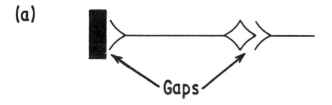

(b)

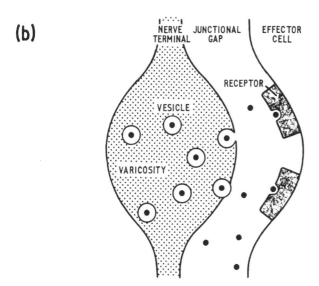

Figure 1.14. (a) Synaptic gaps across which nerve impulses are carried by chemical transmitters. (b) Enlarged view of the synaptic gap showing how the transmitter may be released from a vesicle to diffuse across the junctional gap and bind to a molecular receptor

proven but certainly cyclic nucleotides seem to be implicated in some instances. This is very important in current quantitative pharmacological studies. Presumably the binding of a transmitter (or an agonist) to the receptor causes the enzymes which synthesize cyclic adenosine monophosphate (cAMP) or cyclic guanosine monophosphate (cGMP) to produce cyclic nucleotides. The cyclic nucleotides regulate in turn a family of enzymes, the protein kinases which phosphorylate substrate proteins. The cyclic AMP protein kinase seems to be capable of regulating the synthesis of neuro-transmitter, and above all the actions of the protein which acts as an ion pump. The observed physiological effects of neuro-transmitters depend on the degree of phosphorylation of membrane proteins.

The effects of noradrenaline at some junctions between nerves and smooth muscle are mediated via the stimulation of the enzyme adenylate cyclase, which synthesizes cyclic AMP.

In the case of ganglia the role of cyclic nucleotides on neuronal function is more complicated but gives a high degree of control over the exact nature of the membrane potential produced in the post-synaptic membrane. Studies of the mammalian superior cervical sympathetic ganglion have implicated three types of receptor. The principal effect of acetylcholine release at the ganglion is to give a rapid excitatory potential in the post-synaptic membrane. The sum of several of these gives rise to an action potential. This is a normal nicotinic effect, blockable by hexamethonium. In addition there appears to be a muscarinic receptor, blockable by atropine leading to the production of cyclic GMP and ultimately producing a slow excitatory potential. Further, another muscarine receptor, blockable by atropine produces dopamine which via an interneuron and cyclic AMP produces a slow inhibitory potential. The combination makes for very fine control of the transmitted signal and conductance changes.

Receptors

The idea of a receptor grew from the extreme structural specificity demanded in agonists and antagonists. Even different stereoisomers of the same molecule have very different effects. Originally the model was described as a 'lock-and-key' mechanism. Considerations of molecule–molecule interactions in general, however, leave open or even promote the possibility that either the lock or key or both may be flexible and change shape when interacting. Whatever happens, the structural specificity required leaves the idea of a receptor, possibly a protein with a suitable binding site, as a useful hypothesis.

Returning to the question of what the pharmacologist and medicinal chemist would like to know, we may now rephrase our answer using the idea of a receptor. If the electronic density variation or, almost as useful, the atomic constituents and positions of the atoms in the active site of a particular receptor were known, then it would be much easier to design small molecules to fit and bind with the active site.

To this end much effort has been and is being expended to extract receptors, crystallize them and to look at their three-dimensional form in the solid phase. The work is fraught with difficulty. The density of receptors on a cell surface is not high and it is difficult to be sure just what constitutes a receptor. Nevertheless, much progress has been made and more can be expected although we are still left with the problem of knowing the nature of the receptor site in the working environment. The acetylcholine nicotinic receptor is the best characterized, being a four-subunit protein.

Because of the practical difficulty of isolating receptors and the unknowns remaining concerning its active environment a rather less direct means of characterizing the active site is normally employed. The receptor is studied by synthesizing a range of small molecules to interact with it and concentrating on possible relationships between the structure of the small molecule and the resulting biological activity. The nature of the receptor is thus inferred from the study of naturally occurring active molecules and their agonists

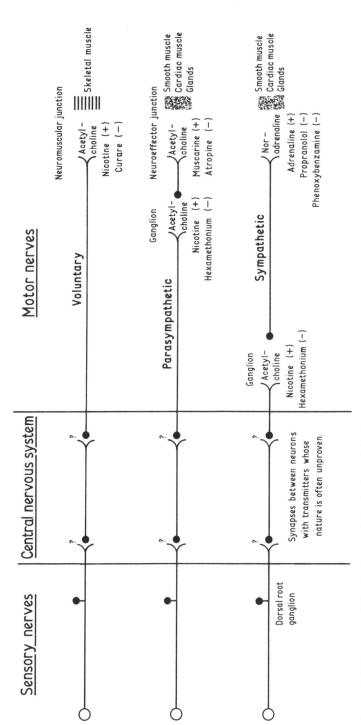

Figure 1.15. Summary of chemical transmission in the peripheral nervous system. Agonists are labelled (+) and antagonists (−)

and antagonists. This use of structure–activity relationships is a very indirect procedure but one which is forced upon us by the nature of the problem. It is, of course, fraught with complexity and possible false conclusions. As Oleg Jardetzky put it, 'it is like trying to decide on the beauty of a woman by looking at photographs of her husband'.

In practice however it is not quite so daunting a prospect. Rather than learning about a woman from details of her husband, the process, thanks to synthetic organic chemists, is much more akin to inferring the nature of a woman given details of several thousand lovers, some of whom were rejected but others accepted to a greater or lesser extent. It is possible to build up a fairly accurate impression.

Summary

The role of small molecules in biology is largely in control systems. Slow response or long-lasting control is achieved using hormones and rapid control by the nervous system. An essential part of nerve impulse transmission, that between cells, is chemical.

In the peripheral nervous system the transmitters are known and are summarized diagrammatically in *Figure 1.15* which also gives a typical agonist and antagonist for each type of junction.

The transmitter diffuses across synaptic or neuromuscular junction gaps and binds with a receptor molecule. The binding may trigger the production of cyclic AMP or cyclic GMP leading to control of the protein kinase enzyme systems which give rise to the observed biological effect of conductance change.

A large part of molecular pharmacology concentrates on the interaction of the neuro-transmitters, their agonists and antagonists, with the receptors. The receptor binding site is highly specific and can be studied by investigating the varying biological or biochemical response to a series of chemically similar substances.

Further reading

BARLOW, R. B. *Introduction to Chemical Pharmacology*, 2nd edn, Methuen, London (1964)
    Particularly strong on chemical aspects such as structure–activity relationships.
BOWMAN, W. O. and RAND, M. J. *Textbook of Pharmacology*, 2nd edn, Blackwells, Oxford (1980)
    A particularly good account of introductory physiology is included.
COTTRELL, G. A. and UNSHERWOOD, P. N. R. *Synapses*, Blackie and Son, Glasgow (1977)
GILMAN, A. G., GOODMAN, L. S. and GILMAN, A. (eds). *The Pharmacological Basis of Therapeutics*, 6th edn, Macmillan Publishing Co., New York (1980)
    Excellent reference work.
GOTH, A. *Medical Pharmacology: Principles and Concepts*, C. V. Mosby Co., St. Louis (1976)
    Links basic and clinical aspects.
KOROLKOVAS, A. *Essentials of Molecular Pharmacology*, Wiley–Interscience, New York (1970)
    Emphasizes molecular aspects.
KUTTLER, S. W. and NICHOLS, J. G. *From Neurone to Brain*, Sinauer, Sunderland, Mass. (1976)
MARTIN, A. R. *Synaptic transmission* in *MTP International Review of Science. Physiology Series I.* Vol 3 pp. 53–80
C. C. Hunt, (ed), Butterworths, London (1975)

Chapter 2

Quantitative pharmacology

Pharmacological measurements

It is very important for a clinician or a theoretician using data provided by a pharmacologist to be aware of the difficulties of pharmacological experimentation. The work is paradoxical in the sense that experimental tests are normally very sensitive but rather inaccurate. For example, it is quite possible using very simple techniques to detect the presence of 10^{-8}g of adrenaline in a solution but typical accuracy is the order of 10 per cent.

A commonly used experimental set-up for *in vitro* experiments is illustrated in *Figure 2.1*. The effect of adding a drug to the solution which surrounds the

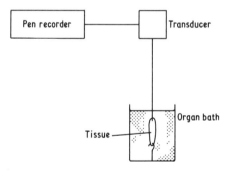

Figure 2.1. Experimental arrangement

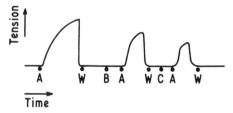

Figure 2.2. Effects of administered drugs on the tension of a strip of muscle. A = acetylcholine administered; W = drug washed out; B, C = drugs B or C administered

19

appropriate tissue is to cause a contraction which can be amplified and recorded either electronically or mechanically by means of a lever working a pen on moving chart-paper or, as was formerly common, a point marking the response on a smoked rotating drum (a kymograph).

Results are thus frequently produced in the form shown in *Figure 2.2*.

Responses

The effect produced by a given drug can be divided into two types. *Graded responses* are given, for example, when the contraction of a piece of smooth muscle is measured as a function of the dose of drug; anything between no contractions at all to the full contraction is possible. The results may be plotted either as dose–response curves or as log dose–response curves. *Figure 2.3* shows such curves for two substances (A and B) which can produce the same maximum response but the substance B requires higher doses. This type of log dose–response curve from *in vitro* experiments produces some of the most useful data for molecular pharmacologists.

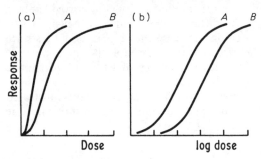

Figure 2.3. Dose–response and log dose–response curves

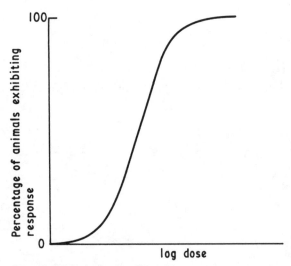

Figure 2.4. Log dose–percentage curve

When working on whole animals (*in vivo*) the response may be *all or none* or *quantal*. A test animal could be just alive or dead as a result of an injection or cured or not cured. Slightly less crude quantal responses have more divisions on the scale than merely binary possibilities but probably no more than four or five levels of observed response. The results of this type of experiment can be plotted as dose–percentage or log dose–percentage curves as in *Figure 2.4*.

From these so-called 'dose–percentage curves' it is frequently the case that a dose called the 'LD50' or the lethal dose for 50 per cent of a sample is defined: that dose which will kill 50 per cent of a test population of animals. The figure is much used in toxicological testing. Slightly less gruesome is a similarly defined ED50: the dose which is effective in some prescribed manner for 50 per cent of a population of test experiments.

For marketed drugs it is clearly desirable to have the LD50 and ED50 values of a compound to be as different as possible to avoid dangers associated with overdose. Thus the ratio LD50/ED50 is taken as the *therapeutic ratio*.

Dose–response curves

The dose–response curve plays a crucial role in molecular pharmacology since it is from these curves that the manner of activity is inferred and any theories of drug action at a molecular level have to be consistent with these primary measurements.

It is, of course, difficult to define the 'dose' with total precision and at the same time have a meaningful quantity. The quantity of a substance administered to a live animal bears only an indirect relationship to the number of molecules which may be in the receptor environment, because of problems caused by absorption, transport, permeability or metabolism of the chemical. Thus, isolated tissue measurements are preferred whenever possible.

Similarly the response, be it an increase in tension of a tissue, of blood pressure or of acid secretion, is only the end result of a complicated series of molecular events involving perhaps whole enzyme systems and complicated controls.

The basis of the interpretation of dose–response curves rests on the idea that in order to provoke a response the small molecule must bind to its specific receptor. In this binding process two factors are considered as

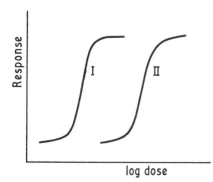

Figure 2.5. Compounds with equal intrinsic activities but differing affinities

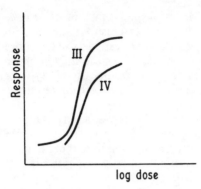

Figure 2.6. Compounds with nearly equal affinities but differing intrinsic activities

separate and essential features. Firstly, there is the *affinity* of the small molecule for the receptor binding site. Affinity is a measure of the binding free energy between the partners. The second factor is less easy to define even though qualitatively it is obvious that even for a given binding energy different molecules may produce effects of widely differing magnitudes. Ariens has called this second factor the *intrinsic activity* of the compound, while Stephenson has used the term *efficacy*. There is some confusion between intrinsic activity and efficacy in the literature. They are not synonymous, Stephenson's concept allowing for the possibility that a drug of high efficacy may give a maximal response when only a fraction of the total receptor population is occupied.

Figure 2.5 illustrates two dose–response curves for molecules I and II which have equal intrinsic activities (judged by having the same asymptotic limits) but the second compound is required in greater concentration and is judged

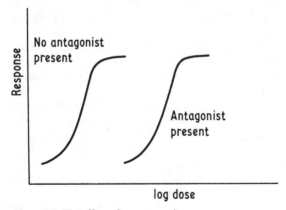

Figure 2.7. The effect of an antagonist

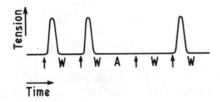

Figure 2.8. Effect of an antagonist on a response: at times indicated by the arrows a natural agonist is applied; W indicates washing out of compounds; antagonist is added at A

to have a lower affinity. The case of near equal affinities of compounds III and IV but differing efficacies is shown in *Figure 2.6*. Compound IV is said to be a *partial agonist*. Partial agonists have affinity and some efficacy but may antagonize the action of other drugs which have a higher efficacy.

Antagonists are thought of as compounds with appreciable affinities for the receptor binding site but with zero efficacy. If administered together with an active molecule, then the antagonist may compete for the available receptor sites so that higher concentrations of the active species are required (*Figure 2.7*). Administered alone they have no effect.

In terms of the experimental set-up described earlier (*Figure 2.2*), these distinctions might show up in the manner illustrated in *Figure 2.8*.

Direct binding studies

One of the most significant and encouraging developments in molecular pharmacology has been the recent introduction of truly molecular direct binding studies which can give affinities in terms of binding constants and activities in terms of cyclic nucleotide production, for example, rather than mere biological response.

If a compound of very high affinity for a receptor is available, radioactive molecules can bind to the receptor and be used to locate, identify and even count the receptor sites. For example, the nicotinic acetylcholine receptor in the electric organ of electric eels and torpedo can be characterized by the binding of radio-labelled polypeptide toxins which bind virtually irreversibly. For other receptors where a fortuitously available highly specific ligand is not known, the binding of more normal antagonists or even agonists can be studied although more care is needed. The labelled molecule may bind not only to the appropriate receptor but also to sites involved in transmitter uptake or storage or even to proteins in a non-specific manner. However the binding of transmitters has been investigated, not only for those involved in the peripheral nervous system but even for most of the postulated transmitters involved in the central nervous system.

The measurement of a small amount of specific binding in the presence of a lot of weak non-specific interactions may be made using labelled compounds of known stereochemistry and very high radioactivity. Preliminary experiments can indicate a suitable quantity of protein to use and settle upon a standard procedure for leaving the labelled compounds in contact with the binding material, separating the radioactivity bound to the protein from that free in solution (for example, by filtration or centrifugation), washing and measuring the remaining activity bound to protein with a scintillation counter. As an example we may consider the binding of opiates to their receptor which is stereospecific for molecules of *l* stereochemistry. First the binding of labelled [^{3}H] *l* opiate in the presence of excess of the unlabelled *d* isomer must be measured. Secondly the binding of the same labelled [^{3}H] *l* compound in excess of unlabelled *l* isomer is measured. Since the receptor is specific for the *l* isomer, the first experiment should reveal the total binding and the second provides the non-specific contribution. Subtraction of the second result from the first yields the true concentration of specifically bound compound and hence a truly molecular measure of affinity.

The necessity of having both d and l isomers can be avoided if preliminary experiments are performed to find a concentration of unlabelled compound which will saturate the small number of specific binding sites without reducing non-specific binding.

For example we may consider the measurement of the binding constant of agonists or antagonists to a particular receptor. The compound, x, in which we are interested, has to be available in a highly radioactive tritiated form. After preliminary experiments to establish the procedures to be used we must first measure the total counts as a function of the concentrations of added x, as in *Figure 2.9*, curve I.

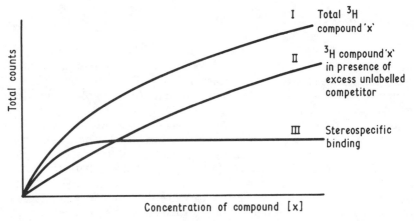

Figure 2.9. Direct binding studies

Curve I which increases indefinitely reveals the total binding, both specific and non-specific. Secondly (curve II), the experiment is repeated in the presence of the predetermined excess of a compound which will swamp the specific receptor binding sites, so that curve II indicates only the non-specific binding. The competitor which will occupy the specific high affinity sites may be a synthetic agonist or antagonist with a high affinity for the site, but experiments are even possible using the natural transmitters in this role since they do have strong affinity for the specific molecular receptor. Curve III is the difference between I and II and thus indicates the stereospecific binding curve from which the concentration of x required to half saturate the specific sites may be read. This concentration is directly related to the binding constant of x.

Once the binding characteristics of drug x have thus been determined the affinities of other related drugs for the binding site which the radioactive ligand x occupies can be found by measuring the displacement of radioactive x by increasing concentrations of the particular drug in question. Results for a typical series of experiments will resemble those shown in *Figure 2.10*. From the figure the IC50s (the concentration of drug at which specific binding is reduced by 50 per cent) can be determined and structure–activity relationships can be deduced.

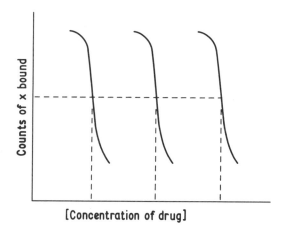

Figure 2.10. Displacement of radioactive compound
x by increasing concentrations of drug

Direct binding assays are now available for most receptors which will be encountered in the following chapters.

The experiments can be performed on whole cells but a cell-free system with only membrane present is probably more significant in molecular terms. Members of a series of compounds which bind at a particular receptor may be compared quantitatively by their ability to compete for the occupancy of sites.

In some direct binding studies where the neuro-transmitter acts by influencing the production of cyclic AMP the binding data may be supplemented by data for stimulation or competitive inhibition of adenylate cyclase present in the same membranes. Whereas the direct binding studies provide a measure of affinity, the intrinsic activity is revealed by the ability to stimulate adenylate cyclase.

In a number of instances there is a good correlation between molecular parameters derived from direct binding and more classical measures of activity from dose–response curves or clinical doses.

Theories of drug action

In any molecular topic there are essentially three modes of approach to understanding: the structural approach, the use of thermodynamics and the use of chemical kinetics. Of these three the structural method, a sort of molecular anatomy, has been the most powerful in molecular biology and is indeed the approach of this book. For complete understanding we would like to know exactly what is going on in molecular terms, as for example it is now possible to discuss the action of certain enzymes. However, for this best approach it is necessary to have a detailed knowledge of the structures of all the molecules involved. Clearly this is still not possible in the realm of pharmacology.

In consequence the less illuminating thermodynamic and kinetic methods have to be employed. These methods will not provide an explanation of events. Instead they can be used to test whether any hypothesis based on experimental observation is a possible mechanism. For drug action the only sets of data which can be taken as experimental facts are the dose–response curves. Thus 'theory of drug action' is a rather grand way of describing an hypothesis which is consistent with the known dose–response curves.

The shape of the simple non-logarithmic dose–response curve is so similar to the Langmuir adsorption isotherm used in heterogeneous catalysis that the obvious first simple theory introduced by Clark parallels simple adsorption ideas.

$$\text{Drug} + \text{Receptor} \rightleftharpoons \text{Complex} \rightarrow \text{Response}$$

The effect will increase as more receptor sites are occupied reaching a limit when they are saturated.

Developments of this basic idea have taken into account the experimental fact that at least in some systems all the accessible receptors need not be occupied to give a maximum response. This fact can be demonstrated by occupying some receptor sites with an irreversible blocking agent (an antagonist with very high affinity) and observing no decrease in maximal response.

There are two main variants on the extension of the simple Langmuir isotherm approach. Both start with a similar mechanism not unlike the enzyme substrate interaction.

$$\text{Drug} + \text{Receptor} \underset{k_{-1}}{\overset{k_1}{\rightleftharpoons}} \text{Complex} \underset{k_{-2}}{\overset{k_2}{\rightleftharpoons}} \ldots \text{Response}$$

The kinetic theory introduced by Paton hypothesizes that the rate of formation of complexes is the factor of importance. The occupation theory on the other hand gives importance to the number of drug–receptor complexes.

Experimentally it is hard to distinguish the two theories since both give plausible shapes for dose–response curves, although the rate theory does conveniently explain why some tissues are very insensitive immediately after treatment with a high dose of drug (tachyphylaxis).

Another phenomenon which theories have to explain is that of desensitization. This is often observed in studies with isolated tissues. Repeated applications of the same concentration of an agonist drug produce smaller responses as time progresses. This has been explained on occupation theory by postulating that a state of the receptor is produced where the drug is bound but does not produce its effect.

Desensitization occurs in a wide variety of systems and may in some instances involve changes in the receptor at sites other than the actual drug–receptor combining point. It is not certain how important the effect is physiologically but it could have a possible protective role.

Changes in receptor sensitivity can occur as circadian rhythms. It is also possible for receptor sensitivity to increase. For instance, if a nerve is cut then the terminal degenerates but the post-synaptic membrane which was enervated becomes more responsive to agonists. This example involves increased numbers of receptors, but it is also possible that changes in sensitivity not involving changes in receptor population can occur. These may play an important part in the actions of drugs which cause changes when administered over long periods.

Recent more elaborate theories of receptors have suggested that the proteins which control ionic conductance of the post-synaptic membrane may be naturally in equilibrium between two conformations, which have been called 'open' and 'closed' states. It is suggested that the action of the drug is to alter this equilibrium. This is in contrast to the simple occupation theory in which the binding of the drug to the receptor was said to cause conformational changes in the membrane. These theories have been elaborated to include evidence which suggests that in some cases more than one drug molecule may be required to produce each unit receptor change.

The actions of antagonists may not involve merely a simple blockade of agonist binding. Evidence for this is the fact that some antagonists have their effect altered by the presence of agonists and by the state of the membrane. This suggests that while some antagonists bind to the unactivated receptor as the simpler theory suggested, others bind to the membrane and alter the conductance change produced by the agonist. These have been called 'open-channel' blocking agents.

Clearly, while the simple occupation theory explained a considerable amount of the experimental evidence the detailed knowledge which is now accumulating is showing that the actions of drugs are far more complex than was first imagined.

It is probable that in reality there are aspects of both theories which are necessary for a full explanation. However, since plausibility of kinetic and thermodynamic schemes can only disprove a theory and never prove one, the most hopeful approach to understanding comes from the structural method. We would like to know what is going on at a molecular level and the combined forces of crystallography, magnetic resonance and theoretical calculations seem most likely to yield useful results.

Quantitative receptor theory

The simple occupation theory describes the combination between drug and receptor according to the law of mass action:

$$\text{drug} + \text{receptor} \underset{k_2}{\overset{k_1}{\rightleftharpoons}} \text{complex} \tag{1}$$
$$\text{with concentrations} \quad x \quad\quad 1-\theta \quad\quad\quad \theta$$

In this and the following equations: x denotes the concentration of agonist; y denotes the concentration of antagonist; x' denotes the concentration of agonist in the presence of antagonist; K_x is the equilibrium constant for agonist k_2/k_1; K is the equilibrium constant for antagonist; θ is the proportion of occupied receptors.

At equilibrium, from equation (1)

$$k_2\theta = k_1x(1-\theta)$$

whence

$$\theta = \frac{k_1x}{k_2 + k_1x} \tag{2}$$

$$= \frac{x}{x + K_x} \tag{3}$$

It is assumed that the response is proportional to the number of occupied receptors. Hence at the concentration of agonist which produces half the maximum response (the ED50 concentration)

$$\frac{\theta}{1-\theta} = 1,$$

but from equation (2) this is also equal to

$$\frac{k_1 x}{k_2 + k_1 x} \bigg/ \left(1 - \frac{k_1 x}{k_2 + k_1 x}\right)$$

$$= \frac{k_1 x}{k_2}$$

$$= \frac{x}{K_x}$$

so that at the ED50, $x = K_x$.

When a competitive antagonist is present, from equation (3)

$$\theta = \frac{x}{x + K_x}$$

If x' is the concentration of agonist which produces the same response as does the concentration x in the absence of antagonist, then a similar equation can be derived for x' and y.

$$\theta = \frac{x'}{x' + K_x\left(\dfrac{y}{K_y} + 1\right)} \tag{4}$$

If equal responses are equivalent to equal occupations of receptor (θ) then from equations (3) and (4)

$$\frac{x}{x + K_x} = \frac{x'}{x' + K_x\left(\dfrac{y}{K_y} + 1\right)}$$

Experimentally this is readily achieved by determining the concentrations which produce equal responses in the presence and in the absence of the antagonist, i.e.,

$$K_y = \frac{y}{\left(\dfrac{x'}{x} - 1\right)}$$

with x'/x being called the dose ratio or DR. Thus

$$K_y = \frac{y}{DR - 1} \tag{5}$$

Using this equation the equilibrium constant for the antagonist may be obtained from the antagonist concentration and the dose ratio.

Equation (5) is used in the calculations of what are called pA values. They describe the effect of competitive antagonists. pA is defined as the negative logarithm of the antagonist concentrations which produces a dose ratio of n.

When $n = 2$, from (5) $K_y = y$

By definition pA $= -\log y$

$$\therefore \text{pA}_2 = -\log K_y \tag{6}$$

Now when DR $= 10$, similarly

$$K_y = \frac{y}{9}$$

$$\therefore \text{pA}_{10} = -\log K_y - \log 9$$

but from (6) $-\log K_y = \text{pA}_2$

$$\therefore \text{pA}_2 - \text{pA}_{10} = \log 9 = 0.95 \text{ (approx)}$$

This is used as a test of competitive antagonism. If $\text{pA}_2 - \text{pA}_{10}$ is close to 0.95 then the antagonism is likely to be competitive.

Specific antagonism gives high pA values. If the action of an antagonist on two different agonists produces similar pA values, it is likely that the agonists are acting at the same receptor.

In some cases there is strong experimental evidence that the simple theory of one drug molecule combining with one receptor site does not account for the results. It may be the case that one initial drug molecule is required to activate the site or that 'cooperativity' occurs, either in the binding or the results of the binding of molecules. In such cases the Hill plot is used to determine the relationship.

If $\Delta = $ response

Δ_{max} is the maximum response.

The assumption is made that the response is proportional to occupancy as before

$$\therefore \theta = \frac{\Delta}{\Delta_{\text{max}}}$$

But then from (3)

$$\frac{\Delta}{\Delta_{\text{max}}} = \frac{x}{x + K_x}$$

$$\therefore \frac{\Delta}{\Delta_{\text{max}} - \Delta} = \frac{x}{K_x}$$

$$\therefore \log \frac{\Delta}{\Delta_{\text{max}} - \Delta} = \frac{\log x}{K}$$

$$= \log x - \log K$$

If $\log \dfrac{\Delta}{\Delta_{\text{max}} - \Delta}$ is plotted against $\log x$, then the slope will be unity if there is a simple one-to-one relationship. However if two molecules of drug combine with the receptor then the slope is equal to 2 because x^2 replaces x in our initial equation (1).

$$\therefore \log \frac{\Delta}{\Delta_{max} - \Delta} = 2 \log x - \log K$$

Non-integral slopes in the Hill plot suggest cooperativity.

Some complications

At the risk of frightening some physical scientists away from the fascinating areas of molecular pharmacology it is necessary to underline some of the complications which arise from the fact that measurements are usually of the dose–response type with no clear knowledge of the molecular mechanism. Perfectly reproducible dose–response data may not give direct information which can be interpreted in molecular terms.

There are numerous complications particularly when the pharmacological experiments have to be performed in whole animals, starting with the mode of administration of the drug. Depending on the route, different types of membrane may have to absorb the drug. For drugs administered by mouth absorption from the stomach or intestines may depend on the ability of the molecule to penetrate the lipid layer of membrane.

For molecules largely present in an ionized form transport may involve the percentage of un-ionized species which is rapidly replenished by rapid proton transfer, or some active transport mechanism involving a carrier. Fat solubility is however often a required property so that if a drug is an acid or base then an un-ionized form must exist (a pK_a of between roughly 4 and 10). The crossing of membranes is also important for drugs administered through any of the bodily orifices as lozenges, pessaries or the suppositories so beloved of continental European physicians.

Quaternary ammonium salts which are permanent cations are only poorly transmitted across membranes. The ability of a drug to cross a membrane may be an essential feature even when experiments are performed on single tissues or even cells.

The central nervous system appears to be separated from the rest of the body by something equivalent to a membrane which prevents ions from passing directly into the system. This hypothesized membrane is called the *blood–brain barrier*.

When a molecule is inside the body it may, of course, be altered by the body's own enzyme and chemical systems and be metabolized. After attack by an enzyme, the product is usually conjugated with some highly acidic group giving a polar compound with a low pK_a which will not penetrate membranes but is filtered by the kidney and is consequently excreted.

Summary

Pharmacologists measure the response of an animal or an isolated tissue to a measured dose of a chemical compound. The shape of the curve of percentage of maximal response against the logarithm of the dose gives some indication of the behaviour of the molecule with the receptor. Dose–response curves do not give a clear indication of the concentration or nature of the active species at the receptor nor the initial molecular response. Both the affinity and efficacy of drugs are important. Labelled binding studies are providing direct measures of affinity and stimulation of the production of cyclic nucleotide manifests efficacy.

Explanations of the mode of action of the drug with its receptor which are thermodynamically acceptable and consistent with the kinetics are possible but a clear structural explanation of the activity in molecular terms remains a goal of molecular pharmacologists.

Further reading

The introductory texts listed at the end of Chapter 1 provide fuller details of some of the material in this chapter. In addition the following may be helpful.

ALEXANDER, R. W., DAVIS, J. N. and LEFKOWITZ, R. J. *Nature, Lond.*, **258**, 437 (1975)
  Direct binding studies including inhibition effects.
BURGEN, A. S. V. *Rev. Pharmac.*, **10**, 7 (1970)
  Receptor mechanisms.
FEWTRELL, C. M. S. *Neuroscience*, **1**, 249 (1976)
GOLDSTEIN, A., ARONOW, L. and KALMAN, S. M. *Principles of Drug Action: The Basis of Pharmacology*, 2nd edn, John Wiley, New York (1970)
LEFKOWITZ, R. J. *et al.*, *Biochim. biophys. Acta*, **457**, 1 (1976)
  The β-adrenergic receptor and adenylate cyclase.
O'BRIEN, R. D. (ed) *The Receptors*, Plenum Press, New York (1979)
RANG, H. P., *Quart. Rev. Biophys.*, **7**, 283 (1974)
  Acetylcholine receptors.
STEPHENSON, R. A. and BARLOW, R. B. in R. Passmore and J. S. Robson (eds), *A Companion to Medical Studies*, Vol. 2, Blackwell Scientific Publications, Oxford (1973)
  An excellent account of quantitative measurements.
WAUD, D. R. *Pharmacol. Rev.*, **20**, 49 (1968)
  Pharmacological receptors.

Chapter 3

Acetylcholine

A perspective drawing of acetylcholine in a stable extended conformation is shown in *Figure 3.1*. Acetylcholine was one of the first transmitters to be identified at the beginning of this century and thus has received much attention. The accessibility, in the peripheral nervous system, of cholinergic synapses has led to their providing much basic information about the mechanisms of synaptic transmission summarized in the schematic diagram below (*Figure 3.2*).

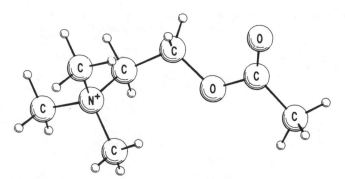

Figure 3.1. Acetylcholine in its crystal conformation

The actions of acetylcholine at the different sites can be mimicked or blocked by many agonists and antagonists but the pattern of action of these drugs is not identical at all synapses. On the basis of these effects the receptors for acetylcholine were classically divided into 'muscarinic' and 'nicotinic' types. Muscarinic receptors are found at parasympathetic neuroeffector junctions (III) and nicotinic receptors at the skeletal neuromuscular junctions (I) and in autonomic ganglia (II). The nicotinic receptors are not identical at these two sites with respect to the actions of drugs but there are similarities.

In any of these systems, drugs may act in a number of different ways to produce a given response. For example drugs may

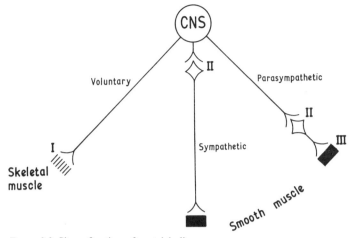

Figure 3.2. Sites of action of acetylcholine

(1) Mimic effects of acetylcholine.
(2) Affect the release of acetylcholine from the stores in nerve endings.
(3) Affect the action of acetylcholine at the receptors.
(4) Affect the enzyme which destroys acetylcholine (acetylcholinesterase) and thus prolong its effect.

We will now consider the action of acetylcholine at each of the three types of junction distinguished in *Figure 3.2*: the neuromuscular junction of voluntary nerves, ganglia, and the neuroeffector junction of parasympathetic nerves and smooth muscle, cardiac muscle or glands. For each type of activity we will give some examples of agonists and antagonists. Acetylcholine also plays an important role in the central nervous system but this aspect will be treated in Chapter 6.

Voluntary nerves: the neuromuscular junction

The neuromuscular junction is the technical term for the junction between the endings of voluntary nerves and skeletal muscle. The sensory nerves which operate in the opposite direction are less well understood and defining response may be difficult. For voluntary motor muscles there is no such problem. The nerve may be stimulated by an electric shock and the response measured as a twitch or contraction.

Skeletal muscle and smooth muscle may be distinguished by the fact that skeletal muscle cells are larger than smooth muscle cells. In skeletal muscle the individual muscle cells may range in length from a few millimetres to over 30 mm and from about 10 to 100 μm in diameter. The cell contains the contractile apparatus, getting its striated appearance from the sets of protein strands which slide into each other on contraction. The nerve joins the muscle at the end-plate region.

Figure 3.3 shows in diagrammatic form the nature of the neuromuscular junction.

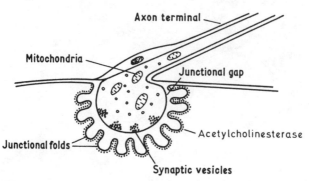

Figure 3.3. The neuromuscular junction

The muscle consists of sets of motor units joined by connective tissue. Each cell will have an end plate similar to that shown above. A single nerve axon will feed a group of cells.

The tip of a microelectrode which may be less than one micron across can be inserted into a muscle cell and record the potential difference (p.d.) between the inside and outside. This p.d. is about 90 mV with the interior being negative. Inside the cell the concentration of K^+ is very much greater than that of Na^+ while the converse is true outside where there is also a small concentration of Ca^{2+}.

When a nerve is stimulated either naturally or electrically a regenerated change in membrane permeability (the action potential, *see* Chapter 1) sweeps along the nerve. When the wave of depolarization reaches the terminal of the axon it causes release of stored acetylcholine. This is triggered by influx of calcium ions due to a temporary increase in permeability of the terminal membrane to this ion. The acetylcholine, released in packets known as 'quanta', diffuses across the synaptic cleft and combines with the receptors on the post-synaptic membrane. Only the end-plate region of the muscle (where it is in contact with the nerve terminal) is sensitive to acetylcholine. Combination of acetylcholine with the receptors leads to a local increase in the permeability of the post-synaptic membrane to sodium, potassium and chloride ions. The resultant local depolarization is known as the end-plate potential (EPP). Spontaneous release of quanta of acetylcholine occurs leading to many small depolarizations of the end-plate, miniature end-plate potentials (MEPPs). The end-plate potential triggers the propagation of action potentials along the muscle, causing contraction.

The acetylcholine combines with the receptor only briefly (of the order of milliseconds). It is rapidly broken down by the enzyme acetylcholinesterase, which lies on the post-synaptic membrane. Inhibition of this enzyme considerably prolongs the effects of acetylcholine.

Agonists

For each of the active molecules which we will consider a considerable number of agonists and antagonists are known. Details of these may be found in any of the pharmacological texts quoted. In the space available here it is necessary to restrict attention to a small range of compounds which illustrate the sensitivity of biological systems to small chemical modifications and highlight the structural questions which have to be answered.

In the typical case of acetylcholine acting as the neuromuscular junction, *Table 3.1* illustrates the variation in activity of agonists as the nature of the onium head is changed. The figures are quoted as equipotent molar ratios. This means, for example, that if a given quantity of acetylcholine produces a response, five times as much of the compound with one ethyl replacing a methyl is required. Thus the more active the compound the smaller the number in terms of the equipotent molar ratio.

TABLE 3.1. Cholinergic agonists (frog rectus)

Molecule	Equipotent molar ratio
$CH_3CO.O.CH_2CH_2N^+Me_3$	1
$-N^+Me_2Et$	5
$-N^+MeEt_2$	300
$-N^+Et_3$	5000

TABLE 3.2. Cholinergic agonists (frog rectus)

Molecule	Equipotent molar ratio
$CH_3CO.O.CH_2CH_2N^+Me_3$	1
$HO.CH_2CH_2N^+Me_3$	700
$Me_3CCO.O.CH_2CH_2N^+Me_3$	7
$PhCO.O.CH_2CH_2N^+Me_3$	50

From this table we see that the size of the groups on the nitrogen is critical, but *Table 3.2* shows that the other end of the molecule is perhaps less sensitive.

An important point which underlines the specificity of the receptor is the effect of methylating acetylcholine carbons α and β to the N^+.

$$CH_3CO\ O\ CH_2\ \underset{\underset{Me}{|}}{CH}\ N^+\ Me_3 \qquad \text{equipotent molar ratio 1}$$

$$CH_3CO\ O\ \underset{\underset{Me}{|}}{CH}\ CH_2\ N^+\ Me_3 \qquad \text{equipotent molar ratio 100}$$

These differences may represent intrinsic effects but could also reflect differences in susceptibility to cholinesterase. Most notable, however, are the effects of the two optical isomers possible in each case. For both cases one of the optically active forms is about one hundred times more active than the other. When whole tissues are used the measured effect of a drug is the result of its ability to penetrate the tissue, its efficacy, and the rate of breakdown or removal by the tissue.

Antagonists

Antagonists or neuromuscular blocking agents are useful compounds to produce muscle relaxation during anaesthesia, preventing the contraction of muscles when they are touched or cut. Merely applying anaesthetics to produce this relaxation is dangerous since very heavy doses are necessary, making recovery from post-operative shock difficult. Good muscle relaxants are also needed in electric shock therapy for profound depression when it is important to prevent massive convulsions.

Experimentally a strip of diaphragm is used. This tissue has the advantage of being thin and easily oxygenated. The frog rectus abdominus is also much used. The sort of result obtained on tissue is illustrated in *Figure 3.4*.

For tests on intact animals the cat is usually preferred, and in man the ability to grip. However, extrapolation from one species to another is a further difficulty of quantitative pharmacology as *Table 3.3* shows.

TABLE 3.3. Comparison of efficacies of drugs in man, cat and rat

Drug	Man	Cat	Rat
		Equipotent molar ratio	
I	1	1	1
II	5	4	50
III	2	2	25
IV	1	1	15
V	0.3	0.1	25
VI	1	10	15

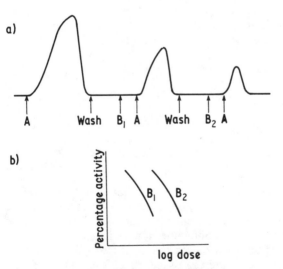

Figure 3.4. (a) Tension of a strip of muscle as a function of time. At point A acetylcholine is administered; B_1 and B_2 are antagonists which reduce the effect of the transmitter as shown in (b)

As may be seen, the cat approximates most closely to man and has the technical advantage of having rather tough blood vessels.

Clinically useful neuromuscular blocking agents act post-synaptically by one of two major mechanisms.

(1) Competition with acetylcholine for the end-plate receptor; so-called non-depolarizing blocking agents.
(2) Prolonged depolarization followed by desensitization to the transmitter despite repolarization, often called depolarizing blockers.

The classic neuromuscular blocking agents are found in South American arrow poisons such as curare. This is only toxic when injected, not when eaten, perhaps because the active parts of the complicated mixture of compounds are quaternary ammonium compounds and cannot traverse membranes, e.g. tubocurarine (*Figure 3.5*).

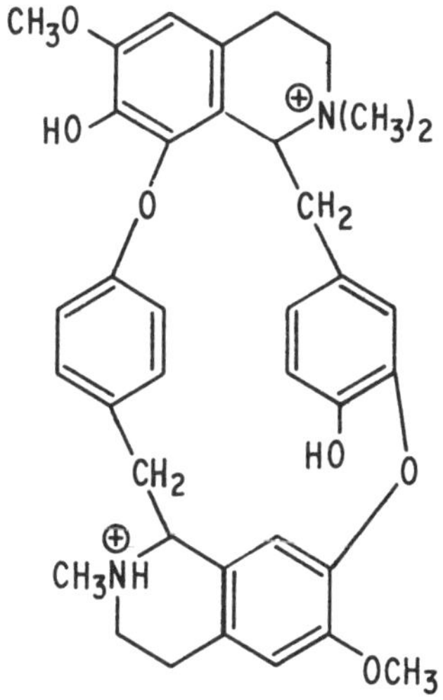

Figure 3.5. Tubocurarine

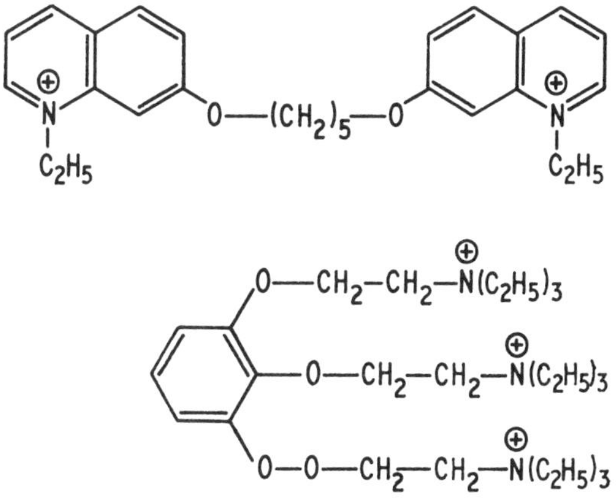

Figure 3.6. Antagonists of acetylcholine at the neuromuscular junction

Tubocurarine acts by competing with acetylcholine for the receptor and thus prevents acetylcholine from depolarizing muscle end plate. (It is a monoquaternary salt not bisquaternary as stated in many texts.)

Synthetic alterations which are also quaternary compounds with aromatic groups include examples shown in *Figure 3.6*.

The simpler compounds $(CH_3)_3N^+ - (CH_2)_n - N^+(CH_3)_3$ are also effective. With $n = 10$-decamethonium, the compound is about as effective as curare. The mechanism in this case is, however, that of a depolarizing block. The actions of competitive antagonists can be reversed by anti-cholinesterase agents as these increase the concentration of acetylcholine. In the case of depolarizing blocking agents the effects are not reversed as increasing endogenous acetylcholine causes further depolarization. Clinically a compound such as succinylcholine is preferred as it is shorter acting because broken down by cholinesterase. This is also a blocking agent of the depolarizing type.

There is of course often some overlap in activity at different sites for synthetic anticholinergics and cholinomimetics. In particular it is noteworthy that hexamethonium is a ganglion blocker while decamethonium is a neuro-muscular blocker.

Autonomic ganglia

The main transmission through ganglia is by cholinergic nicotinic receptors but there is a complex neuronal network within the tissues involving several different transmitter systems which regulates transmission.

Transmission of a nerve impulse by acetylcholine across the synaptic gap in a ganglion is in many ways similar to the transmission at the neuromuscular junction in the voluntary system just discussed. There are miniature synaptic potentials rather similar to miniature end-plate potentials and the release of acetylcholine seems to be quantal from vesicles. It is possible that many measurements merely reflect the ability of a compound to gain access. Aryl groups may increase activity by rendering the compound more lipid-soluble.

The most commonly used preparation is the superior cervical ganglion of the cat which is situated in the neck and is involved in the control of the nictitating membrane or third eyelid. Strips of guinea-pig ileum are used in tests of the activity of drugs on parasympathetic ganglia. The rise in blood pressure of the cat was also used in ganglionic tests with the effects of acetylcholine at the nerve endings blocked by atropine.

Recent developments in the study of antagonist actions at the neuro-muscular junction and at ganglia, using recording techniques for measuring the parameters of ion channel opening, have shown that some antagonists have another effect as well as binding to the receptor site. They appear to bind to sites within the channels, after these have been opened by agonist-receptor combination, and so block ion movements.

Agonists

The simplest agonist molecules are tetra-alkyl ammonium ions. *Table 3.4* gives a selection of results which yet again illustrate how sensitive receptors

TABLE 3.4. Ganglion stimulant agonists of acetylcholine

Molecule	Equipotent molar ratio with respect to tetramethyl ammonium
$Me - N^+Me_3$	1
$Et - N^+Me_3$	4
$nPr - N^+Me_3$	20
$nBu - N^+Me_3$	1

are to the nature of the interacting molecule. Again we must remember the difficulty of ensuring that activity differences represent true differences in intrinsic activities and not different susceptibility to enzymic attack.

Nicotine (*Figure 3.7*) which mimics acetylcholine at the ganglionic junction as well as at the neuromuscular junction is especially noteworthy since it can stimulate and ultimately block the transmission of ganglia. Its blocking action at high dose levels was in fact used to locate the actual anatomical positions of the various ganglia. The equipotent ratio with respect to acetylcholine is 0.1; the high activity probably is due to the failure of acetylcholinesterase to destroy it.

Other related compounds which act as agonists include leptodactyline and some tropine derivatives (*Figure 3.8*).

A simplistic rationalization of the structural requirements for agonist activity postulates the necessity of having a partial positive charge a few

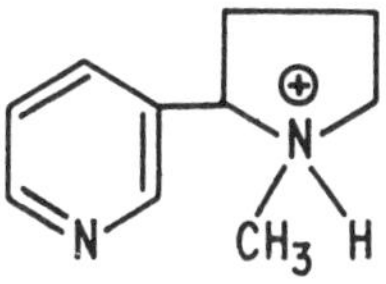

Figure 3.7. Nicotine ion

(a)

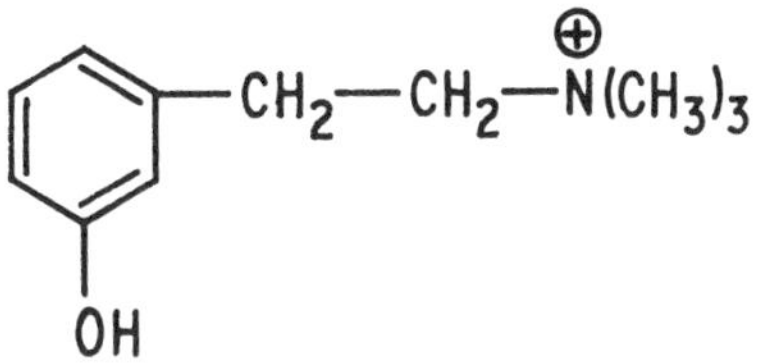

(b)

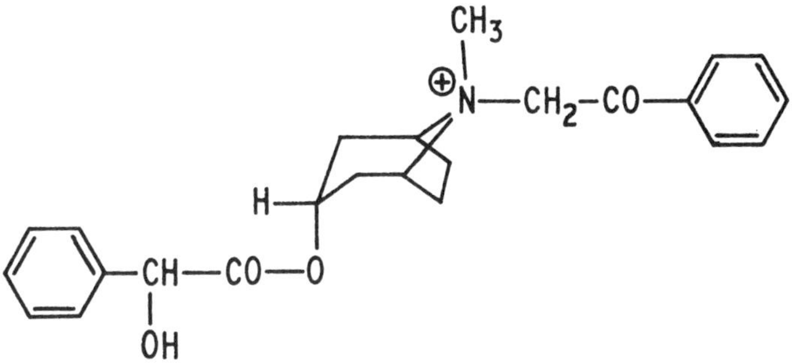

Figure 3.8. (a) Leptodactyline. (b) Phenactropinium

Ångströms from a quaternary nitrogen although this is a problem ripe for detailed study.

Antagonists

Ganglionic transmission can be blocked either by prevention of the depolarizing action of acetylcholine or by drugs which produce persistent depolarization.

As is so frequently the case, the antagonists can be very similar to the agonists as they should be if they need affinity for the same site. Hence tetraethyl ammonium is a blocker. The major effect of ganglionic blocking is a fall in blood pressure. It is for this reason that nicotinic agonists were once sought.

Although not as impressive as its action at the neuromuscular junction, tubocurarine is fairly active at ganglia.

Bis-onium salts are very effective and in particular hexamethonium (*Figure 3.9*).

$$(CH_3)_3 \overset{\oplus}{N} - (CH_2)_6 - \overset{\oplus}{N}(CH_3)_3$$ *Figure 3.9*. Hexamethonium

However, as usual quaternary ammonium compounds are only poorly absorbed and are consequently clinically rather inconvenient. The chance finding that mecamylamine (*Figure 3.10*), a secondary amine, is active led to an intensive search for tertiary bases. Out of some thousands of compounds screened drugs such as pempidine (*Figure 3.11*) were developed. This is smoothly absorbed and builds up in lipid layers. It is nonetheless striking that so many compounds had to be tested before hitting on a suitable compound.

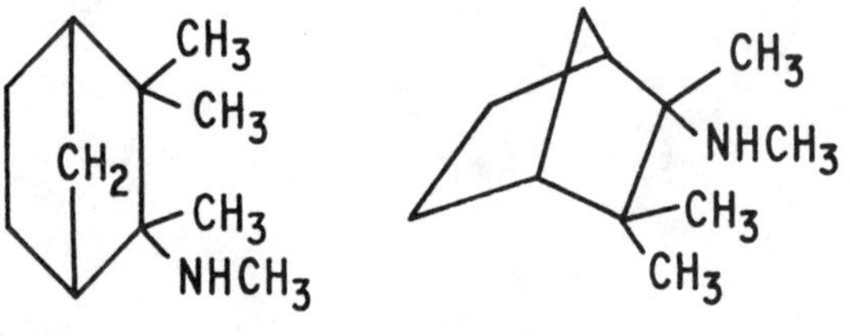

Figure 3.10. Mecamylamine

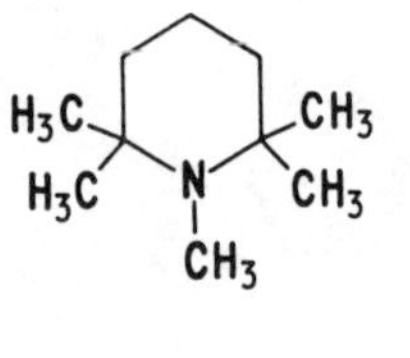

Figure 3.11. Pempidine

Post-ganglionic nerve endings

Acetylcholine is the transmitter at the nerve endings of parasympathetic nerves where they innervate smooth muscles and cardiac muscles. Smooth muscles keep organs 'toned', that is constantly under some tension. Smooth muscle cells are only about one ten-thousandth the size of skeletal muscles and are frequently organized into sheets but with wide variations between different organs. There is no observed end plate and the precise anatomy is not clearly understood.

Transmission at such sites as the heart, stomach or intestines is markedly different from that which takes place at the voluntary neuromuscular junction and in ganglia. The events are much longer lasting and less precise; tension appears to be continuously variable rather than quantal. There is an action potential between the inside and outside of smooth muscle cells which is attributed to the changes in permeability of the membrane to Ca^{2+} and other ions. From the behaviour of agonists and antagonists it is inferred that the receptors in both the heart and other smooth muscle are similar; again an inference about receptors from the behaviour of the small molecules which combine with them.

Agonists

Muscarine (*Figure 3.12*) is the analogue of nicotine in the case of parasympathetic nerve endings and such activity is frequently referred to as 'muscarinic activity'. Many of the possible isomers and analogues of muscarine have been studied, showing large differences due to configuration, reflecting the requirement of the receptor. *Figure 3.13* shows the most active configuration.

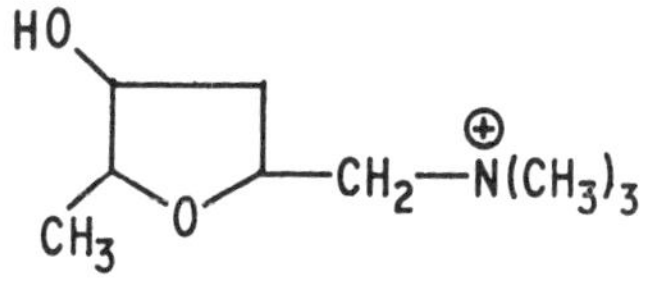

Figure 3.12. Muscarine

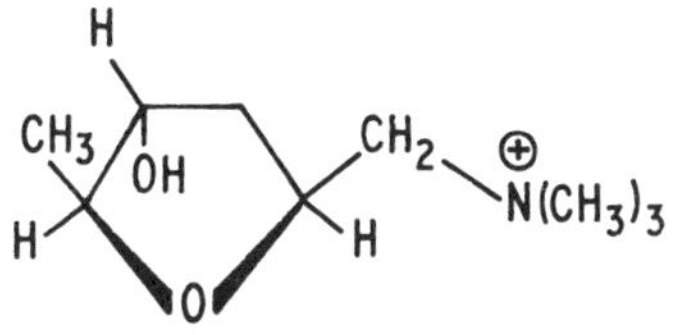

Figure 3.13. The most active isomer of muscarine

Marked activity is restricted to those compounds in which the arrangement of the hydroxyl and methyl groups and the onium side-chain is the same as muscarine.

Antagonists

The classic antagonist of acetylcholine at the neuroeffective junction is atropine (*Figure 3.14*), only one optical isomer of which is so active.

Antagonists are frequently developed from agonists as illustrated in *Figure 3.15* for alkyl trimethyl ammonium salts.

More complex blockers include those developed from atropine such as those shown in *Figure 3.16*.

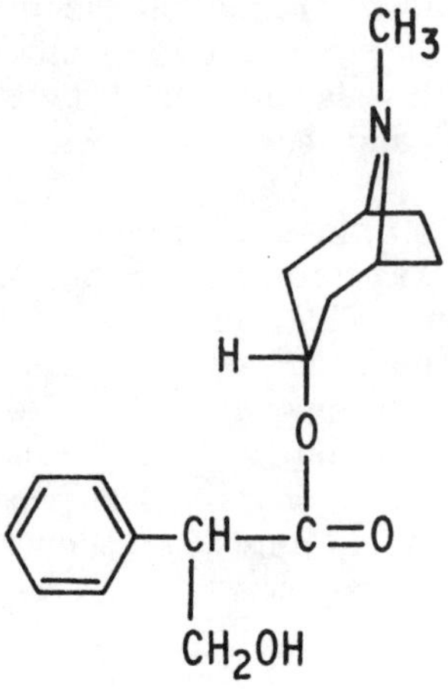

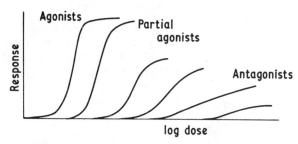

CH_3

N

$H-$

O

$-CH-C=O$

CH_2OH

Figure 3.14. Atropine

Response

Agonists

Partial agonists

Antagonists

log dose

Figure 3.15. Dose–response curves which distinguish agonists from antagonists. Affinity and efficiency increase with increasing alkylation of alkyltrimethyl ammonium salts

Atropine, scopolamine and related antagonists find important applications in ophthalmology, anaesthesia and cardiac and gastro-intestinal diseases, but in addition to peripheral anticholinergic effects most of these drugs act in the central nervous system.

Other blockers have come from the study of acetylcholine analogues and include the benzilic ester drawn in *Figure 3.17*. Unlike atropine this compound, being a quaternary ammonium derivative, will not readily penetrate the central nervous system through the blood–brain barrier and as a result does not cause central nervous effects such as hallucinations caused by atropine.

Anticholinesterases

Compounds which interfere with cholinesterases and inhibit the destruction of the transmitter produce higher concentrations of acetylcholine and may also potentiate the action of administered choline esters. These cholinesterase inhibitors are of significant medical interest and have been used in the treatment of myasthenia gravis and the control of glaucoma. They are also used as insecticides.

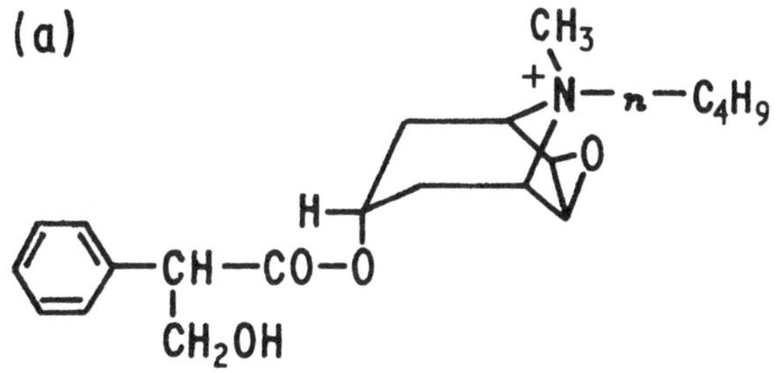

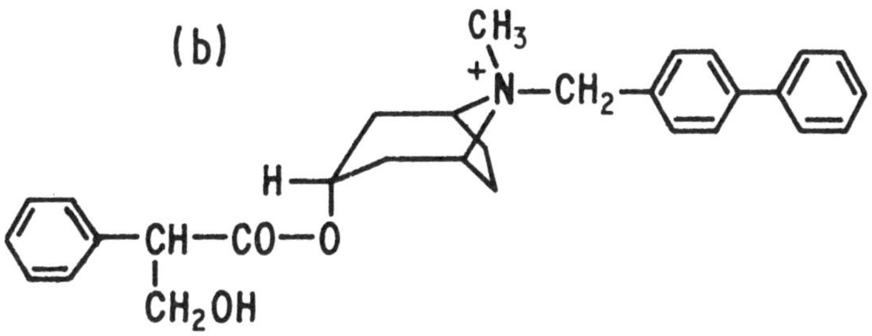

(a)

(b)

Figure 3.16. (a) Buscopan. (b) Gastropin

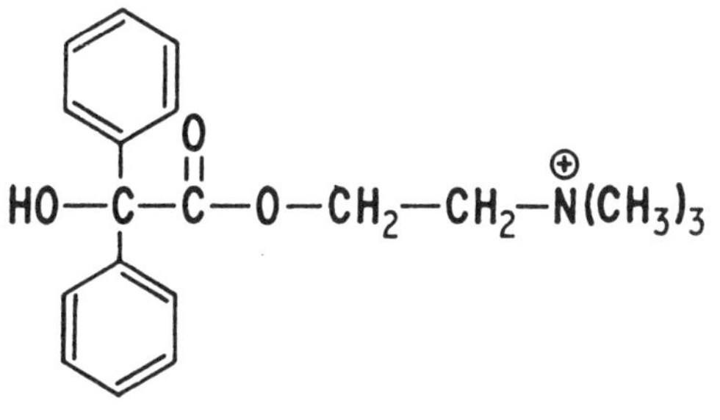

Figure 3.17. Benzilic ester

Investigation of the natural product calabar led to the development of physiostigmine and neostigmine (*Figure 3.18*). The affinity of these compounds for cholinesterase is of order 10^4 greater than that of acetylcholine. These compounds bind to both sites on the enzyme to which acetylcholine binds and then are slowly hydrolysed so that they block the hydrolysis of acetylcholine. These sites have been called the 'esteratic' and 'anionic' sites. Some drugs may bind to only one site, for example tetramethylammonium ion (anionic site). The organophosphorus inhibitors, such as dytros (which combines only at the esteratic site) are effectively irreversible, synthesis of new enzyme being necessary for return of function. These compounds form a stable phosphorylated compound with the enzyme.

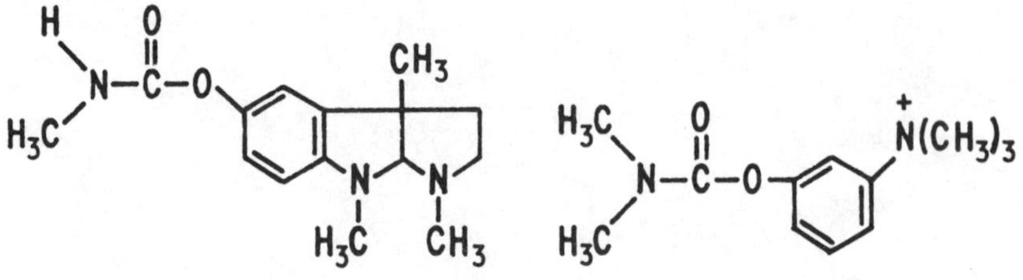

Figure 3.18. Physiostigmine and neostigmine

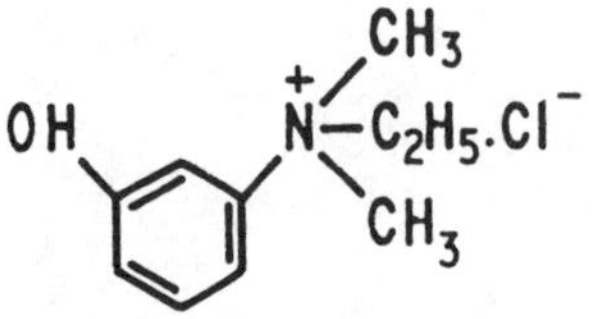

Figure 3.19. Edrophonium chloride

The drug edrophonium (*Figure 3.19*) is an antidote to curare, but its action is probably a direct one at the receptor rather than a cholinesterase inhibitor.

Acetylcholine release

Certain drugs are known to act by interfering with acetylcholine release. A well known example of these is botulinus toxin, produced by the bacteria *Clostridium botulinum*, the most powerful bacterial toxin known. This selectively prevents the release of acetylcholine and thereby causes paralysis, 'botulism'.

Hemicholinium decreases acetylcholine release by competing with choline for the uptake mechanism in the presynaptic terminal thus decreasing the synthesis of acetylcholine. Several drugs have been shown to increase acetylcholine release, as well as possessing other pharmacological actions, for example carbachol (also a direct cholinergic agonist) and tetraethylammonium (a ganglion blocking agent).

Isolation of acetylcholine receptors

Considerable progress has been made in the isolation and characterization of nicotinic acetylcholine receptors particularly from the electric tissues of the eel *Electrophorus electricus* and of the fish *Torpedo*, but also from skeletal muscle. The receptors may be labelled selectively with a high molecular weight compound α-bungarotoxin isolated from snake venom.

An homogenate of tissue from the electric organ of *Torpedo* of which 50 per cent of the surface is synapse can be treated with radioactive α-bungarotoxin and the labelled proteins purified by chromatography.

The receptor appears to be a protein of molecular weight about 350 000 made up from four constituent polypeptides with molecular weights approximately 40 000, 50 000, 60 000 and 65 000. Although it is a membrane protein it does seem possible to keep it intact in an aqueous environment and to make preliminary binding studies.

Current views suggest that the receptor is a five or six subunit complex each with two binding sites, themselves composed of two regions of binding. The complex does appear to be capable of translocating ions.

Similar work on the more dilute and hence difficult skeletal muscle junction uses denervation to provoke an increase in the number of receptors. Results from these studies suggest that there are 20–25 000 receptors per square micron at folds in the post-synaptic membrane. Electron micrographs indicate that the receptors are located directly opposite the acetylcholine-releasing vesicles.

It is tremendously encouraging that the molecular nature of receptors is becoming better and better defined. However the crystal structure or knowledge in atomic detail of the binding sites remains for the future even if prospects are good.

Summary

Acetylcholine is the transmitter in voluntary motor nerves at the end plate between nerve and skeletal muscle. It is also the transmitter at the ganglia of both sympathetic and parasympathetic autonomic nerves and the junction between parasympathetic nerves and smooth muscle or cardiac muscle. The actions at the neuromuscular junction of voluntary connections and in the ganglia in the parasympathetic and sympathetic nerves of the autonomic nervous system are imitated by nicotine and blocked by curare alkaloids but not atropine; they are called *nicotinic* effects. At the neuroeffector junction of parasympathetic fibres with smooth muscles the effects are said to be *muscarinic*, imitated by muscarine, blocked by atropine but not by curare alkaloids.

Although there are many similarities, the different behaviour of agonist and antagonist molecules suggests that there are differences between the receptors in the three main subdivisions with possible further variations for specific synapses.

In no case is the nature of the molecular process involved in the binding of acetylcholine, its agonists or antagonists, understood in any detail. In part this is due to the difficulty of the pharmacological experiments but a detailed investigation of all the information available has yet to be undertaken particularly at a sub-molecular level. Perhaps the most encouraging prospect is the detailed structural picture which should emerge from isolated purified protein receptors and more direct thermodynamic and kinetic data from labelled binding studies.

Acetylcholine is also of considerable importance in the central nervous system and many anticholinergic effects are often unwanted side effects from other drugs, particularly those used in the CNS.

Further reading

In addition to chapters in general text books, the following reviews give fuller details.

BRIMBLECOMBE, R. W. 'Drug actions on cholinergic systems', in P. B. Bradley (ed.), *Pharmacology Monographs*, University Park Press, Baltimore (1974)

COHEN, J. B. and CHANGEUX, J. P. *A. Rev. Pharmac.*, **15**, 83 (1974)
  The cholinergic receptor protein in its membrane environment.
HUBBARD, J. I. and QUASTEL, D. M. J. *A. Rev. Pharmac.*, **13**, 199 (1973)
  Micropharmacology of vertebrate neuromuscular junction.
GOLDBERG, A. M. and HARRIS, I. (eds) *Biology of Cholinergic Function*, Raven Press, New
  York (1974)
KUBA, K. and KOKETSU, K. 'Synaptic events in sympathetic ganglia', in *Progress in
  Neurobiology*, *11*, 77 (1978)
MACINTOSH, F. C. and COLLIER, B. in E. Zaimis (ed), *Handbook of Experimental
  Pharmacology*, Vol. **42**, 99–228, Springer Verlag (1976)
  The neuromuscular junction.
RAFTERY, M. A. *et al.*, in L. Jaenicke (ed.), *Biochemistry of Sensory Function*, Springer
  Verlag, New York (1974)
  The isolation of the cholinergic receptor protein.
VOLLE, R. L. *Pharmacol. Rev.*, **18**, 839 (1966)
  Modification by drugs of synaptic mechanisms in autonomic ganglia.

Chapter 4

Catecholamines

The catecholamine noradrenaline (*Figure 4.1*) is the neuro-transmitter at the sympathetic nerve ending with smooth muscle, cardiac muscle and glands. Adrenaline (*Figure 4.1*), a secondary amine with one proton of noradrenaline replaced by a methyl group is not thought to be a peripheral neuro-transmitter but is produced by the adrenal medulla and reaches receptor sites producing effects similar to noradrenaline. (It should be noted that in the USA, 'Adrenaline' is a trade name so that the synonyms epinephrine and norepinephrine are used.) The main function of noradrenaline appears to be the contol of smooth muscle tone and the adjustment of circulation while adrenaline is an emergency hormone preparing for fight or flight.

Dopamine, which is similar to noradrenaline but lacks the hydroxyl on the beta carbon atom, is an important transmitter in the central nervous system. This will be considered along with other transmitters of the central nervous system in Chapter 6.

This chapter concentrates on catecholamines in the peripheral nervous system.

The catecholamines are formed from the amino acid tyrosine (*Figure 4.2*). They are ultimately broken down to a series of complex products some of which may be active. The initial uptake and rapid disappearance is associated with enzymic O-methylation to metanephrine (*Figure 4.3*), and with monoamine oxidase which can remove all the catecholamines (*Figure 4.4*).

There are enzyme-inhibiting chemicals which will block these enzymes but even in their presence the effects of noradrenaline are rapidly terminated. It has been shown that noradrenaline is rapidly inactivated through its recapture by the sympathetic nerves, an energy-requiring mechanism. This recapture is highly selective and may be the most general mechanism for the inactivation of neuro-transmitters.

The classification of receptors

The effects of the sympathetic transmitter can be divided into at least two broad categories. The classification is now based on the sensitivity to different

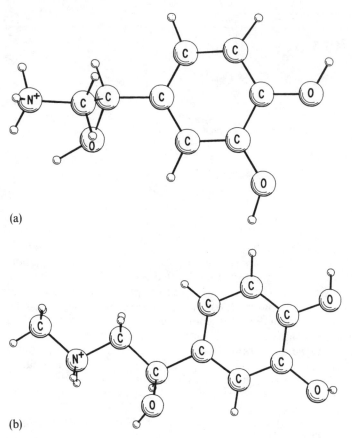

(a)

(b)

Figure 4.1. Ions of (a) noradrenaline and (b) adrenaline in their
crystal conformations

agonists, in particular, noradrenaline, adrenaline and isoprenaline (which
is similar to adrenaline except that the N-methyl is replaced by an isopropyl
group).

For α effects, noradrenaline greater or approximately the same as
   adrenaline > isoprenaline in agonist activity
For β effects, isoprenaline > adrenaline > noradrenaline.

The behaviour of specific agonists supports the broad classification, but
further subdivisions and additional classifications have been made.

β-receptors are of two types. β_1-receptors are responsible for cardiac
stimulation and lipolysis. β-receptors mediate adrenergic bronchodilatation
and vasodepression so that β_2-agonists are especially useful in the treatment
of asthma, having only slight effects on the heart. β_1-receptors have an
affinity for isoprenaline which is four times that for noradrenaline while
in the case of β_2-receptors isoprenaline has one hundred times the affinity
of noradrenaline.

A summary of the classification of adrenergic receptors is given in *Table*

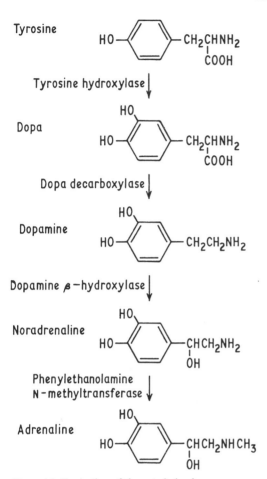

Figure 4.2. Formation of the catecholamines

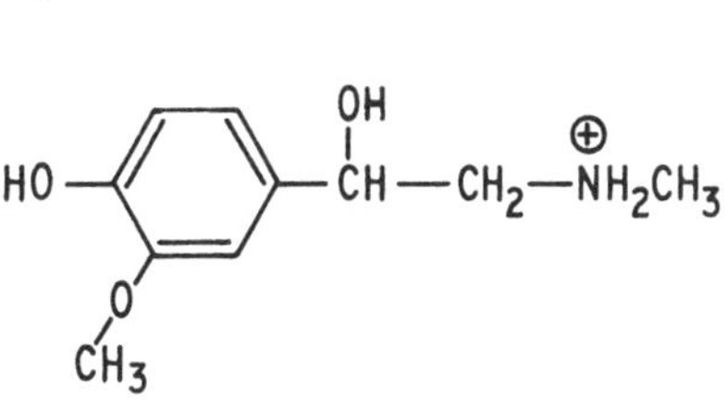

Figure 4.3. Metanephrine

4.1. β-receptors are located on the outer surface of target cells. Interaction between the catecholamines and receptors usually stimulates adenylate cyclase to produce cyclic AMP from adenosine triphosphate.

Recently the α-receptors have also been divided into two types following the discovery that the release of noradrenaline is controlled by a feedback mechanism involving receptors apparently located in the presynaptic terminal. Study of the effects of agonists and antagonists on these receptors showed that they are not identical to the post-synaptic α-receptors (now called α_1). They have been called 'presynaptic' or α_2-receptors and have also

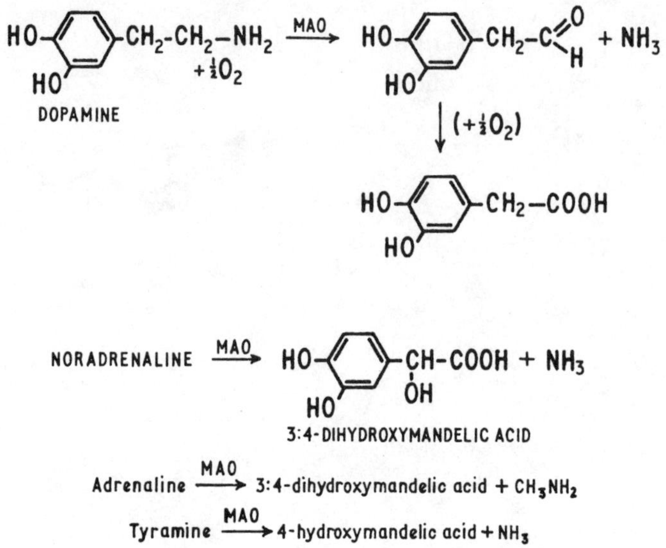

Figure 4.4. Removal of catecholamines by monoamine oxidase (MAO)

TABLE 4.1. Receptors mediating adrenergic effects

Effector organ	Response	Receptor
Heart	Increase in rate, contractility, excitability	β_1
Blood vessels (coronary, pulmonary, skeletal muscle, abdominal viscera)	Dilatation	β_2
(to skin)	Contraction	α
Lungs	Relaxation of bronchial muscle	β_2
Uterus	Relaxation	β_2
Kidney	Stimulation of renin release	β_1
Gastrointestinal tract	Relaxation of smooth muscle	β
	Contraction of stomach and intestine	α
Eye	Relaxation of ciliary muscle	β
	Contraction of radial muscle	α
Skeletal muscle	Decreased tension and degree of fusion of incomplete tetanic contractions of slow muscle. Stimulation of glycogenolysis,	β_2
	lactate production	β_2
Adipose tissue	Stimulation of lipolysis	'β_1'
Pancreas	Increased insulin secretion	β_2
Blood	Increase in factor 8 levels and fibrinolysis and decrease in whole blood clotting time. Increase in platelet aggregation	β_2

been found at other sites, e.g. cerebral cortex, ganglia, platelets. Unlike the α_1-receptors they appear to be coupled to adenyl cyclase as their activation causes inhibition of this enzyme.

Pharmacological preparations

Isolated preparations used experimentally to study α-receptors include the vas deferens of the rat or guinea pig. For β_1-effects the guinea-pig atrium has been used while for β_2-effects the relaxation of bronchial muscle studied with an isolated calf trachea has been used.

It is now also possible to distinguish α_1, α_2, β_1 and β_2-effects in whole animals providing effects other than the one under investigation have been blocked by specific antagonists.

Agonists

Drugs which are agonists of noradrenaline are called sympathomimetics. They may act directly on α- and β-receptors or indirectly by releasing catecholamines. Other drugs have combined properties and give a mixed action.

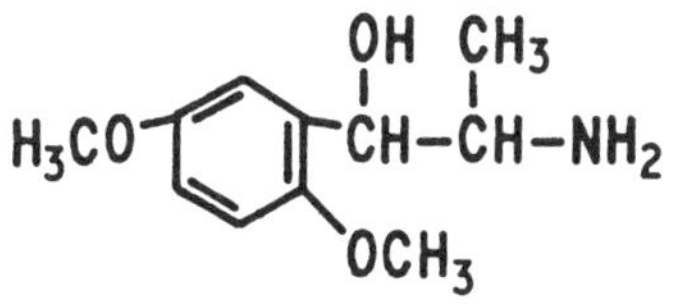

Figure 4.5. Methoxamine

Methoxamine (*Figure 4.5*) is a direct acting α_1-agonist which has virtually no cardiac effect. Tyramine and amphetamine on the other hand act indirectly.

Sympathomimetic compounds produce a rise in blood pressure. However, it is difficult to be clear as to the significance of measurements on blood pressure, for instance we may consider the activities listed in *Table 4.2*.

All the compounds do produce a rise in blood pressure but not necessarily by identical mechanisms. Cocaine potentiates the effects of adrenaline and noradrenaline as it blocks the neuronal uptake mechanism. Supersensitivity can be produced by denervation, which leads to increases in the number of receptors. Depletion of monoamine stores by reserpine causes noradrenaline and adrenaline to give larger rises in blood pressure but the effects of indirectly acting amines, such as tyramine, are prevented. Replenishment of stores by adrenaline or noradrenaline restore the capacity of tyramine to raise blood pressure.

The conclusion which has been drawn from experiments is that only compounds very like adrenaline do act directly. The following skeleton seems to be essential (*Figure 4.6*).

The optimum arrangement of the molecule for sympathomimetic action is when there is a two-carbon chain between the ring and the amino group.

TABLE 4.2. Sympathomimetic compounds (blood pressure)

Molecule	Equipotent molar ratio relative to noradrenaline
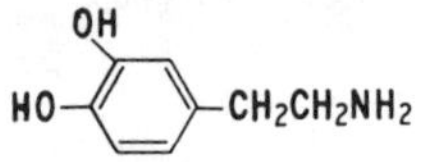 OH HO—⟨⟩—$CH_2CH_2NH_2$	10
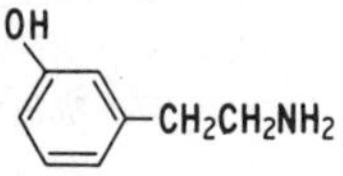 OH ⟨⟩—$CH_2CH_2NH_2$	10
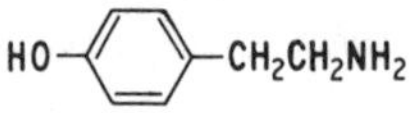 HO—⟨⟩—$CH_2CH_2NH_2$	100
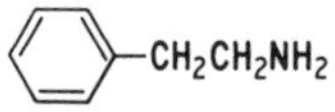 ⟨⟩—$CH_2CH_2NH_2$	100
$CH_3CH_2CH_2NH_2$	1000

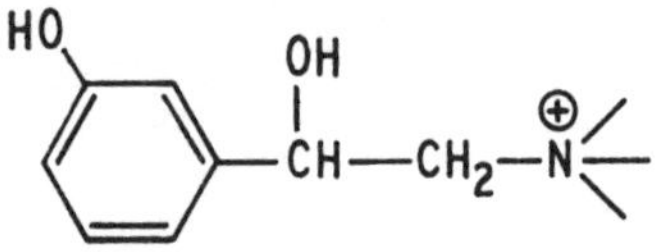

Figure 4.6. The essential molecular skeleton for direct sympathomimetic activity

Activity at β-receptors is found when the molecules possess large N-alkyl substituents but $\beta_1:\beta_2$-selectivity is conferred by other substituents.

Methoxamine has a selective agonist action at α_1-receptors, while chloridine, which is used in hypertension, has more action at α_2 than α_1 sites.

Action at central α_2-receptors is thought to be the basis of chloridine's production of hypotension.

Isoprenaline, more commonly named isoproterenol in the USA, is the typical direct acting β-agonist, acting on both β_1- and β_2-receptors. Salbutamol is a β_2-selective agonist producing bronchodilation with little, or no, effect on the heart.

Ephedrine (*Figure 4.7*) has a mixed action on β-receptors and also acts

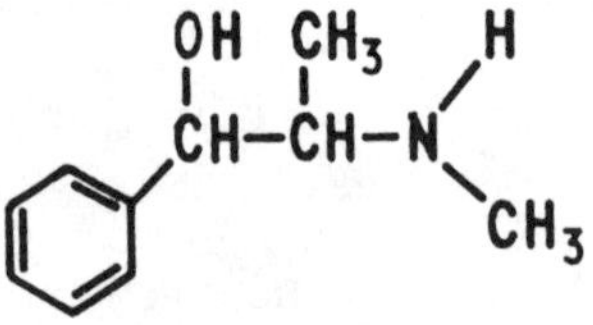

Figure 4.7. Ephedrine

indirectly on α-receptors. It is widely used in the treatment of bronchial asthma and is thought to act in part by releasing catecholamines from their storage vesicles. Amphetamine, which is a drug of abuse, is an indirectly acting sympathomimetic. The molecule is hydrophobic and therefore enters the brain causing central stimulation.

α-Receptor antagonists

α-Blockers are no longer considered to be important therapeutic agents but they do have some use diagnostically for tumours which secrete adrenaline.

Broadly, blockers of α-effects fall into two categories. In one group are competitive antagonists such as ergot alkaloids. The presence of these drugs shifts dose–response curves but does not alter the ultimate response.

The major problem in the use of ergot is the intense vasoconstrictor effect. This is not present in 9, 10-dihydroergotamine which nonetheless retains the valuable anti-adrenaline quality while having much less vasoconstrictor and oxytocic activity.

Recent studies have suggested that α-adrenergic receptors may be identified by the binding of dihydroergocryptine to smooth muscle. Typical of the second category are the β-haloamines which produce very persistent α-blockage. The simplest such compound is illustrated in *Figure 4.8*. This compound is a long-acting blocking agent but is no longer used clinically.

Many variants have been studied leading to the definition of required characteristics for compounds to act like phenoxybenzamine. It appears that

(a)

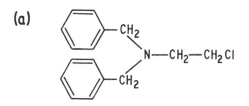

(b)

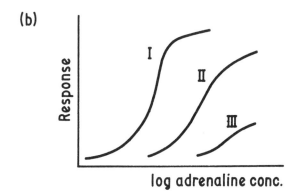

Figure 4.8. (a) Dibenamine. (b) Effects of increasing concentration (I, II and III) of dibenamine on response

compounds need to have a tertiary or quaternary nitrogen—at least one β-haloalkyl group and an unsaturated ring with ring substituents coplanar with the ring.

The rationale of this set of limitations is the notion that the active intermediate is an ethylene iminium ion (*Figure 4.9*), which is stabilized by delocalization of charge. The long-lasting activity is explained by the suggestion that this intermediate alkylates the receptor, a suggestion supported by the fact that the thiosulphate ion, which will react with ethylene iminium ions, removes the activity.

Selective α-receptor antagonists have been found, for example prazosin

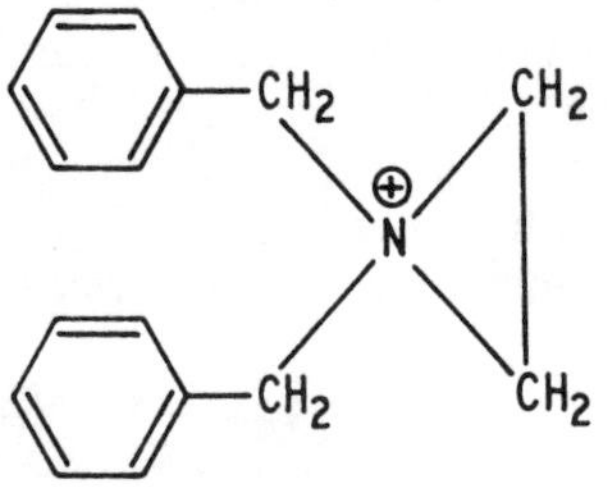

Figure 4.9. Ethylene iminium ion

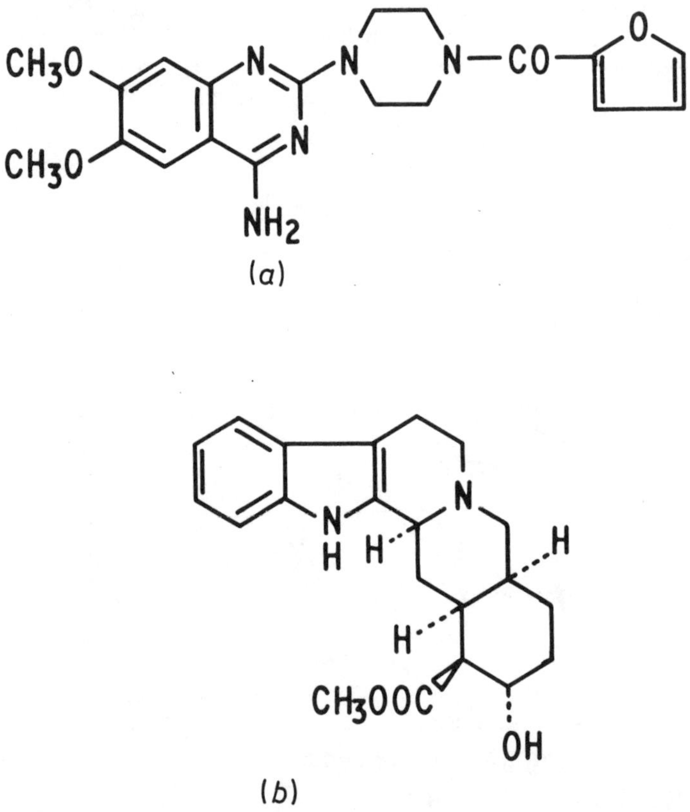

(a)

(b)

Figure 4.10. (a) Prazosin. (b) Yohimbine

has a greater action at α_1-than α_2-receptors; yohimbine is an antagonist at α_2-receptors, with less α_1-action (*see Figure 4.10*).

β-Receptor antagonists

Because cardiovascular problems are a major cause of death in western society much effort is being expended in the search for drugs to alleviate these conditions. The blocking of *β*-effects on the heart is useful for sufferers of cardiac arrhythmias or angina, and hypertension.

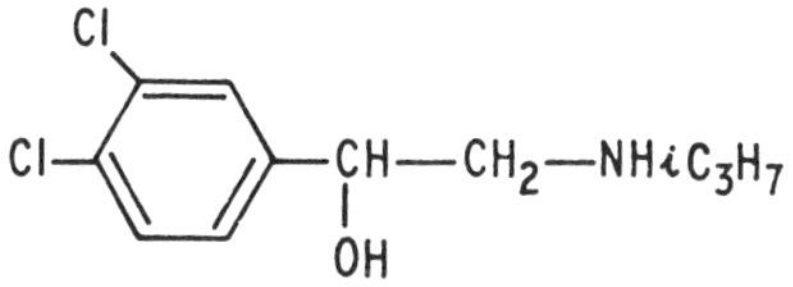

Figure 4.11. Dichlorisoprenaline (dichlorisoproterenol)

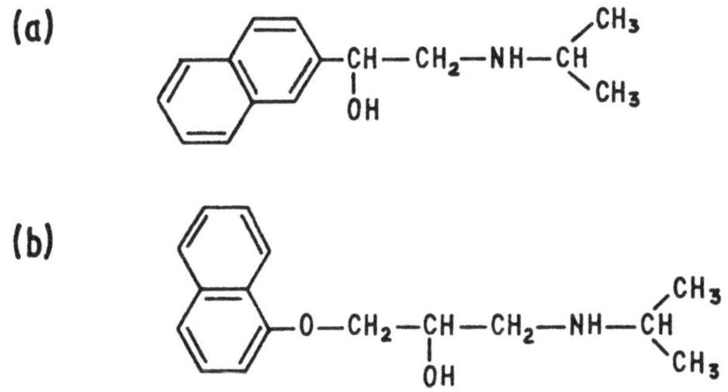

(a)

(b)

Figure 4.12. (a) Pronethol. (b) Propanolol

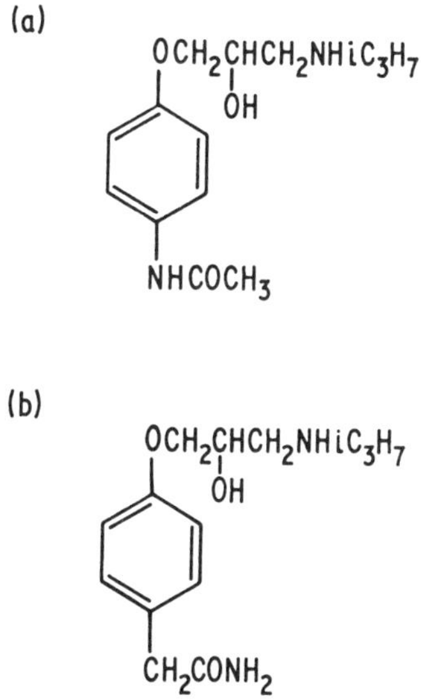

(a)

(b)

Figure 4.13. (a) Practolol. (b) Atenolol

Most β-blockers are structural analogues of isoprenoline and were discovered as a result of systematic research. The first β-adrenergic blocking agent discovered was dichlorisoprenaline (dichlorisoproterenol), shown in *Figure 4.11*. It is a partial agonist, retaining some intrinsic sympathomimetic activity in addition to the capacity to block the β-receptor.

The related compound propanolol (*Figure 4.12*) is clinically useful and does not retain any agonist effects.

Recent drugs include compounds which are selective in blocking β_1- and β_2-receptors, supporting the subdivision into two β-categories. Practolol (*Figure 4.13(a)*) is selective for β_1-receptors. Unfortunately practolol has had to be withdrawn owing to adverse side effects, but a more recent β_1- selective agonist is atenolol (*Figure 4.13(b)*). It is even more cardioselective than practolol. Although β-blockers are extremely valuable as in the relief of hypertension and have the advantage of being usable with asthmatic patients who need a β-blocking drug, the mechanism by which they produce their effect is not fully elucidated. It is easier to understand their effect on the heart rate which is through direct β-blockade.

Selective β_2-blockade is possible with butoxamine (*Figure 4.14*).

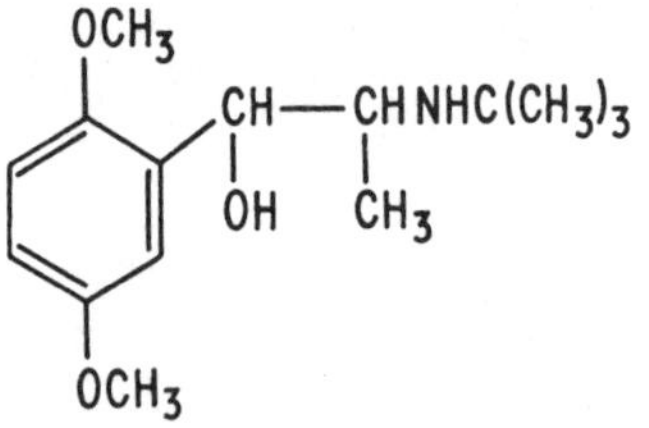

Figure 4.14. Butoxamine

The β-adrenergic receptor and adenylate cyclase activity

The effect of occupancy of β-sites is to stimulate adenylate cyclase to produce the second messenger cyclic AMP. The cyclic nucleotide production matches β-responses measured in more classical pharmacological procedures.

The β-receptors can be labelled with high specific activity, high affinity β-antagonists. These receptor sites have all the characteristics to be expected of β-receptors such as high specificity, including stereospecificity. It has been possible to compare direct binding studies and cyclic AMP production.

The important practical result of this is that β-adrenergic effects may be assayed in molecular terms by measurement of the cyclic AMP production. The details of the actual molecular mechanism remain obscure. Although catecholamine plus receptor causes the enzyme to produce cyclic AMP other factors may be essential such as the presence of Ca^{2+}, cyclic GMP or even adenosine.

Agonists of noradrenaline or adrenaline cause a high production of cyclic AMP, whereas antagonists have a high affinity as measured in labelled binding studies, but a low production of cyclic AMP. In this way both affinity and efficacy can be determined in molecular terms and such studies offer the most attractive type of data for a theoretician to use as the basis of any rationalization of structure–activity relationships.

Blockage of release and uptake

Some drugs appear to act, not by binding to the adrenergic receptor, but by preventing the release or uptake into temporary stores of the transmitter. Reserpine (*Figure 4.15*), an alkaloid derived from *Rauwolfia serpentina*, has been used therapeutically in various conditions since ancient times. It is taken up by the noradrenaline storage vesicles and impairs the uptake of mono-amines. This results in depletion of stores and loss of transmission. It affects the storage of dopamine and 5-hydroxytryptamine as well as noradrenaline, and affects the CNS and periphery. It is now used predominantly as a research tool, its therapeutic applications in hypertension and as a major tranquillizer being limited by its ability to cause severe depression.

The drug bretylium (*Figure 4.16*) blocks sympathetic nerves but does not block sensitivity of the tissue to injected adrenaline. It is thus believed to prevent the release of transmitter from the nerve ending.

Guanethidine (*Figure 4.17*) on initial injection causes a stimulation of sympathetic nerves followed by a blockage of nervous activity, although

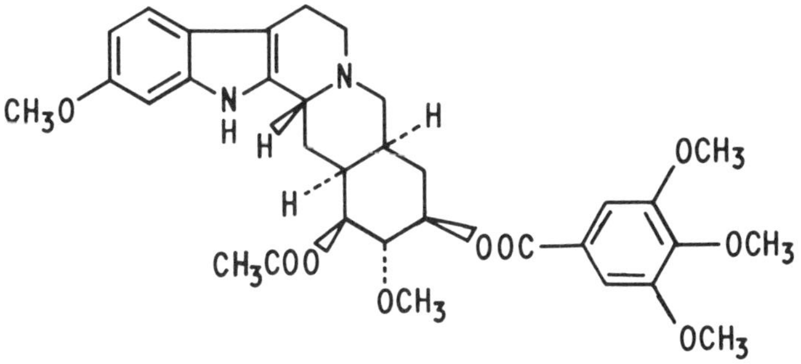

Figure 4.15. Reserpine

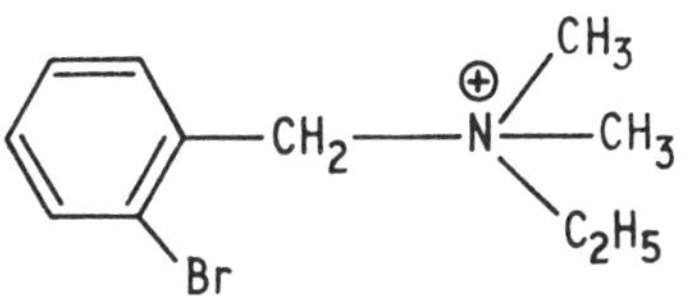

Figure 4.16. Bretylium

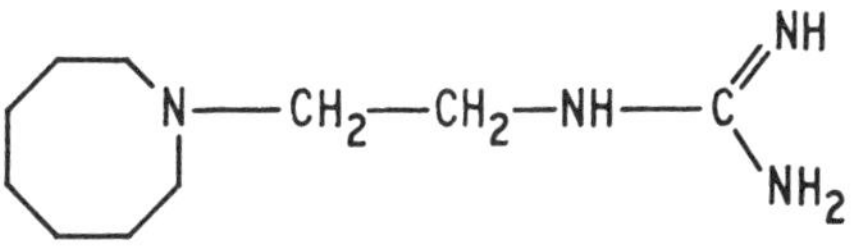

Figure 4.17. Guanethidine

injection of adrenaline will still stimulate so that it must be the nerve which is being affected rather than the muscle. It is thought that the prolonged block produced by guanethidine is caused by a depletion of peripheral stores of adrenaline since the initial action is to produce a large outflow.

Transport of the neuro-transmitter into the presynaptic nerve terminals is the primary mechanism for reducing the concentration of catecholamines in the synaptic gap. The uptake of noradrenaline into cells (this is different from that into storage vesicles) has been found to consist of two processes. The uptake into neurons, known as uptake (1), is active at low concentrations of noradrenaline and is saturable. Uptake (2) is thought to be into extra-neuronal tissues and operates mainly at high concentrations. The structural requirements for drugs taken up by these two processes are different and they are blocked by different inhibitors. Uptake (1) takes up the indirectly acting amines, such as amphetamine or tyramine, so that these drugs decrease noradrenaline removal. It is also inhibited by cocaine (an action not possessed by other local anaesthetics) and by the tricyclic antidepressants (see Chapter 7). Inhibitors of uptake (1) potentiate the effects of administered catecholamines and sympathetic stimulation but prevent the actions of indirectly acting sympathomimetics.

Uptake (2) is linked with the metabolism of noradrenaline by catechol-o-methyl transferase (COMT). It has been suggested to have a physiological role only at high monoamine concentrations but in some tissues may have greater importance. It takes up all catecholamines. Uptake (1) does not take up isoprenaline and is inhibited by pyrogallol, certain steroids and β-haloalkylamines.

Monoamine oxidase (MAO) inhibitors

Just as blockers of cholinesterase can modify the actions of acetylcholine, inhibitors of monoamine oxidase can raise the concentrations of catecholamines even though enzymic degradation is not the major mechanism of destruction.

The serious disadvantage of MAO inhibitors is that they increase the likelihood of adverse reactions to amines in diet or to drugs which release amines in the body. Thus foods with a high content of tyramine such as cheese and beef concentrates have caused hypertensive emergencies in patients undergoing a course of treatment with MAO inhibitors (see Chapter 6).

Summary

The catecholamine noradrenaline is the neuro-transmitter at the sympathetic nerve endings. The receptors can be classified broadly into two types α and β, with each being further subdivided into subclasses. Drugs can affect noradrenergic transmission by altering the release, uptake or storage of catecholamines.

Further reading

BLASCHKO, H. and MUSCHOLL, E. (eds) *Handbook of Experimental Pharmacology*, Vol **33**, (1972)
  Catecholamines.
BURNSTOCK, G. and COSTA, M. *The Adrenergic Neurone*, Chapman and Hall, London (1975)
SHORE, P. A., *Ann. Rev. Pharmac.*, **12**, 209 (1972)
  Storage and uptake of catecholamines.
WESTFALL, T., *Physiological Reviews*, **57**, 659 (1977)
  Local regulation of noradrenergic transmission.

Chapter 5

Histamine

The drawing of the histamine monocation (*Figure 5.1*) shows how histamine, like acetylcholine and the catecholamines, is a 1:2 disubstituted ethane with a basic nitrogen atom at one end of the molecule and a delocalized electron system at the other. The similarities do not end with these facts since, as we shall see, histamine is also able to interact with two types of receptor which are capable of being blocked by distinct specific antagonists. The precise nature of its role in normal physiology remains obscure, but it plays a part in inflammation, anaphylaxis, allergies and drug reactions. It may also have a neuronal function in the central nervous system.

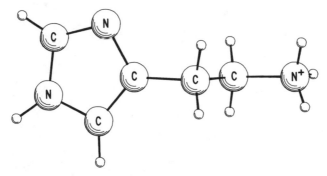

Figure 5.1. The histamine monocation

Occurrence

Histamine is present in fairly large quantities widely distributed in the body. It is produced by the decarboxylation of the amino acid histidine and is stored in an inactive form bound to the mucopolysaccharide heparin in 'mast' cells. These cells are distinguished by their high content of granules composed of the basic histamine bound to the acidic heparin.

Mast cells are found throughout the body, but concentrated at the interface between the body and the outside environment: the skin, the lungs, the gut and viscera, although less in the liver. There is a wide species variation, some animals having far more than others.

In the blood histamine is present in white cells (basophil leucocytes) and in platelets where it appears to be associated with adenosine triphosphate or diphosphate rather than with heparin.

Histamine given orally does not contribute to the stores of the amine but is excreted as imidazole acetic acid after first being methylated.

Physiological and pathological effects

The effects of histamine release are normally unpleasant and produce the following effects:

(1) Contraction of smooth muscles, e.g. gut, bronchi and uterus. Effects include restriction of the passage of air into and out of the lungs. Asthmatics are particularly vulnerable to a dose of histamine.
(2) Dilation of blood vessels with a consequent fall in blood pressure.
(3) Increase in capillary permeability producing oedema and a loss of blood fluid.
(4) Increased secretion by many glands notably the acid-secreting glands of the stomach, the mucus-secreting glands of the respiratory passages and tear glands, so familiar to sufferers of hay-fever.

Histamine release

Histamine may be released directly in tissue damage; for example, when one is cut, scratched or burned. The molecule may be physiologically active in inducing the removal of products of cell damage since most cells are concentrated in the skin of those parts of the body most frequently damaged: the feet, snout and ears.

The most serious circumstance causing the release of histamine is, however, as part of the allergic response, which again suggests that it is part of the body's protection against invasion by foreign matter.

When foreign proteins (antigens) invade the body the immunological system acts as the defence. Antibody proteins are formed to bind with the invader, be it a bacterial toxin or a protein of the bacterial cell wall. The aggregate of antigen and antibody is then degraded by the phagocytic cells.

This defence system deals not only with harmful bacteria but also with any foreign protein, including those such as dust or pollen or animal dander which enter through the nose, lungs or eyes and even through an abnormally permeable gut wall. Some of the antibodies formed become attached to the surface of cells and the tissues are then sensitized so that a further exposure to the antigen and antibody–antigen combination provokes the release of histamine. This is the allergic reaction. It does not take place if so much antibody is produced that the combination takes place in the blood stream or if very little is produced as is the case when the antigen is only weakly absorbed into the body or alternatively rapidly broken down. Sodium chromoglycate prevents the release of histamine after antibody–antigen combination and is very useful in allergies.

Many bases can also release histamine from its ionically bound stores and this release does show some chemical specificity. An effect of this type has been noticed when guanidines are used in treatment.

Curare, morphine and possibly heroin are histamine releasers which can be observed by the fact that they cause itching. Addicts can accustom themselves to normally lethal doses of drug but death may be caused by histamine release. The dangerous use of quinine in abortion again produces histamine release.

Pharmacological testing

The two distinguishable pharmacological actions of histamine are designated as H1 and H2. The H1 receptor mediates contraction of smooth muscle of the small intestines and bronchi. H1 receptor activity is normally determined by the effect on the isolated guinea-pig ilium. Effects on the permeability of cells, such as those of the skin, may be measured by injecting a suitable dye which will penetrate and stain tissues whose permeability has been increased, or by observing a wheal on human skin.

H2 receptors mediate acid secretion in animals. *In vitro* H2 effects are shown by the inhibition of contractions of the rat uterus and by increasing the rate of beating of the guinea-pig atrium. H2 receptors are also found in the central nervous system.

The two types of receptor may be defined pharmacologically by antagonists which selectively block responses of the appropriate preparation to histamine stimulation. The differentiation of the two types of receptor is also reflected in the relative agonist activities of some analogues.

Agonists

Even amongst molecules which are structurally very similar to histamine, there are a number of compounds which are relatively selective agonists at the two types of receptor. Some examples are given in *Table 5.1*. It is not certain whether the molecules act in the uncharged, free base form or ionized, but monocations are the most abundant species at physiological pH, as shown in *Table 5.2*.

For H1 activity it appears that structural features such as outlined in *Figure 5.2* are required.

Similarly some functional aspects which seem to be prerequisites for agonism at H2 receptors are displayed in *Figure 5.3*.

Of the H2 agonists, impromidine is striking in that it is more potent than

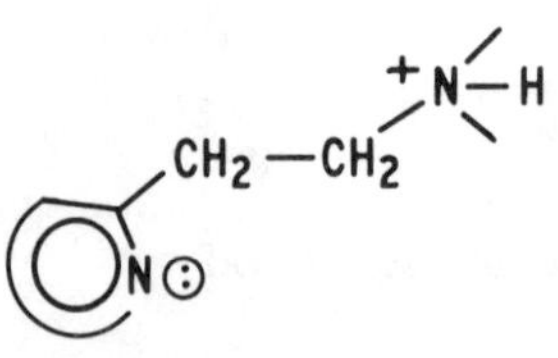

Figure 5.2. Functional groups required for histamine H1 agonism: side chain cation and N–H; heterocyclic basic N: in ortho position; ring rotation or 'essential' conformation

TABLE 5.1. Relatively selective agonists at histamine receptors

H1 Selective

2-methylhistamine

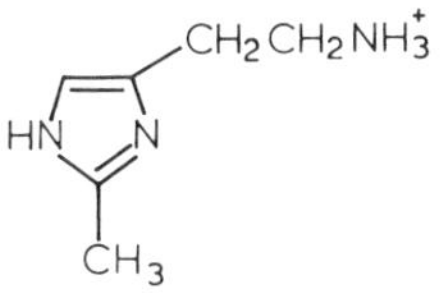

2-pyridylethylamine

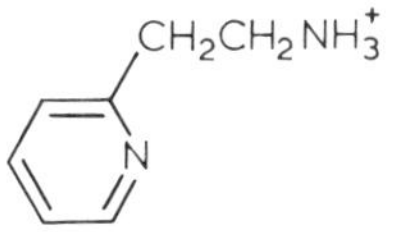

2-thiazoylethylamine

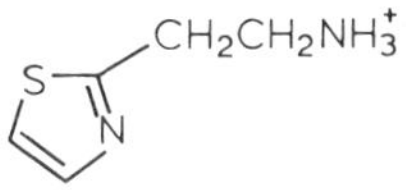

H2 Selective

4-methylhistamine

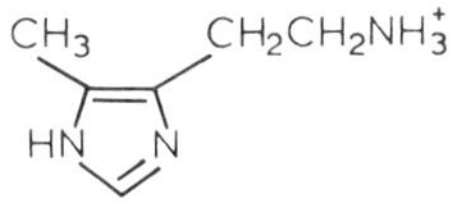

Betazole

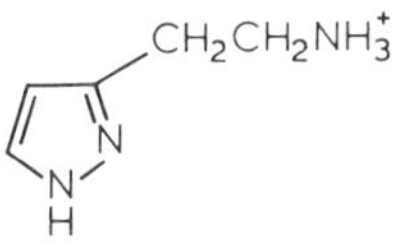

Dimaprit

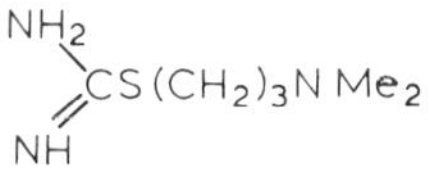

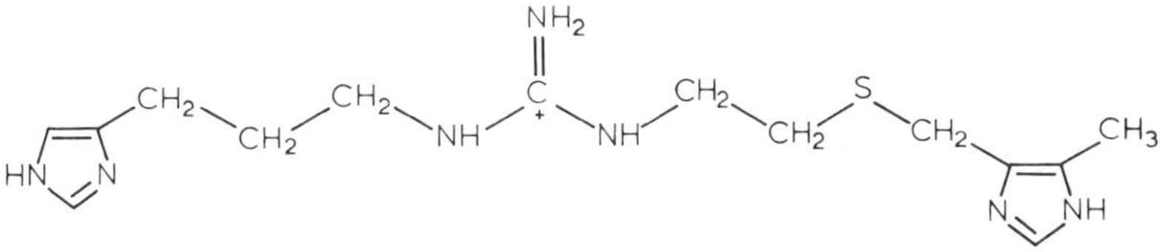

Impromidine

TABLE 5.2. Population of histamine species in aqueous solution at pH = 7.4 and at pH = 5.4 expressed as mole fraction, n [data from *J. med. Chem.*, 18, 905 (1975)]

Species	n	
	pH = 7.4	pH = 5.4
Dication	0.025	0.715
Monocation	0.966	0.285
Neutral	0.01	0.001
Anion	2.5×10^{-6}	2.5×10^{-8}

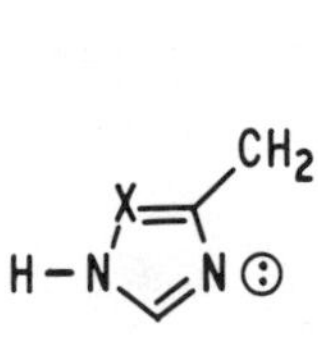

Figure 5.3. Functional groups required for histamine H2 agonism: side chain cation and N–H; N–H tautomer and amidine system; function as a proton transfer agent

histamine itself. Again dimaprit presents intriguing puzzles. In the first place if, as has been suggested, the ring has its function as a protein transfer agent in a charge relay system, then just how can dimaprit perform this role? The two possibilities are amplified in *Figure 5.4*. Although the second alternative looks structurally closely akin to histamine this demands the use of sulphur in a lone-pair donation which is both extremely rare in chemistry and unlikely on theoretical grounds. In addition, whilst dimaprit is a potent agonist with three carbons between the sulphur atom and amino-nitrogen, the analogues with two and four carbons respectively are not active. This ought to be some clue to the conformational requirement for agonism.

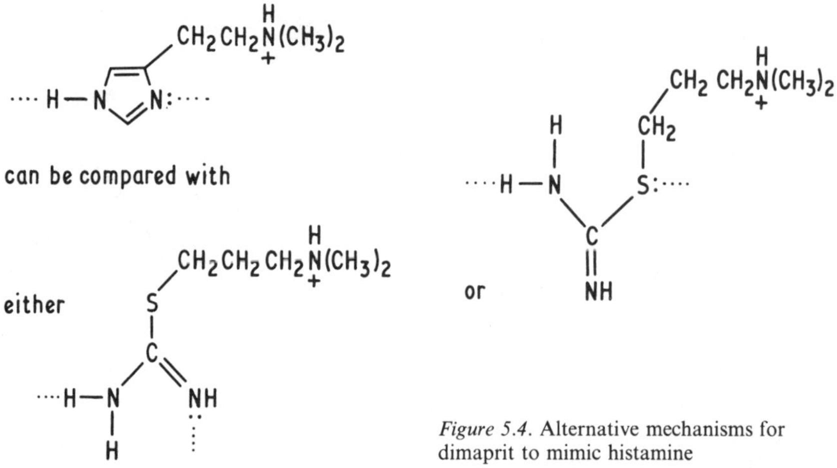

Figure 5.4. Alternative mechanisms for dimaprit to mimic histamine

H1 Antagonists

The effects of histamine release are so unpleasant that considerable effort has been expended in finding suitable antagonists. Until recently all the successes were in the discovery of antagonists of H1 activity, commonly called antihistamines.

Histamine-blocking activity was first detected by Bovet and Staub in 1937. The subsequent search has followed the familiar pattern of screening substances for activity, altering the structure and testing the new compound. By a combination of good organic chemical intuition and sheer hit-and-miss testing, a number of useful compounds have emerged.

If the side-chain nitrogen atom is loaded up with large groups, we do

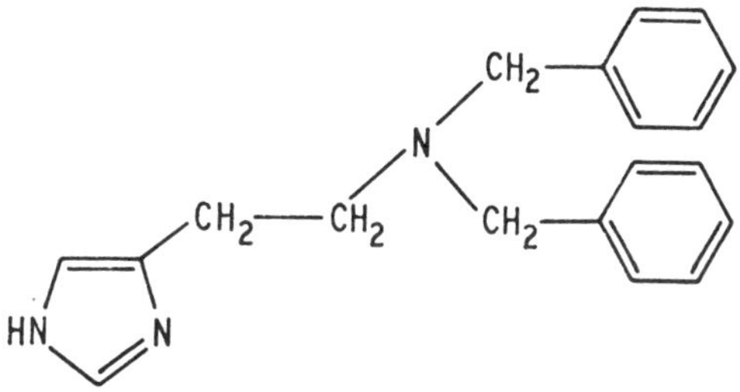

Figure 5.5. An H1 antagonist

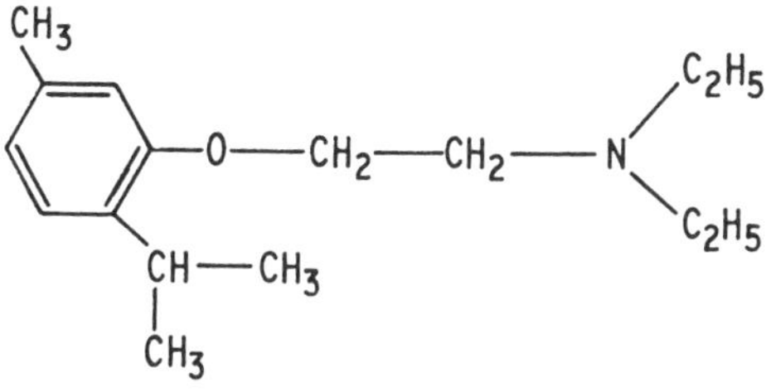

Figure 5.6. The antihistamine F929

obtain a compound which will block histamine H1 activity. The compound shown in *Figure 5.5* is an example.

After much search, the compound illustrated in *Figure 5.6* was found. It was designated F929 after Fourneau the chemist who prepared it. It was originally synthesized and screened as a potential oxytocic substance.

The basic structure of the anti H1 histamine can be represented as a substituted ethylamine.

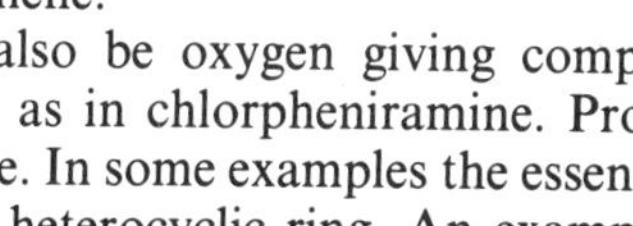

In most cases the *R* groups are methyls.

When the *X* in the formula is nitrogen the resulting compounds may be considered to be derivatives of ethylenediamine. Examples include tripelennamine and methapyrilene.

The atom *X* may also be oxygen giving compounds such as diphenhydramine, or carbon as in chlorpheniramine. Promethazine contains the phenothiazine structure. In some examples the essential ethylamine structure is incorporated into a heterocyclic ring. An example is cyclizine. All these examples are illustrated in *Figure 5.7*. They fall into five broad categories with many examples of each type.

Anti H1 histamines are used in cases of allergic rhinitis, urticaria and stings where they block obvious results of histamine release, but also for some types of asthma and motion sickness.

Antihistamines also produce noticeable effects on the central nervous system, particularly drowsiness.

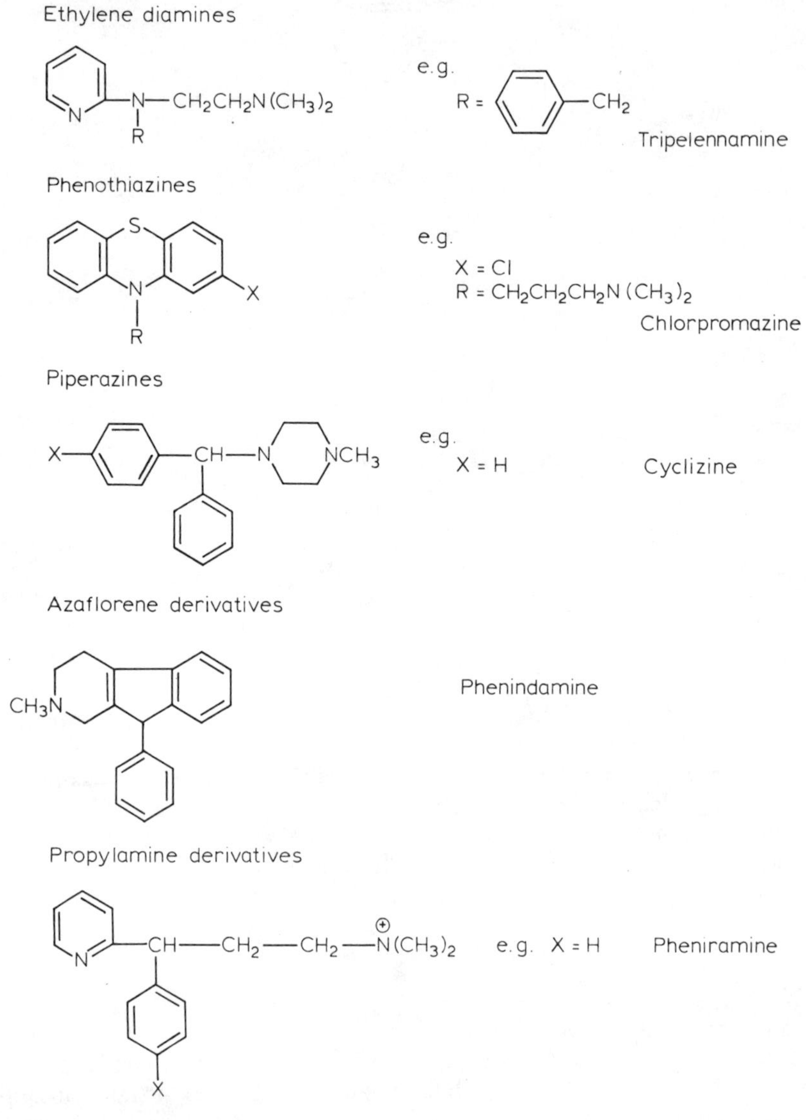

Ethylene diamines

e.g.

R = —CH$_2$

Tripelennamine

Phenothiazines

e.g.
X = Cl
R = CH$_2$CH$_2$CH$_2$N (CH$_3$)$_2$

Chlorpromazine

Piperazines

X——CH—N—NCH$_3$

e.g.
X = H

Cyclizine

Azaflorene derivatives

CH$_3$N

Phenindamine

Propylamine derivatives

—CH—CH$_2$—CH$_2$—$\overset{\oplus}{N}$(CH$_3$)$_2$

e.g. X = H   Pheniramine

Figure 5.7. The categories of H1 antihistamines with examples

H2 Antagonists

With the discovery of an H2 receptor antagonist by Black and his colleagues many of the puzzling aspects of histamine pharmacology can be clarified. The availability of H2 antagonists is thus of major scientific as well as medical importance. Clinically H2 blocking drugs are widely used in cases of peptic ulceration and other gastric hypersecretory states.

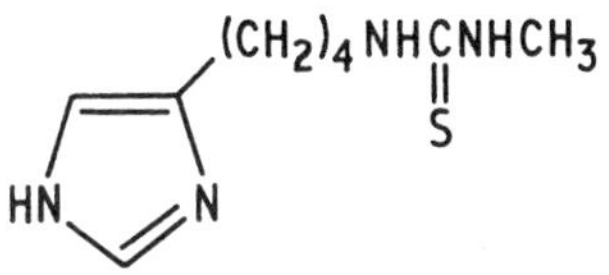

Figure 5.8. Burimamide

The antagonists are structurally similar to the natural agonist and were developed from it in a systematic scientific manner.

The first antagonist discovered was burimamide (*Figure 5.8*). When used alone this compound blocks the responses to histamine which cannot be blocked by H1 antagonists such as mepyramine. Histamine responses such as hypotension, which can only be antagonized partially by mepyramine alone, can be blocked completely by combination of the two drugs.

Metiamide (*Figure 5.9*) is structurally similar to burimamide but is a more potent H2 antagonist. It does have some undesirable side effects which are not found, however, in the very successful cimetidine (*Figure 5.10*) in which the thiourea is replaced by cyanoguanidine. Some other H2 antagonists are shown in *Figure 5.11*.

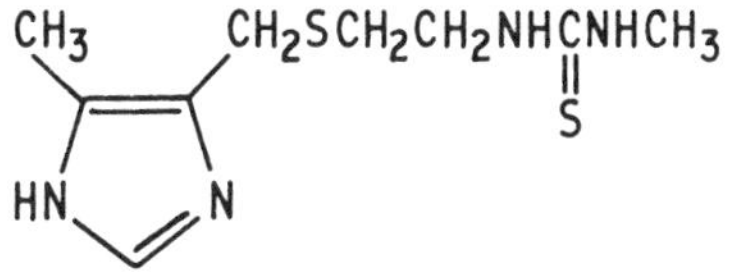

Figure 5.9. Metiamide

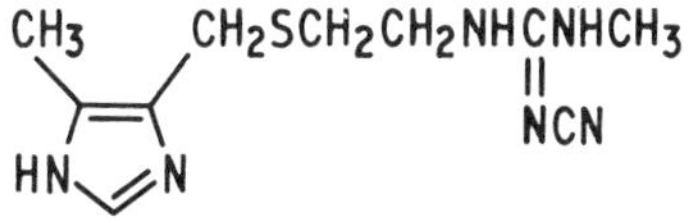

Figure 5.10. Cimetidine

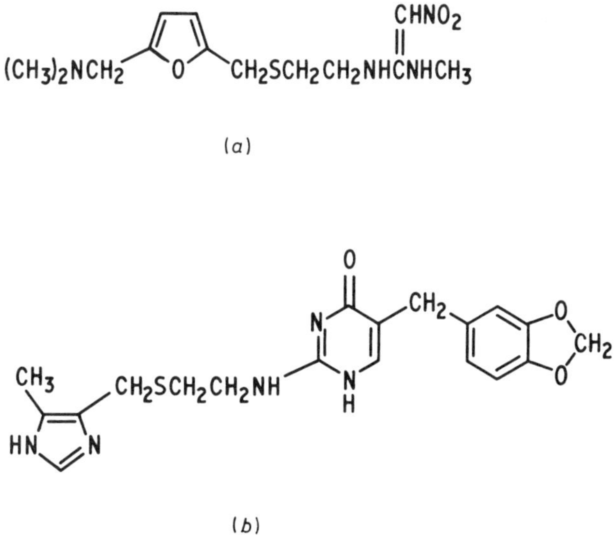

(a)

(b)

Figure 5.11. (a) Ranitidine. (b) Oxmetidine

The discovery of these drugs is a perfect example of just how scientific the research for new medicinal compounds has become. The unkind epithet 'molecular roulette' which is often used to describe the process of pharmaceutical research has no place in this study which was a textbook example of the application of pure science to a medicinal problem.

Summary

Histamine, like the transmitters met earlier, acts at two distinguishable receptors, probably as a monocation. An amino–ethyl side chain attached to an unsaturated ring appears to be necessary for interaction with the receptors. Distinct antagonist molecules are known for both the H1 and H2 activities but very little is known about the details of the receptors or the biochemical results of receptor binding.

Further reading

BLACK, J. W. *et al. Nature, Lond.*, **236**, 385 (1972)
  Definition and antagonism of histamine receptors.
BURLAND, W. L. and SIMPKINS, M. A. (eds). *Cimetidine, Excerpta Medica*, Amsterdam (1977)
DOUGLAS, W. W. in L. S. Goodman and A. Gilman (eds), *The Pharmacological Basis of Therapeutics*, 5th edn, Macmillan, New York (1969)
  Chapter 29 Histamines and anti-histamines.
DURANT, G. J., GANELLIN, C. R. and PARSONS, M. E. *J. med. Chem.*, **18**, 905 (1975)
  Chemical differentiation of histamine receptor agonists.
GANELLIN, C. R. *J. med. Chem.*, **24**, 913 (1981)
  Structure–activity analysis in the discovery of H2 antagonists.
GANELLIN, C. R. and DURANT, G. J. in M. E. Wolff (ed), *Burger's Medicinal Chemistry*, 4th edn, Wiley–Interscience, New York (1979–81)
GREEN, J. P. and WITIAK, D. T. in M. E. Wolff (ed), *Burger's Medicinal Chemistry* Part 2, 3rd edn, Wiley–Interscience, New York (1970)
  Chapters 64 and 65.

Chapter 6

Central nervous system
I. Monoamines and acetylcholine

Even though there remain many unsolved problems concerned with the peripheral nervous system, the situation as regards the central nervous system is infinitely more complex. Despite this, it is an area of considerable scientific interest and excitement.

The central nervous system consists of the spinal cord and the brain. The brain itself is a mass of cross-connected nerves, there being approximately 10^{10} nerve cells, each of which may be capable of multiple connections. The individual nerve cells are anatomically independent but functionally connected by the transmitter chemicals which enable signals to cross synaptic gaps.

As illustrated in *Figure 6.1* some areas of the brain are concerned with specific functions. Many other areas are involved in coordination and organization. The cortex and other so-called 'higher' centres are thought to be responsible for intellectual processes, while 'lower' areas such as the

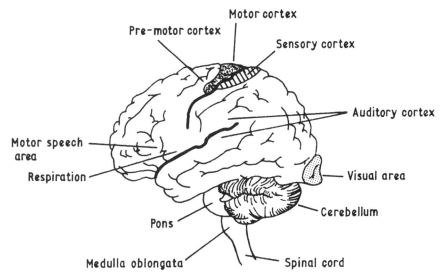

Figure 6.1. The human brain

medulla and brainstem control vegetative functions. There is a multitude of neuronal pathways linking the different areas. Each neuron within the brain receives input from thousands of other cells. By lesioning and studying changes in behaviour some information has been obtained about the complex circuitry but much remains unknown.

Much of current belief about the mechanisms of synaptic transmission in the brain is based on analogy with the peripheral system because of the difficulty of research on the brain. It is, for example, very difficult to devise satisfactory *in vitro* experiments. Further it is very difficult to measure quantitatively or even reproducibly some of the higher functions of the central nervous system such as emotions. It is also extremely hazardous to associate biochemical properties determined by *in vitro* experiment with function. The brain is not homogeneous and specific neurons are very inaccessible. With *in vivo* experiments on animals the time taken to extract parts of the brain and the associated chemicals must complicate any interpretation. All these obstacles mean that the knowledge of central nervous system transmitters is far less complete than for the peripheral system.

What does not seem to be in doubt is that transmission is by chemical neuro-transmitters.

Much more information about the distribution of chemicals in the brain has been obtained in recent years using radioimmuno-assay techniques.

Chemical transmitters

In Chapter 1 the list of pieces of evidence required to establish the identification of a transmitter was given. The mere fact that a substance is present in the brain and can produce a response is insufficient. By these criteria none of the postulated central nervous system transmitters is as clearly defined as is acetylcholine in the external system.

The type of study used to identify putative transmitters starts with identification of the substances in the brain, and usually by fluorescent studies the location of concentrations in specific regions. As with peripheral neurohormones the behaviour of agonists and antagonists can lend considerable support to the identification. For most of the postulated compounds it has been possible to show that enzymes and cofactors are present for their synthesis and possibly their destruction; metabolites are found. Perfusion experiments may show that transmitters are released in specific areas and micro-iontophoretic experiments can show that putting a transmitter into a precise location reproduces the effect of natural transmitter. Perhaps the most important criterion for identification of central transmitters is that of 'identity of action'—the demonstration that the substance produces exactly the same ion conductance changes in the post-synaptic membrane as does the endogenous substance.

Recently it has become apparent that some chemical messengers act as 'modulators' rather than producing rapid post-synaptic responses such as those seen in the periphery. Many substances, including some peptides, produce slow changes in the cell membranes and are probably involved in controlling the 'background' excitability.

Some of this work will be mentioned as the substances which are generally accepted as neuro-transmitters in the brain are discussed individually.

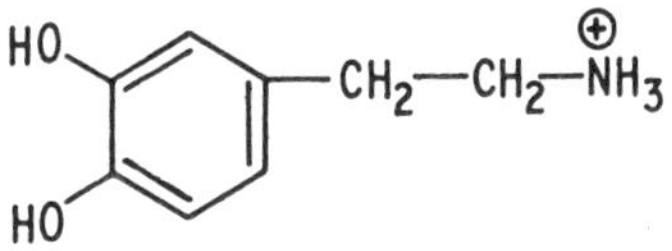

HO—⟨benzene ring⟩—CH_2—CH_2—$\overset{\oplus}{N}H_3$

Figure 6.2. Dopamine

Catecholamines

In some respects more is known about brain catecholamines than any other neuro-transmitters. Fluorescence photomicrography and the use of drugs which selectively destroy nerves containing the catecholamines noradrenaline and dopamine (*Figure 6.2*) have made it possible to locate the cell bodies and to trace the pathways of their axions and nerve endings.

Noradrenergic neurons innervate the hypothalamus, cortex, limbic system and many other areas. The cell bodies are mostly confined to the locus ceruleus of the pons and part of the reticular system. Noradrenergic transmission is thought to be involved in control of alertness, movement, mood, many endocrine functions and control of blood pressure, temperature and reproduction.

In the case of noradrenaline (and adrenaline) direct binding studies have identified receptors of the β-type: binding is stereospecific and affinity is highest for potent β-adrenergic antagonists. These β-receptors seem to mediate catecholamine-induced cyclic AMP formation in the brain. The role of β-receptors in the brain is not clear. There are also central α-receptors whose role is clearer. Central α-receptors are thought to be important in the central control of blood pressure. Thus α-methyl dopa and clonidine are thought to be hypotensives through their central α_2-agonist effects.

Cocaine blocks the uptake of noradrenaline and consequently magnifies its effects. Some antidepressant drugs have the same effect. Amphetamine both blocks uptake and promotes release of noradrenaline and is a psycho-motor stimulant. Many drugs used in the treatment of hypertension also affect the storage and release of noradrenaline. Monoamine oxidase in-hibitors prevent destruction of the transmitter and consequently potentiate its effect. It is widely believed that mental depression is associated with decreased availability of brain catecholamines. Further details of drugs which may produce their effect by acting on monoamine transmission are given below.

In addition to noradrenaline there is some evidence that adrenaline is a central nervous system transmitter. Nerves containing adrenaline have been found in the brain stem.

Although in the periphery dopamine is a precursor of noradrenaline it is thought to have a transmitter role of its own in the central nervous system. It is specifically localized in the basal ganglia, which are concerned with movement; in the limbic system, which is associated with mood and emotion; the olfactory tubercle and parts of the hypothalamus and cortex.

The dopamine-containing tracts play an important role in the integration of movements; making up a dopamine deficiency by administering dopa is used in the treatment of Parkinson's disease which is thought to arise from the imbalance between acetylcholine and dopamine.

In the extrapyramidal system, cholinergic neurons are excitatory and synapse with dopaminergic neurons which are of an inhibitory nature. Parkinson's disease is caused by a progressive atrophy of these dopaminergic neurons and the corresponding release of the excitatory cholinergic system results in the characteristic tremor, rigidity and akinesia associated with the disease.

It has been found that the symptoms are considerably alleviated by the administration of *l*-dopa, which is the precursor of dopamine and which crosses the blood–brain barrier while the latter does not.

Direct binding studies have been made of the stereospecific binding of labelled compounds to the dopamine receptors. This binding can be inhibited by a variety of antipsychotic drugs with inhibitory potencies which correlate well with clinical doses used for controlling schizophrenia.

Homogenates of the appropriate regions of rat brains also contain an adenylate cyclase which is activated by small contractions of dopamine. This stimulatory effect can be blocked by dopamine antagonists including effective antipsychotic drugs and stimulated by some agonists. In *Figure 6.3* the concentrations of antipsychotic drugs which reduce the stereospecific component of the binding of tritiated haloperidol (a potent dopamine antagonist and clinically useful antipsychotic drug) by half (IC_{50}) are plotted against average doses used in the treatment of schizophrenia. The correlation is compelling. Amphetamines can produce psychoses rather like schizophrenia which is thought to result from excess dopamine release.

A subclassification of dopamine receptors has been suggested. D_1-receptors are those which stimulate adenyl cyclase and D_2-receptors are those which

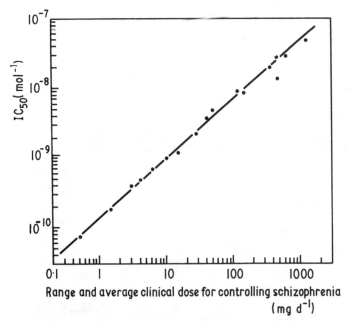

Figure 6.3. Correlation between IC_{50} values of antipsychotic drugs and clinical doses used in cases of schizophrenia

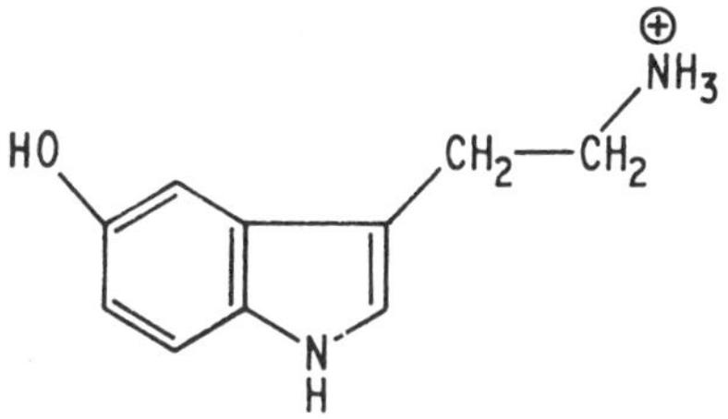

Figure 6.4. 5-Hydroxytryptamine

do not do this. Distinctions such as these may provide the answer to some of the mysteries of drug actions on the central nervous system and will result in more selectively acting drugs.

Tryptaminergic neurons based on 5-hydroxytryptamine or serotonin (*Figure 6.4*) are found in certain mid-brain nuclei (the 'raphe' nuclei) and pathways extend to the limbic system, cortex, mid-brain and other areas. Among other functions they are thought to be involved in the control of sleep.

Drugs with structural similarities to 5-hydroxytryptamine, such as LSD, can produce vivid hallucinations. Several antagonists are known such as LSD, but it appears possible that some of these compounds act at pre- rather than post-synaptic serotonin receptors. A direct binding 5-hydroxytryptamine assay is available. Many clinical useful drugs (e.g. tricyclic antidepressants) affect 5-hydroxytryptamine uptake mechanisms but the relevance of this to their clinical effect is uncertain. Drug structures are given later.

Histamine

Histamine is found in the brain as is specific histidine decarboxylase and the metabolizing enzyme imidazole N-methyl transferase. Antihistamines appear to have some effect on the central nervous system. The firing rate of certain neurons in the brain is depressed by histamine and H2 antagonists such as metiamide specifically block this depression. Histamine also raises cyclic AMP levels in brain slices.

The role of histamine in the central nervous system is less clear than that of the compounds described above.

Acetylcholine

The distribution of acetylcholine in the brain is inferred from the location of synthesizing and degrading enzymes. The transmission mechanism is thought to be similar to that at the neuromuscular junction or ganglionic sites.

Binding sites with a high affinity and specificity for tritiated quinuclidinyl benzilate have been found in brain homogenates. These binding sites resemble those of muscarinic cholinergic receptors. Muscarinic agonists and antagonists will displace the labelled compound while nicotinic compounds are ineffectual.

The actions of acetylcholine at Renshaw cells are, however, blocked by curare and mimicked by nicotine and are thus thought to contain nicotinic receptors.

This is the clearest example of cholinergic transmission in the central nervous system but pathways have been described, for example in the cortex, hippocampus and thalamus.

Many behavioural effects of cholinergic drugs have been described and cholinergic pathways are thought to be involved in control of several functions.

Central nervous system drugs

Although in some of the cases of postulated central transmitter it is possible to discuss agonist and antagonist activity as with peripheral transmitters,

TABLE 6.1. Phenothiazine derivatives

Phenothiazine nucleus		
		Aliphatic side-chain
Chlorpromazine	(2) Cl	(10) $CH_2CH_2CH_2N(CH_3)_2$
Triflupromazine	(2) CF_3	(10) $CH_2CH_2CH_2N(CH_3)_2$
		Piperidine side-chain
Thioridazine	(2) SCH_3	(10)
Mesoridazine	(2) $\overset{O}{\overset{\uparrow}{S}}CH_3$	(10)
Piperacetzine	(2) $COCH_3$	(10) $CH_2CH_2CH_2N$—CH_2CH_2OH
		Piperazine side-chain
Prochlorperazine	(2) Cl	(10) $CH_2CH_2CH_2N$——NCH_3
Trifluperazine	(2) CF_3	(10) $CH_2CH_2CH_2N$——NCH_3
Butaperazine	(2) $CO(CH_2)_2CH_3$	(10) $CH_2CH_2CH_2N$——NCH_3
Perphenazine	(2) Cl	(10) $CH_2CH_2CH_2N$——NCH_2CH_2OH
Fluphenazine	(2) CF_3	(10) $CH_2CH_2CH_2N$——NCH_2CH_2OH

it is not so in all cases and there is not complete agreement on such a classification. Thus we will follow the common practice of discussing central nervous system drugs on the basis of use rather than the more satisfying rationalization with respect to molecular mechanism.

Antipsychotics

Antipsychotics or neuroleptics were formerly called major tranquillizers. They reduce psychotic symptoms of various aetiologies without excessive sedation and without causing addiction. The symptoms of schizophrenia are ameliorated, but parkinsonian symptoms may be produced as a result of antagonizing dopamine. There is considerable evidence that schizophrenia may be related to hyperactivity of dopaminergic systems although the 'lesion' as such may be at an earlier stage in the control system which is finally manifest as hyperactivity of the dopamine system.

Amphetamine, which releases dopamine, can produce symptoms which resemble paranoid schizophrenia, while potent antipsychotics will block dopamine receptors.

Chlorpromazine was discovered through clinical observation on structurally related antihistamines which produced prolongation of barbiturate-induced sleep. The antipsychotic activity was 'tuned-up' by chemical manipulation, giving some of the many variations on the chlorpromazine structure listed in *Table 6.1*. There is a general relationship between the potency of the various antipsychotic drugs and their ability to block dopamine receptors in binding experiments (see above), but they also have antagonist actions at cholinergic, noradrenergic and histaminergic receptors.

A second major class of antipsychotic drugs which are dopamine antagonists are the thioxanthene derivatives (*Table 6.2*). Structurally they are, of course, closely related to chlorpromazine and the phenothiazines.

A third category of dopamine-blocking antipsychotic drug which is structurally very different is the substituted butyrophenones (*Table 6.3*).

The butyrophenones show many of the pharmacological effects of the phenothiazines and they do antagonize dopamine, but the profile of pharmacological action is not identical.

TABLE 6.2. Thioxanthene derivatives

Thioxanthene nucleus

Examples: Chlorprothixene; $R_1 = Cl$

$R_2 = CHCH_2CH_2N(CH_3)_2$

Thiothixene; $R_1 = SO_2N(CH_3)_2$

$R_2 = CHCH_2CH_2NNCH_3$

TABLE 6.3. Butyrophenones and related compounds

Haloperidol	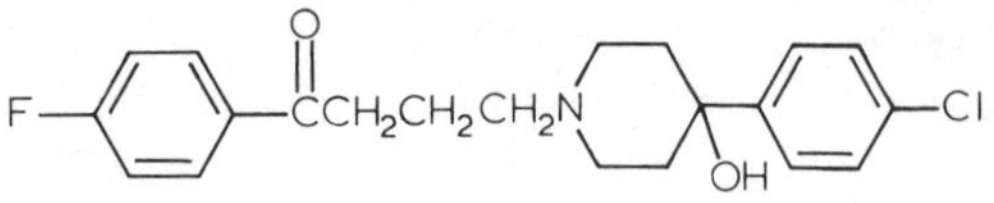
Pimozide	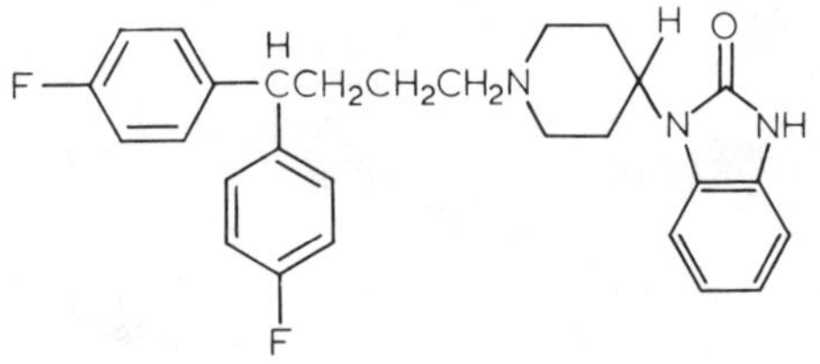
Penfluridol	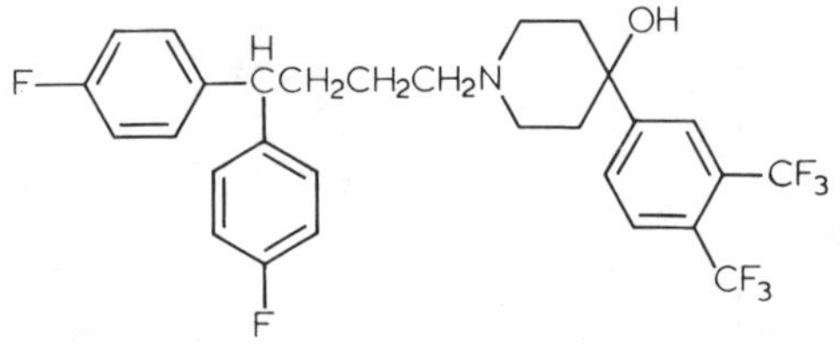

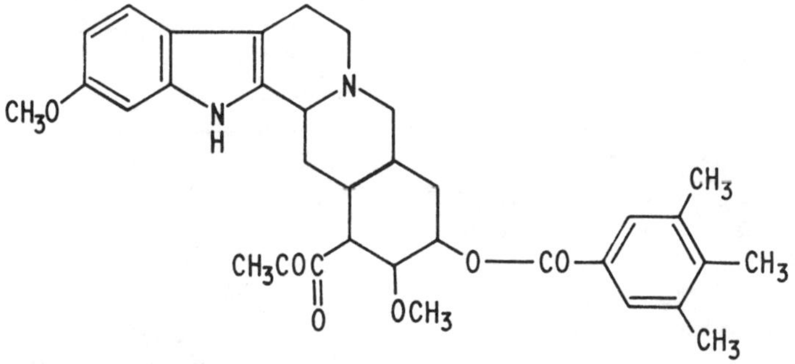

Figure 6.5. Reserpine

A very early example of a 'major' tranquillizer is reserpine (*Figure 6.5*) which has been used in the treatment of mental illness in India for centuries. In the peripheral nervous system it depletes the stores of catecholamines, while in the central nervous system both catecholamines and serotonin are depleted. It cannot be considered as a dopamine antagonist, being more of a chemical sledgehammer producing both antipsychotic and sedative effects.

Antidepressants

There are two major categories of antidepressants; the monoamine oxidase inhibitors (MAO inhibitors) and the tricyclic antidepressants. The former are no longer widely used because of the toxic hazards mentioned earlier.

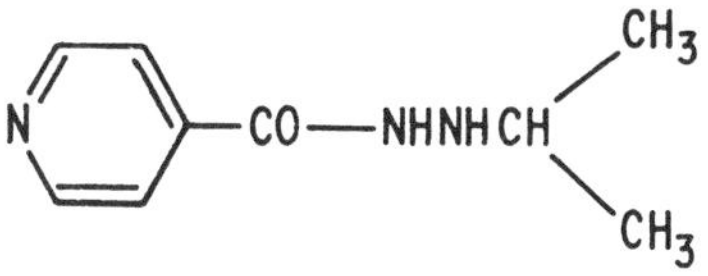

Figure 6.6. Iproniazid

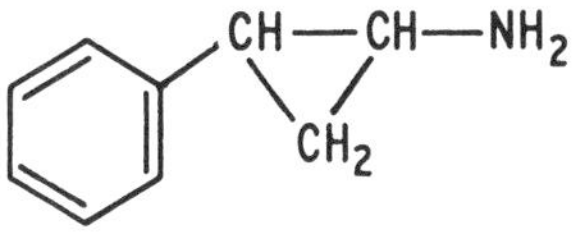

Figure 6.7. Tranylcypromine

TABLE 6.4. Antidepressants

TRICYCLIC TYPE

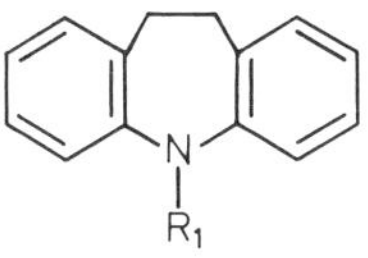

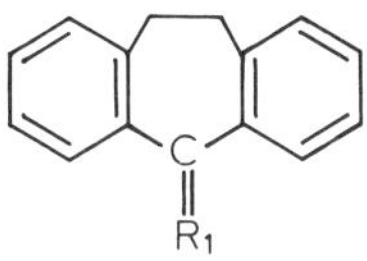

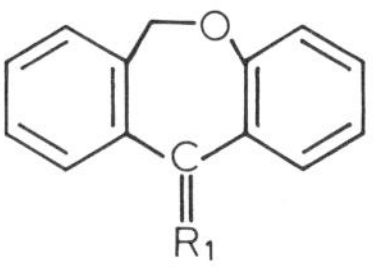

R$_1$ = CH$_2$CH$_2$CH$_2$N(CH$_3$)$_2$
Imipramine

R$_1$ = CH$_2$CH$_2$CH$_2$NHCH$_3$
Desipramine

R$_1$ = CH$_2$CH(CH$_3$)CH$_2$N(CH$_3$)$_2$
Trimipramine

CHCH$_2$CH$_2$N(CH$_3$)$_2$
Amitriptyline

CHCH$_2$CH$_2$NHCH$_3$
Nortriptyline

CH$_2$CH$_2$CH$_2$NHCH$_3$
Protriptyline

CHCH$_2$CH$_2$N(CH$_3$)$_2$
Doxepin

MONOAMINE OXIDASE INHIBITORS

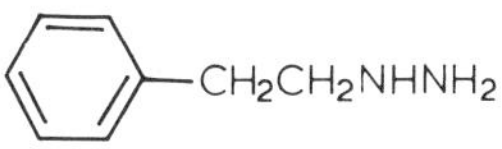

Phenelzine

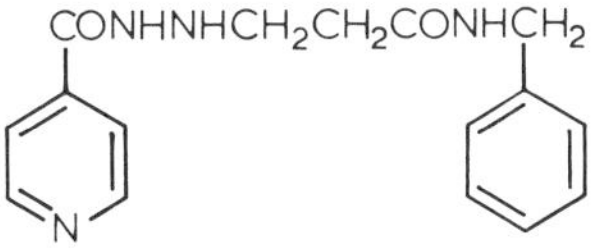

Nialamide

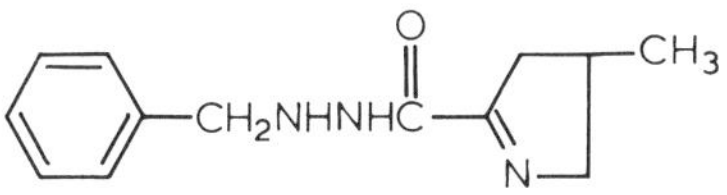

Isocarboxazide

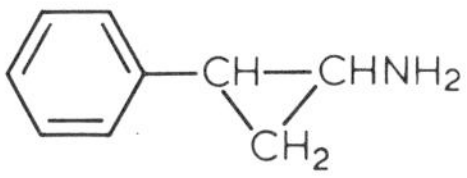

Tranylcypromine

Work on monoamine oxidase inhibitors stemmed from the discovery that the antitubercular drug iproniazid (*Figure 6.6*) also possesses both antidepressant activity and inhibits monoamine oxidases. Ideally such compounds should inhibit the brain enzyme causing an elevation of noradrenaline concentration but not at the same time affect the enzyme in such organs as the liver, whose damage may produce serious side effects.

Tranylcypromine (*Figure 6.7*) is a potent nonhydrazine enzyme inhibitor which also produces stimulation like amphetamine. It is thus a bimodal antidepressant giving a rapid action by virtue of stimulation of amine receptors and a longer lasting action by blocking the enzyme used to destroy the natural transmitter.

As already mentioned, monoamine oxidase inhibitors also have a disadvantage in that problems may be caused to patients who eat foods such as cheese which are rich in the amino acid tyramine.

Because of these problems the tricyclic antidepressants have become more widely used in treatment of depression. When searching for new tranquillizers among the phenothiazine derivatives the compound methotrimeprazine was discovered. This compound produced beneficial effects in depressed patients. Structural variation and screening led to more active compounds such as imipramine (*Table 6.4*).

The mechanism of action of the tricyclic antidepressants is not clear but all drugs which have effective clinical antidepressant action interact in some way with monoamine transmission.

The tricyclics are known to block re-uptake of noradrenaline and of 5-hydroxytryptamine, the tertiary amines having more effect on 5-hydroxytryptamine uptake and the secondary amines more effect on noradrenaline. It is thought however that the therapeutic benefit is due to adaptive changes following this uptake blockade, as the clinical improvement takes 2–3 weeks before it is manifest.

The tricyclics possess cholinergic blocking action which is responsible for many of the side effects.

Several new antidepressant drugs have been developed recently which do not bear much structural resemblance to the tricyclics and which differ in their pharmacological properties (*Table 6.5*). This implies that blockade of monoamine re-uptake is not a necessary feature for effective antidepressant action, although interference with monoamine transmission is still implicated. None of the newer compounds have superior clinical efficiency compared with the older drugs but they do have fewer side effects, especially those due to anticholinergic activity.

Psychomotor stimulants

D-Amphetamine (*Figure 6.8*) is a central and motor stimulant. It has been used to relieve fatigue, the classic example being that of bomber pilots on

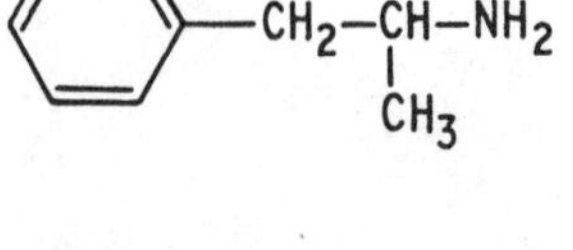

Figure 6.8. Amphetamine

TABLE 6.5. New antidepressant compounds

	Pharmacological properties which may be relevant

Maprotilene

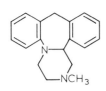

$(CH_2)_3NHCH_3$

Inhibits noradrenaline re-uptake

Trazodone

Agonist and antagonist
actions on 5-hydroxytryptamine receptors
α_2-antagonist and releases
noradrenaline

Mianserin

Blocks 5-hydroxytryptamine receptors
α_2-antagonist, releases noradrenaline

Nomifensine

Inhibits noradrenaline and dopamine re-uptake

Zimelidine

Inhibits 5-hydroxytryptamine re-uptake

wartime operations. It also elevates mood, but there are inevitably rebound effects and it is of little value in the clinic as an antidepressant. D-Amphetamine is a releaser of dopamine and noradrenaline from presynaptic nerve terminals. Hence there is a rationale for the fact that overdosage can give rise to psychotic episodes which resemble paranoid schizophrenia. D-Amphetamine is also a centrally acting anorexic agent and there is evidence to support the view that the biological effects are mediated through dopaminergic mechanisms. Thus the anorexic effects of amphetamine in laboratory animals can be blocked by haloperidol, but a derivative of amphetamine, 'fenfluramine', has more specific anorexic actions, which have been suggested to be due to interaction with tryptaminergic transmission.

The use of amphetamine has been greatly curtailed in recent years because of street abuse.

Other sympathomimetic stimulants are shown below in *Table 6.6*.

TABLE 6.6. Sympathomimetic stimulants

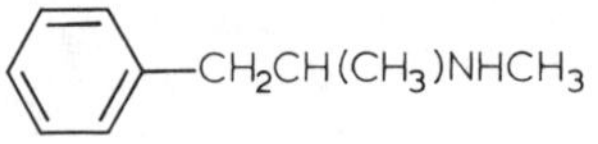

Methamphetamine

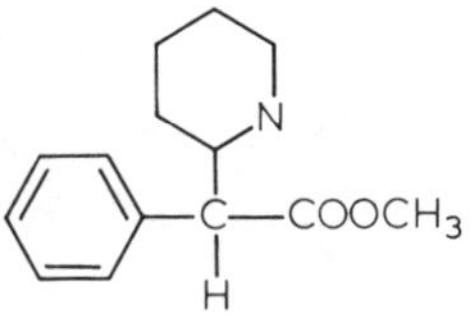

Methylphenidate

Hallucinogens

These compounds can produce psychoses or maladjusted behaviour and may be psychedelic; that is they produce heightened perceptions. They have little clinical value and are most widely known through abuse. They are often 5-hydroxytryptamine antagonists.

It is very difficult to devise objective tests of such compounds and the effects are hard to follow in animals.

LSD or lysergic acid diethylamide (*Figure 6.9*) has been the object of a number of direct binding studies. It produces hallucinations at extremely low doses.

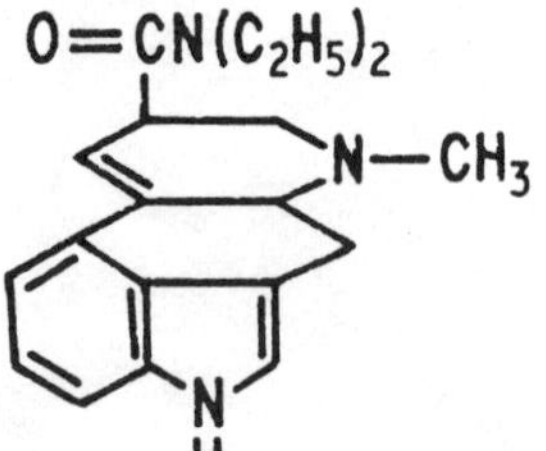

Figure 6.9. LSD (lysergic acid diethylamide)

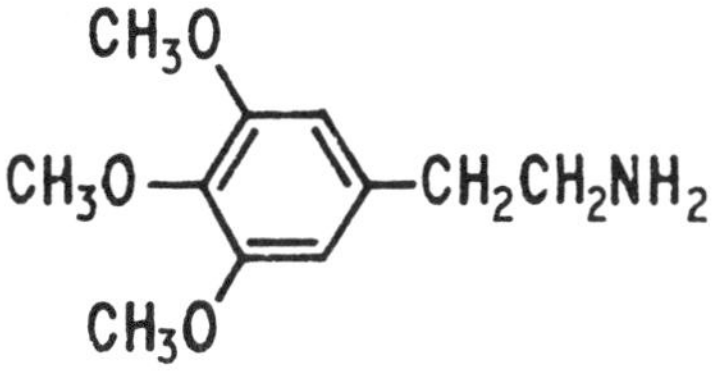

Figure 6.10. Mescalin (3,4,5-trimethoxyphenylethylamine)

Another famous naturally occurring hallucinogen is mescalin (*Figure 6.10*) which is the active principle of the juice from the peyote cactus. Its mechanism of action is uncertain. It is not very potent in the sense that large doses are required, but it gives strong visual hallucinations.

Of cannabis very little is known about its mode of action. The main active ingredient is tetrahydrocannabinol (*Figure 6.11*). One interesting feature of this compound, which makes it rare among the compounds discussed in this book, is the fact that it does not contain a nitrogen atom.

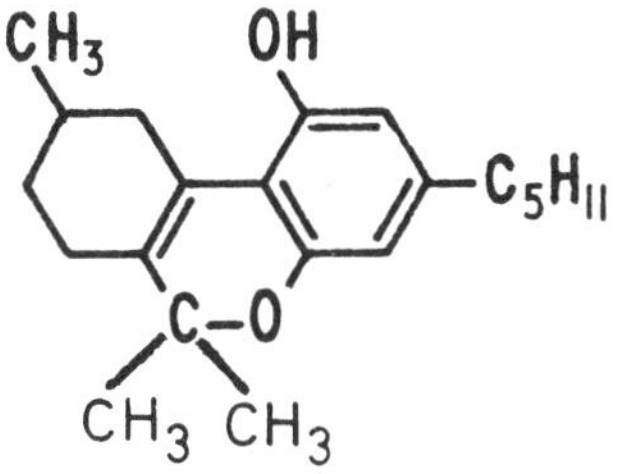

Figure 6.11. Tetrahydrocannabinol

Summary

Despite impressive recent advances there is still much to be learned about central nervous system transmitters, their agonists and antagonists. There is evidence that transmitters do have distinguishable receptors, possibly more than one type for each transmitter. Drugs are classified by their effects rather than by a certain basis of molecular behaviour.

Further reading

COOPER, J. R., BLOOM, F. E and ROTH, R. H. *Biochemical Basis of Neuropharmacology,* Oxford University Press (1978)
GREEN, A. R. and COSTAIN, D. W. in E. S. PAYKEL and A. COPPER (eds), *Psychopharmacology of Affective Disorders,* Oxford University Press (1979).
The biochemistry of depression.
HORNYKIEWICZ, O. *Neuroscience,* 3, 773 (1979).
Psychopharmacological implications of dopamine and dopamine agonists. A critical evaluation of current evidence.
KEBABIAN, J. W. and CALNE, D. B. *Nature, Lond.,* 277, 93 (1979).
Multiple receptors for dopamine.

Chapter 7

Central nervous system
II. Amino acids and peptides

Both amino acids and peptides are now generally believed to be central nervous system transmitters.

Amino acids

Amongst the amino acids the strongest evidence for a transmitter role is for γ-aminobutyric acid (GABA), *Figure 7.1*. Specific labelling suggests that it is a major neuro-transmitter in the brain. It is synthesized from glutamate and information concerning its role has been obtained from binding studies and iontophoretic application, as well as from the actions of drugs which inhibit its synthesis or breakdown. It is metabolized by the enzyme GABA-transaminase but the major method of termination of its synaptic action is thought to be the high affinity uptake mechanism which has been described earlier.

It is an inhibitory transmitter and produces hyperpolarization of neurons by increasing the chloride conductance of the post-synaptic membrane.

Its physiological role has been difficult to elucidate as it is present in most cells because it is an intermediate in metabolism. However, much evidence

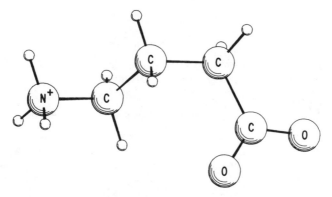

Figure 7.1. γ-aminobutyric acid

now exists to show that it is the inhibitory transmitter used by interneurons in many areas throughout the brain. It is thought to be involved in most post-synaptic inhibitory activity in areas above the spinal cord and in pre-synaptic inhibition within the cord.

Specific antagonists of GABA transmission are known, for example bicuculline (*Figure 7.2*) and picrotoxin (*Figure 7.3*). These are potent con-vulsants, illustrating the importance of the inhibitory role of GABA. Bicuculline binds to GABA receptor sites and is thought to be a competitive antagonist, but picrotoxin does not bind directly to the receptor. It probably binds to the ionophore and prevents the increase in chloride conductance which follows receptor activation. This illustrates the variety of different mechanisms of drug action which are being discovered. Certain barbiturate drugs have been shown to prolong the chloride conductance change caused by GABA and this probably adds to their non-specific general anaesthetic action described in Chapter 8.

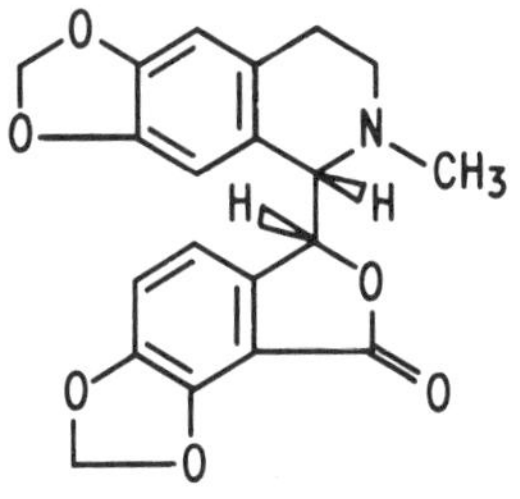

Figure 7.2. Bicuculline

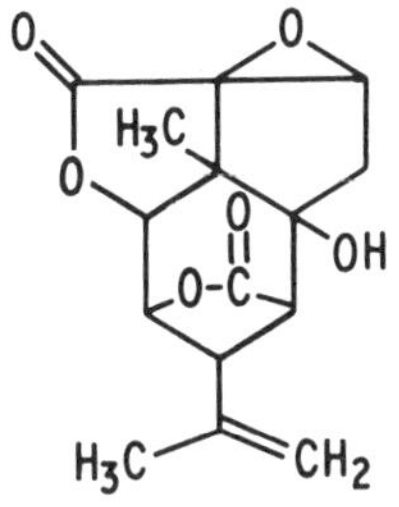

Figure 7.3. Picrotoxin

Another inhibitory transmitter of importance is glycine (*Figure 7.4*). This is thought to be responsible for inhibition in the spinal cord. It also in-creases chloride conductance and produces hyperpolarization. Strychnine is a specific antagonist of glycine and this drug also produces convulsions, but these are characteristically different from those caused by the GABA antagonists described above.

There are no useful therapeutic drugs which interfere with glycine trans-mission but it may be implicated in certain spastic conditions. The location of glycine receptors can be indicated by the use of labelled strychnine.

For all the amino acid neuro-transmitter candidates, the high affinity uptake systems for the acids are highly dependent on sodium ions being present.

Amino acids which have been suggested to be involved in excitatory trans-mission in the central nervous system are L-glutamic acid and aspartic acid.

84

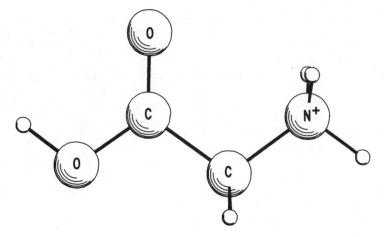

Figure 7.4. Glycine in its crystal conformation (note one hydrogen atom is hidden)

TABLE 7.1. Anti-anxiety drugs

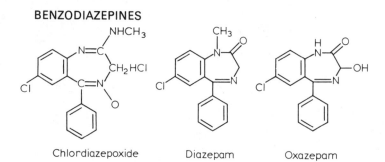

BENZODIAZEPINES

Chlordiazepoxide   Diazepam   Oxazepam

GLYCEROL DERIVATIVES

$NH_2COOCH_2CCH_2OCONH_2$

CH_3

C_3H_7

$C_4H_9NHCOOCH_2CCH_2OCONH_2$

CH_3

C_3H_7

Meprobamate   Tybamate

As with GABA, the determination of the role of these compounds is complicated by their involvement in metabolism and their widespread distribution. Glutamic acid has a powerful excitant action on almost all neurons in the central nervous system so that it is difficult to detect specific pathways and its transmitter status is still uncertain. The situation would become much clearer if specific antagonists of these compounds could be found, but none are yet available.

Anti-anxiety drugs

The name 'anti-anxiety drugs' is currently used for what were formerly described as minor tranquillizers, and prescribed for nervousness or tension in both normal and neurotic individuals. The major groups of anti-anxiety drugs with some examples are displayed in *Table 7.1*.

The benzodiazepines are mildly sedative at the clinically useful doses and most are hypnotic at higher doses. They are well on the way to replacing the barbiturates as minor tranquillizers and hypnotics, one reason being that they are virtually suicide-proof as they have a very high therapeutic index.

Much work has been carried out recently on the mechanism of action of the benzodiazepines. The results of early binding studies on the glycine receptor (displacement of strychnine binding) suggested that the benzodiazepines produce their clinical effects through interaction at this receptor. This interpretation has not gained general acceptance and may reflect the pitfalls in relating direct binding studies to the particular principal mechanism of biological effects.

It is now known that there are specific binding sites in the central nervous system for the benzodiazepines, commonly, but not exclusively, adjacent to GABA receptors. It has been suggested that action at these receptor sites increases the effect of GABA at its receptor and, by this or other mechanisms, they are known to increase the effects of endogenous GABA.

Recently studies have involved a search for an endogenous ligand which may be acting at these sites, to control GABA transmission. Results so far have proved inconclusive. A new specific antagonist of the benzodiazepine action has been reported. It binds to the same receptor site, but has little effect on normal animals. Its actions should prove very interesting when full details of its effects in various conditions are available.

Many thousands of benzodiazepine drugs have been synthesized but the profile of pharmacological action is very similar for all of them, despite attempts to separate the different actions. The main differences between the different structures are pharmacokinetic (see *Table 7.2*) and these are important when they are being prescribed.

The main pharmacological effects of all the structures are an anxiolytic effect, central muscle relaxation and anticonvulsant activity. They may sometimes produce a mild dependence and withdrawal symptoms have been described but they are considerably safer in this respect than the barbiturates.

TABLE 7.2. Benzodiazepines

Structure		Half-life

1,4-substituted
  e.g. Diazepam (Valium)
  Flurazepam (Dalmane)
  Nitrazepam (Mogadon)
  Chlordiazepoxide
    (Librium)
		30–100 h
		metabolized to
		active compounds

3-OH,1,4-substituted
  e.g. Temazepam
  Lorazepam
		10–20 h
		no important
		metabolites

1,5-substituted ˙ e.g. Clobazam		18 h long-acting metabolite

Anti-epileptic drugs

Many drugs are effective in the different types of epilepsy but little is known about the mechanisms of action. Some of those which are widely prescribed are listed in *Table 7.3*.

Peptides

The case for peptides being central nervous neuro-transmitters is quite the reverse from the usual pattern. Long before the existence of the transmitter was postulated compounds which can act at the receptor were known. The compounds in question are morphine and its analogues, which have been known as analgesics for many years. Only much more recently has a natural agonist known as enkephalin been isolated.

Enkephalin activity is due to two pentapeptides: H-Tyr-Gly-Gly-Phe-Met-OH (methionine enkephalin) and H-Tyr-Gly-Gly-Phe-Leu-OH (leucine enkephalin). The terminal tyrosine residue can adopt conformations similar

TABLE 7.3. Anti-epileptics

Drug	Use	Possible mechanisms of action
Phenytoin	Grand mal Psychomotor epilepsy	Decreases post-tetanic potentiation. Increases GABA transmission in invertebrates
Phenobarbitone	Grand mal Psychomotor epilepsy	Increases threshold for excitation, limits spread of seizure
Sodium valproate $(CH_3CH_2CH_2)_2CHCOONa$	Grand mal Petit mal	Potentiates GABA transmission
Carbamazepine	Psychomotor and other forms of epilepsy	?
Ethosuximide	Petit mal	?
Diazepam	Given intravenously in status epilepticus	Potentiates GABA transmission by action at benzodiazopine receptors

to key portions of the morphine structure (*see* below). Enkephalins also inhibit the stereospecific binding of a tritiated morphine antagonist naloxone in brain homogenates.

The distribution of the enkephalins parallels that known for opiate receptors, high concentrations being found in the limbic system, thalamus, striatium, hypothalamus, mid-brain and spinal cord, as well as in peripheral sites such as the intestine.

'Peptidergic' pathways of neurons containing the enkephalins have been described and the use of radioimmune methods has been particularly useful here. Peptide release on stimulation has been described and there are a variety of peptidase enzymes. The actions of administered enkephalins are very rapidly terminated by these enzymes and recently specific inhibitors of the enzymes have been described.

The discovery of the enkephalins has not materially altered the therapeutic use of opiates (see below) as they have been found to produce the same pattern of pharmacological actions as the synthetic drugs and to produce a similar tolerance and addiction. Manipulations of the natural transmission, possibly involving the use of enzyme inhibitors, may however yet provide more useful drugs.

Action at opiate receptors, whether by exogenous or endogenous compounds does result in inhibition of adenyl cyclase activity and decreases in cyclic AMP concentrations but the relationship between this and the pharmacological activity is not entirely clear. However, changes in this system may be responsible for the tolerance and addiction observed.

One of the most interesting aspects of the discovery of the enkephalins has been the demonstration that, as well as being involved in control of pain, they may be implicated in other systems, such as control of appetite, thirst and other aspects of emotion and behaviour. This has opened up many possibilities for research.

The opiate receptors have now been divided into at least three types and this may explain some of the variation of action, and lack of effect of the antagonist naloxone (*Figure 7.5*) in some situations:

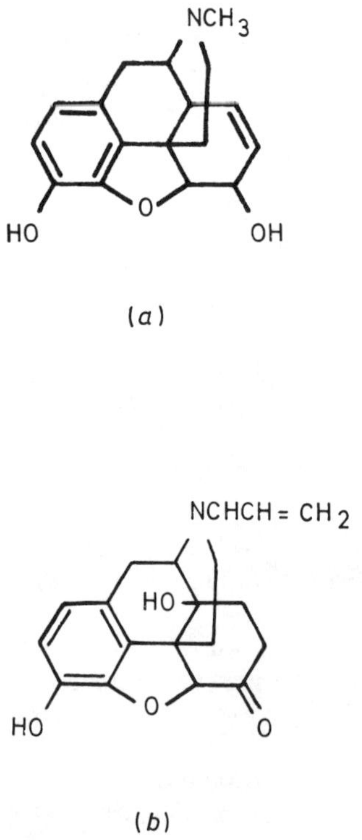

(a)

(b)   *Figure 7.5.* (a) Morphine. (b) Naloxone

(1) 'μ'—classical morphine-like actions.
(2) 'K'—prototype drug is ketocyclazocine; does not substitute for morphine; produces dependence; produces some classical opiate actions.
(3) 'σ'—mediates different pharmacological actions; prototype drug is N-allylnorcyclazocine; may involve interaction with dopamine transmission.

Naloxone is less effective as antagonist at the latter two receptor types.

Several other peptides are also now thought to be neuro-transmitters. For example substance P (an undecapeptide) is found particularly in the spinal cord (as well as other areas) and may be a transmitter in sensory input pathways.

A number of other putative peptide transmitters have been suggested which illustrates the enormous scope for research in this field, particularly perhaps the receptors to the peptide β-endorphin.

Analgesics

Drugs which relieve pain without causing general anaesthesia are called analgesics. Perhaps the most important one with a central nervous action is the alkaloid morphine (*Figure 7.5*) which is derived from opium. From the point of view of molecular pharmacology this molecule is exceedingly important since the essential structure (*Figure 7.6*) is held in a rigid form and it is known that only one optical isomer is active.

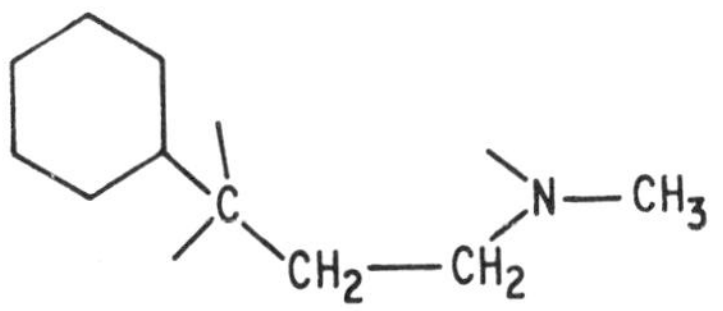

Figure 7.6. The 'essential' structure of morphine

This detail tells us something about the receptor but we may still obtain striking variations in activity merely by changing the nature of the alkyl group attached to the basic tertiary nitrogen atom. The relationship between structure and activity in this area is a large and complex topic. For example in benzomorphans a phenolic OH is essential whereas in pethidine it is not required.

Considerable research effort has been and is being expended in the search for compounds which have the beneficial effects of morphine without having narcotic properties but so far separation of the various pharmacological properties has not been achieved. All the drugs possess respiratory depressant as well as analgesic properties and are liable to produce tolerance and dependence. Some partial agonist opiates are used as analgesics, such as pentazocine (*Figure 7.7*) but they produce their own problems of dependence.

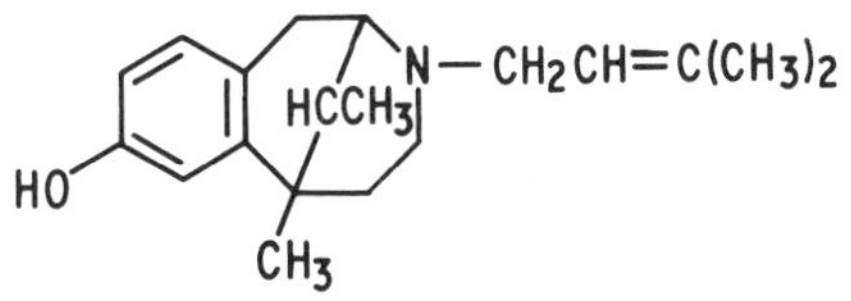

Figure 7.7. Pentazocine

One interesting new synthetic compound in this field is buprenorphine (*Figure 7.8*) which has partial agonist activity and very high lipid solubility. It has been said to cause some tolerance but not as severe physical dependence as the other opiates.

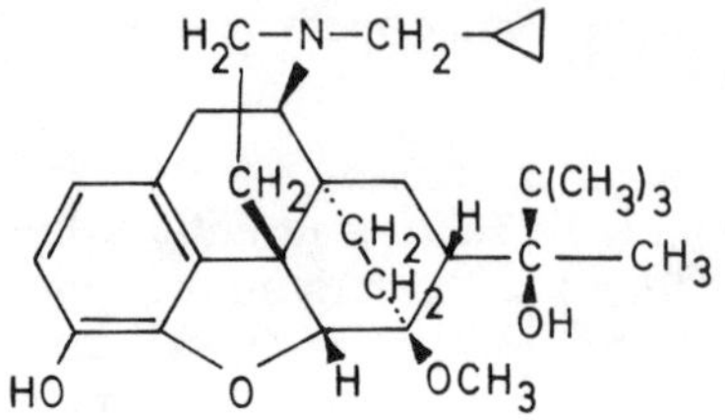

Figure 7.8. Buprenorphine

Summary

New discoveries involving γ-aminobutyric acid (GABA) have given a much clearer molecular picture of the mechanism of this transmitter. Other amino acids seem also to be involved as transmitters. The field of peptide transmission is one of the most actively investigated at the present time but the molecular picture is again far from clear.

Further reading

ANDREWS, P. R. and JOHNSON, G. A. R. *Biochem. Pharm.*, **28**, 2697 (1979)
  GABA agonists and antagonists.
de FEUDIS, F. V. *Trends in Pharmacological Sciences*, **2**, VI (1981)
  GABA studies; therapeutic perspectives.
GARNIER, H. (ed), *Peptides in Neurobiology*, Plenum Press, New York (1977)
MOHLER, H. *Trends in Pharmacological Sciences*, **2**, 116 (1981)
  Benzodiazepine receptors: are there endogenous ligands in the brain?
OLSEN, R. W. *J. Neurochemistry*, **37**, 1 (1981)
  GABA-benzodiazepine-barbiturate receptor interactions.
PARKHOUSE, J., PLEUVRY, B. J. and REES, J. M. H. *Analgesic Drugs*, Blackwells, Oxford (1979)

Chapter 8

Anaesthetics

General anaesthetics are a class of drugs which depress the central nervous system while local anaesthetics produce a reversible blockade of conduction in nerves.

Both classes have obvious intrinsic importance but from the viewpoint of this book they are different from the topics discussed so far because their activities do not show high specificity as regards chemical structure. Their actions seem to depend on physical properties rather than intimate chemical structure.

General anaesthetics

A general anaesthetic produces a reversible loss of consciousness permitting surgical operations to be carried out. Most are inhaled. Non-volatile general anaesthetics are injected intravenously and are often used as basal anaesthetics to produce drowsiness before entering an operating theatre and as induction agents. Four stages of anaesthesia are recognized:

(1) Disorder of perception, impaired consciousness.
(2) Unconsciousness, delirium, reflexes still work.
(3) The surgical plane when muscles begin to relax, progressive loss of reflexes.
(4) Respiratory failure—the toxic phase.

Experimentally the effects of a potential anaesthetic are measured by the loss of some facility or the sleeping time induced. Mice are most often used as experimental animals, but experiments have been performed on goldfish, tadpoles and even bacteria.

Given a sufficient dose almost any small molecule will produce narcosis; even the inert gases will produce anaesthesia at high enough pressures (a hazard in diving).

Most anaesthetics actually used are simple aliphatic compounds. As we ascend an homologous series the compounds are found to be increasingly potent. Very roughly, the addition of an extra $-CH_2-$ group has a threefold effect in terms of equinarcotic concentrations in many series.

The increasing efficacy as the molecular mass increases does not go on indefinitely and a cut-off point is reached. This same type of behaviour is found in a number of physical properties such as solubility, vapour pressure, ability to lower surface tension and partition coefficient between oil and water. This suggests that we are dealing with a phase phenomenon. The activity merely reflects the ratio between the actual concentration of a substance and the concentration required to produce saturation.

Since colligative properties are all interdependent it is possible to produce a wealth of correlations between activity and some property. Lipid solubility is frequently used in this context.

A correlation, however, does not necessarily lead to a molecular picture or mechanism of the anaesthetic effect. On the question of mechanism there is not complete agreement.

Table 8.1 gives some examples of inhalation anaesthetics which are used.

TABLE 8.1. Inhalation anaesthetics

Chemical formula	Comment
Nitrous oxide N_2O	Used in conjuction with other anaesthetics; very weak and is not a good muscle relaxant; useful analgesic
Cyclopropane $CH_2 - CH_2$ with CH_2 above	Disadvantage mainly explosiveness; potent, with few side effects
Diethyl ether $C_2H_5OC_2H_5$	Explosive; produces nausea and vomiting
Trichlorethylene $CCl_2{=}CHCl$	No skeletal muscle relaxation; analgesic properties
Halothane $CF_3 - CHBrCl$	Little nausea or vomiting but depresses circulation and respiration
Methoxyflurane $CH_3 - O - C - CH - Cl_2$ with F above and F below the C	Non-explosive and relaxes skeletal muscles; toxic metabolites
Chloroform $CHCl_3$	Can produce liver and kidney damage; seldom used; can cause cardiac arrest
Ethyl chloride $CH_3 - CH_2Cl$	Depresses circulation and respiration; can produce liver damage

The intravenous anaesthetics include the sodium salts of the very short-acting barbiturates. Thiopental is barbituric acid with the 5 position substituted with an ethyl group and a l-methyl butyl group. It is used to provide rapid pleasant induction. Barbiturates depress respiration and cause severe dependence.

Other intravenous anaesthetics in use include alphaxalone ('Althesis'), which has a steroid structure, and ketamine, which produces a 'dissociative' anaesthesia (*Figure 8.1*).

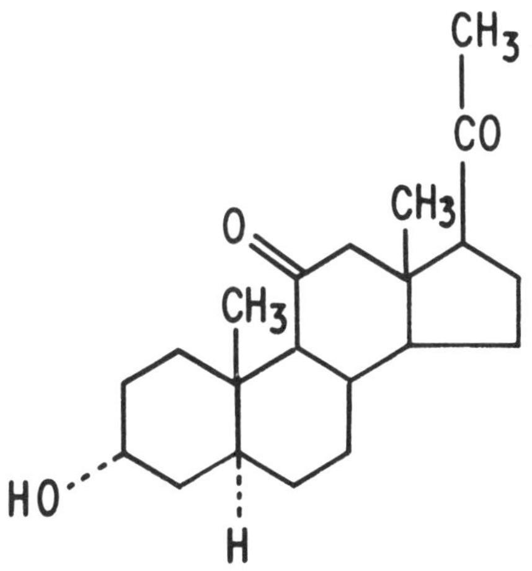

(a)

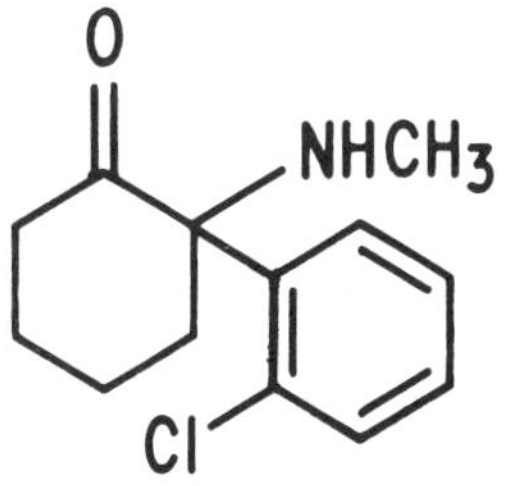

(b)   *Figure 8.1.* (a) Alphaxalone. (b) Ketamine

Theories of general anaesthesia

The theories of general anaesthesia have as their aim the definition of the environment of action rather than a detailed molecular mechanism.

The most general theory due to Ferguson does not even achieve this, although it does provide correlations between the pressure of gas required for anaesthesia and physical properties of the substance. It takes no account of any mechanism of interaction of molecular species but simply relates anaesthetic potency with thermodynamic activity. It is true that the thermodynamic activities of anaesthetics calculated on a Raoult's law basis do lie in a narrow range while concentrations may vary widely. On the other hand a number of agents do not fit this hypothesis, notably CF_4 and SF_6 and the theory cannot lead to any mechanism of molecular interaction or binding.

Two alternative theories which do include some notional molecular aspects are the aqueous and lipid phase approaches.

The hydrate theories of Pauling and Miller focus on the ability of small molecules to stabilize water structure by forming clathrates. The ordered water is then believed to stabilize nerve membranes and their protein components, producing narcosis. Quantitatively reasonable correlations between hydrate dissociation pressures and activity can be produced, but molecules such as SF_6 again do not fit. Furthermore several well-known anaesthetics such as ether and halothanes do not form hydrates.

The most successful correlations are between lipid solubility and anaesthetic potency. These quite striking correlations, albeit of the log–log type (*Figure 8.2*), are convincing enough for it to be generally believed that the site of action is hydrophobic in nature.

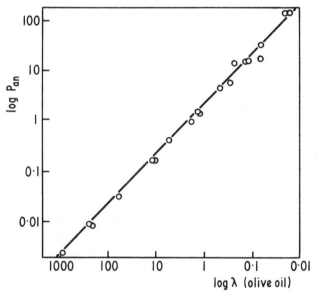

Figure 8.2. Correlation of anaesthetic pressure with oil–gas partition coefficient in olive oil

One important discovery with regard to the actions of anaesthetics *in vivo* was the finding that high pressure (helium or hydrostatic) reverses general anaesthesia. Helium alone produces a hyperexcitability syndrome rather than anaesthesia—probably because its low lipid solubility means that the effects of pressure *per se* are seen before sufficient dissolves in the membrane to produce anaesthesia. The physiological basis of this 'pressure reversal of anaesthesia' is not known.

The effects of anaesthetics on synaptic transmission are many and varied and there is no single action which can be identified as the basis of anaesthesia *in vivo*. Normally higher concentrations of anaesthetics are required to block axonal conduction than to block synaptic transmission. So far no effect of anaesthetics on synaptic transmission shows the 'pressure reversal' seen *in vivo* although partial reversal of the blockade of axonal transmission has been demonstrated. The varied effects of general anaesthetics on synaptic transmission have led many workers to suggest that they produce anaesthesia in a variety of different ways rather than by the same basic mechanism, although physico-chemical studies suggest some common factor. Detailed studies of the effects of anaesthetics, especially on the ionic conductance changes which take place during neuronal transmission, may throw more light on this problem.

Local anaesthetics

A loss of sensation or motor power in a particular region of the body results from the application of a local anaesthetic. The compounds used are neither very specific as regards structure or organ nor very potent. Solutions of strengths of the order of 10^{-2} molar are employed.

Experimental testing most often employs a 'guinea pig wheal' test or a 'rabbit's cornea' test.

The structural elements common to most local anaesthetics are:

(1) An aromatic ring often with electron-donating substituents.
(2) A short chain of about 4 carbon atoms containing a dipolar group.
(3) A tertiary base.

Table 8.2 gives some examples.

The fact that the active compounds are tertiary bases poses the question as to whether the free base or the ionized form is active. Since the appropriate pH for the active environment is not known, the pK_a of the compounds is not sufficient to decide upon this question. For example, in the case of procaine at pH = 7.5 about 10 per cent of the compound would be present as free base and at pH = 8.7 half of the molecule would be protonated. Thus at any reasonably guessed active environmental pH, both forms must be present in significant amounts.

It is possible as in other areas of pharmacology that a free base is required for penetration to the active environment where the ionic form is actually effective.

The mechanism of action is thought to involve the block of nerve conduction by inhibiting the transient increase in permeability of excitable membranes to sodium ions by binding to the channels.

Summary

Local anaesthetics seem to require certain chemical features but are not thought to act by binding to specific receptors. General anaesthesia can be produced by most small molecules in sufficient concentration and efficacy is related to physical properties. In neither the local nor the general case are there satisfactory molecular explanations of the phenomena.

TABLE 8.2. Local anaesthetics

Chemical formula	Comment
Cocaine	

| | Too toxic to be injected; topical anaesthesia; causes vasoconstriction; central stimulant. |

Procaine

Duration about 1 hour; rapid onset; metabolized by plasma cholinesterase.

Lignocaine

More potent than procaine; metabolized in liver.

Bupivacaine

Longer lasting than lignocaine.

Dibucaine

Very potent; long duration of action.

Further reading

COVINO, B. G. *N. Engl. J. Med.*, **286**, 975, 1035 (1972)
  Local anaesthesia.
HALSEY, M. J., MILLER, R. A. and SUTTON, J. A. (eds), *Molecular Mechanisms in General Anaesthesia, a Glaxo Symposium*, Churchill Livingstone, London (1974)
FINK, B. R. (ed) *Progress in Anesthesiology*, Raven Press, New York, Vol I (1975) and Vol II (1979)
MILLER, J. C. and MILLER, K. W. in H. Blaschko (ed), *M. T. P. International Review of Science. Biochemistry Series I*, **12**, 33 (1975)

Approaches to the mechanism of action of general anaesthetics.
MILLER, K. W. and SMITH, E. B. in R. M. Featherstone (ed), *A Guide to Molecular Pharmacology and Toxicology*, Dekker, New York (1973)
Intermolecular forces and the pharmacology of simple molecules.
NARAHASHI, T. and FRAZIER, D. T. *Neurosciences Research*, **4**, 65 (1971)
Site of action and active form of local anaesthetics.
RITCHIE, J. M. *British Journal of Anaesthesia*, **47**, 191 (1975)
Mechanisms of action of local anaesthetics and biotoxins.

Chapter 9

Chemotherapy

The era of chemotherapy began in 1935 when it was discovered that some azo dyestuffs containing the sulphanilamide residue (*Figure 9.1(a)*) had *in vivo* antistreptococcal activity in mice. Prontosil, the red dye (*Figure 9.1(b)*), is active against bacteria *in vitro* but is metabolized *in vivo* to the active species, sulphanilamide.

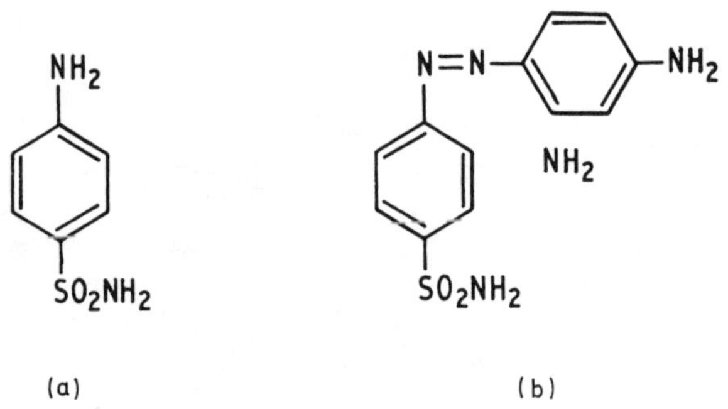

Figure 9.1. (a) Sulphanilamide. (b) Prontosil

Following this observation numerous sulphanilamide derivatives were synthesized and it became possible to control many systematic infections.

The success of sulphanilamides led to interest in antibiotics, the compounds produced by some micro-organisms that inhibit the growth of others. In particular penicillin was shown to be very active and non-toxic and its success led to the development of newer antibiotics which increased the range of antibacterial chemotherapy.

The basic principle of chemotherapy is 'selective toxicity'. This means that drugs can inflict damage on one type of living matter, such as bacteria, without injuring adjacent tissue. The actions of these drugs are therefore on sites at which differences between the organisms can be found. Examples are the cell walls of bacteria which differ from those of higher animal tissues, or differences in metabolic pathways.

Most antibacterial chemotherapeutic agents act by one of the following basic mechanisms:

(1) Competitive antagonism of a metabolite.
(2) Inhibition of bacterial wall synthesis.
(3) Action on cell membranes.
(4) Inhibition of protein synthesis.
(5) Inhibition of nucleic acid synthesis.

TABLE 9.1. Sulphonamides

Basic structure		
Examples:	R_1	R_2
Sulphadiazine		H
Sulphamerazine		H
Sulphamethazine		H
Sulphisomidine		H
Sulphacetamide	$-COCH_3$	H
Sulphioxazole		H
Sulphamethizole		H
Succinylsulphathiazole		
Phthalylsulphathiazole		

Sulphonamides

The structural formulae of some of the more important sulphonamides are given in *Table 9.1*. They compete with *p*-aminobenzoic acid for incorporation into folic acid susceptible bacteria. There is a relationship between the activity of sulphonamides and the pK_a values of the $-SO_2NH_2$ group, maximum activity being at about $pK_a = 6.5$.

Structual differences between the sulphonamides result in compounds which are useful at different sites. For example the neutral sodium salt of sulphacetamide is useful for eye infections; the poorly absorbed succinyl and phthalyl derivatives (*Table 9.1*) are used for decreasing intestinal bacterial flora.

The sulphonamides act by inhibiting the synthesis of folic acid, which is necessary for nucleic acid synthesis. Man, unlike the bacteria, can use pre-formed folic acid and so is less susceptible to this action. The sulphonamides are structural analogues of *p*-aminobenzoic acid, which is used as in *Figure 9.2*.

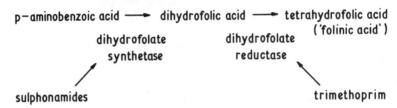

Figure 9.2. The action of sulphonamides

As with many other antibacterial compounds the occurrence of resistant strains of bacteria has decreased the usefulness of the sulphonamides. The combination of a sulphonamide with trimethoprim shows a synergistic effect resulting from the two sites of attack (*see Figure 9.2*) and has proved extremely useful.

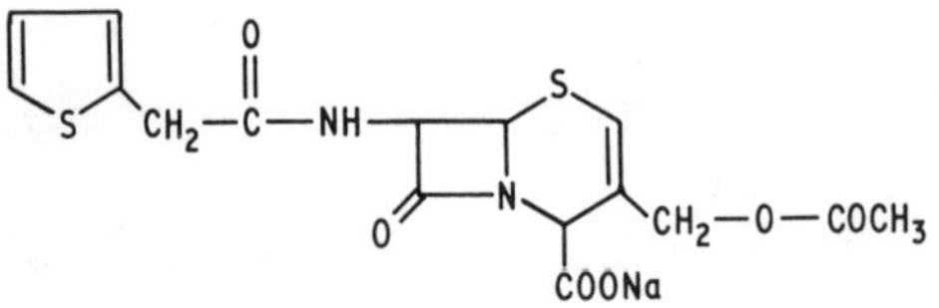

Figure 9.3. Cephalothin

Antibiotics

Antibiotics can be subdivided into those which affect cell membranes (penicillins, cephalosporins and bacitracin), those which affect protein bio-synthesis (streptomycin, erythromycin, tetracyclines and chloramphenicol) and those which act as inhibitors of aminobenzoic utilization in folic acid biosynthesis (the sulphonamides). Alternatively they can be classified chemically, for example as β-lactams, tetracyclines, aminoglycosides, macrolides and sulphonamides.

Some examples of penicillins are given in *Table 9.2*.

The mechanism of action of penicillin is on the bacterial transpeptidase used in the synthesis of the cell wall. This accounts for the relative lack of toxicity to man, the main problem being a high incidence of hypersensitivity.

One mechanism by which bacteria are resistant to the action of penicillins is that of production of an enzyme penicillinase which breaks down the drug.

A major step forward was provided by the discovery of semi-synthetic penicillins which are resistant to penicillinase, and a further advance was

TABLE 9.2. Penicillins

Basic structure

Examples:	R	Acid stable	Penicillinase resistant
Penicillin G		no	no
Penicillin V		yes	no
Methicillin		no	yes
Oxacillin		yes	yes
Nafcillin		no	yes
Ampicillin		yes	no

the introduction of antibiotics produced by the cephalosporium moulds which are again relatively resistant to staphylococcal penicillinase. An example is given in *Figure 9.3*. Certain penicillins, such as ampicillin, have a broad

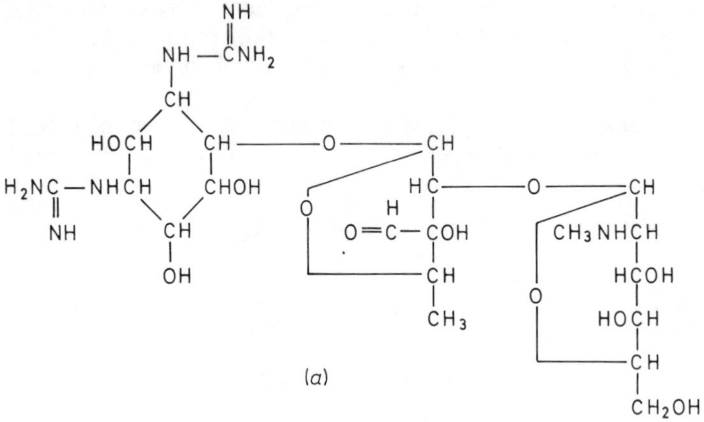

(a)

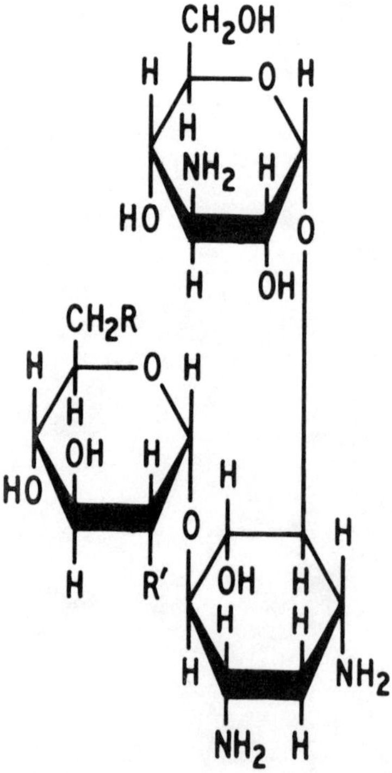

(b)

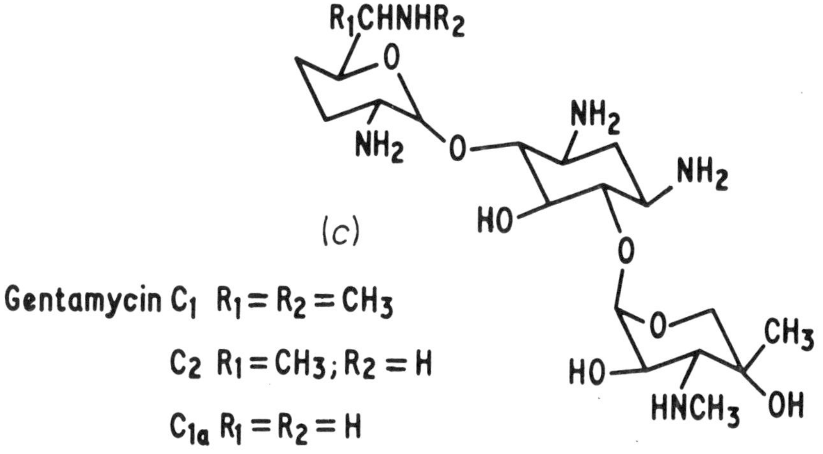

Gentamycin C_1 $R_1 = R_2 = CH_3$

C_2 $R_1 = CH_3; R_2 = H$

C_{1a} $R_1 = R_2 = H$

Figure 9.4. (a) Streptomycin. (b) Kanamycin constituent. (c) Gentamycin

spectrum of action, including Gram-negative bacteria. Some are degraded by acids of the pH of gastric juice and therefore have little activity when given orally (*see Table 9.2*).

Streptomycin (*Figure 9.4*) is an organic base rather than an acid. It is one of a group of antibiotics known as aminoglycosides, which also includes kanamycin which is a mixture as is gentamycin. Streptomycin is mainly used

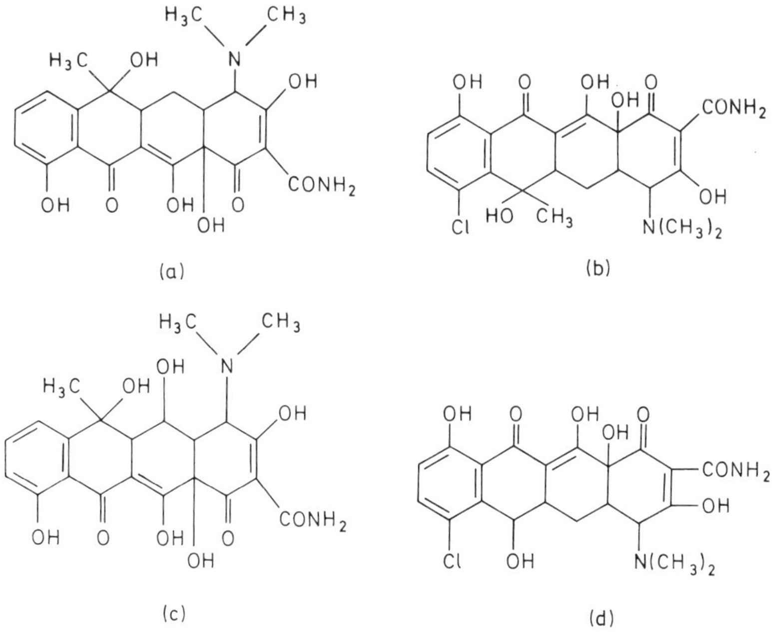

Figure 9.5. (a) Tetracycline. (b) Chlortetracycline. (c) Oxytetracycline. (d) Dimethylchlortetracycline

in the treatment of tuberculosis or in combination with penicillin. The disadvantages of streptomycin are that there is a tendency of bacteria to develop resistance to it and it is also toxic, producing vestibular and auditory side effects. The aminoglycosides inhibit protein synthesis by action at the ribosome, preventing the transcription of the genetic code.

The tetracyclines are a group of four structurally related antibiotics illustrated in *Figure 9.5*. They inhibit protein synthesis by preventing the binding of tRNA to the RNA–ribosome complex so that the addition of amino acids to the peptide chain cannot take place. Bacterial protein synthesis is affected by lower concentrations of the drugs than is the mammalian process so that these are a useful group of drugs. Resistance does however occur, and among the side effects are those due to the action of the drugs in chelating calcium ions—causing accumulation in bones and teeth.

Chloramphenicol, shown in *Figure 9.6*, is a broad spectrum antibiotic with a potency similar to the tetracyclines. It is biochemically unusual in that it contains an $-NO_2$ substituent on the benzene ring. Its use involves a risk of producing fatal aplastic anaemia and so is restricted to life-threatening diseases such as typhoid fever. It acts by preventing protein synthesis by binding to the 50S subunit of the ribosome.

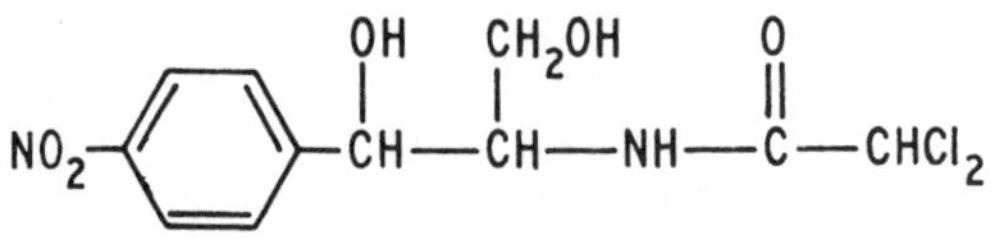

Figure 9.6. Chloramphenicol

The tremendous range of chemical structures amongst the antibiotics extends as far as Bacitracin which is a mixture of polypeptides and is valuable for topical application.

Antimalarials

Malaria is caused by infection with protozoan parasites. Despite public health measures aimed at eradicating the insect vector, the anopheles mosquito, there is still a great need for chemotherapy.

Antimalarial drugs may act at various points in the life cycle of the parasite.

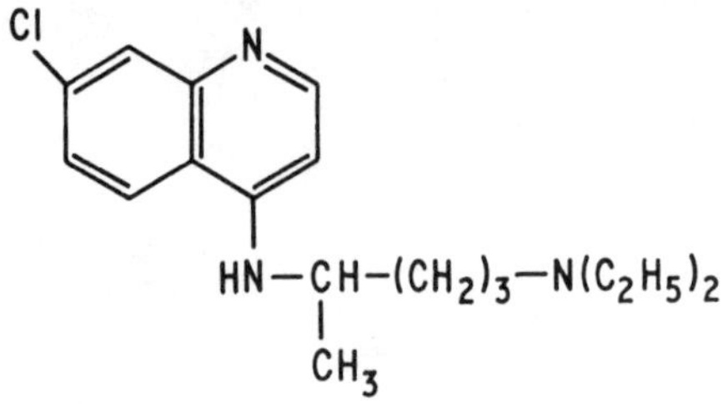

Figure 9.7. Chloroquine

The centuries-old treatment with quinine in the form of chinchona bark has now been superseded by less toxic aminoquinoline derivatives.

Chloroquine (*Figure 9.7*) is highly effective against parasites. Many other antimalarials have some structural similarities; examples are illustrated in *Figure 9.8*.

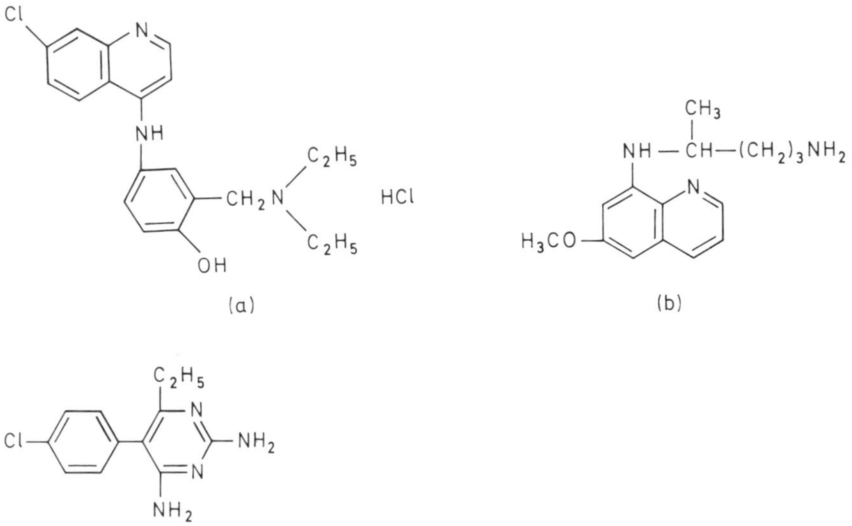

Figure 9.8. (a) Amodiaquin. (b) Primaquine.
(c) Pyrimethamine

Antiviral agents

Chemotherapy has not so far been very successful against virus infections, owing to the fact that the viruses live inside the host cells, making selective attack extremely difficult.

Compounds which inhibit nucleic acid synthesis or block virus penetration can however be effective in the chemotherapy of viral diseases. Two examples, idoxuridine and amantadine are shown in *Figure 9.9*. Idoxuridine is extremely effective by topical application in herpetic keratitis and amantadine

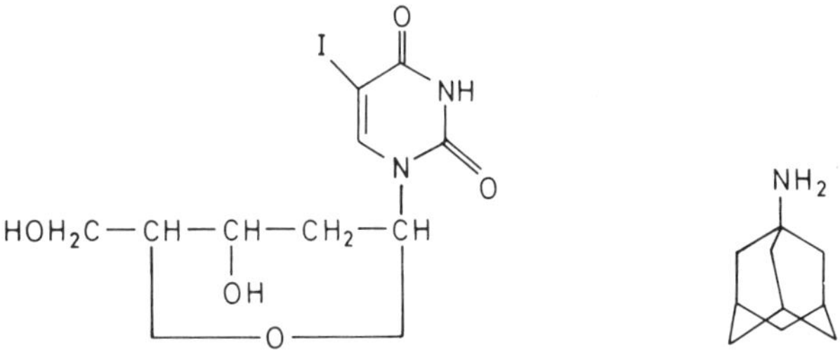

Figure 9.9. (a) Idoxuridine. (b) Amantadine

has been used in the prevention of influenza, blocking penetration of the virus into the host cell.

Cells also have a natural defence against viruses, producing an antiviral protein, interferon. Recently it has been shown that such substances as double-stranded RNA of synthetic origin can induce interferon production. New methods are also being developed for the production of interferon from bacteria, possibly using techniques of bioengineering.

Cancer chemotherapy

Cancers are groups of cells which multiply rapidly and grow in an un-controlled manner. There are few metabolic differences between these and normal cells and so points of chemical attack are difficult to find. The main difference is that they multiply more rapidly than do the majority of normal cells so most of the drugs used are those which interfere with cell division.

Mustard gas, used as a First World War poison gas and the nitrogen mustards (*Figure 9.10*) possess similar properties, acting as alkylating agents. They are believed to alkylate DNA, particularly guanine and thus have a preferential toxicity for rapidly multiplying cells, but are cell cycle non-specific.

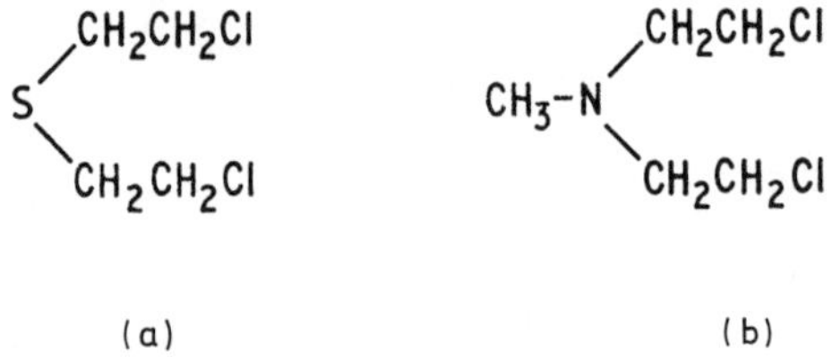

(a)   (b)

Figure 9.10. (a) Mustard gas. (b) Nitrogen mustard

Other currently used alkylating agents include methchlorethanamine and cyclophosphamide (*Figure 9.11*). Cyclophosphamide is broken down in the body to give the active alkylating moiety.

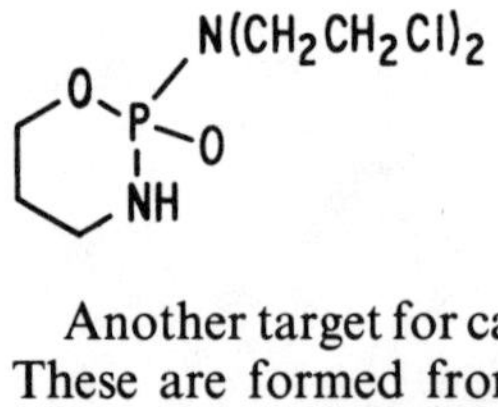

Figure 9.11. Cyclophosphamide

Another target for cancer chemotherapy is the synthesis of DNA and RNA. These are formed from a series of purine and pyrimidine bases and there are many drugs which interfere with these pathways. For example, inhibition of folic acid synthesis by methotrexate affects the reactions which involve transfer of methyl groups. 6-Mercaptopurine and its derivative azathiopurine are incorporated into the purine synthesis pathway and inhibit reactions.

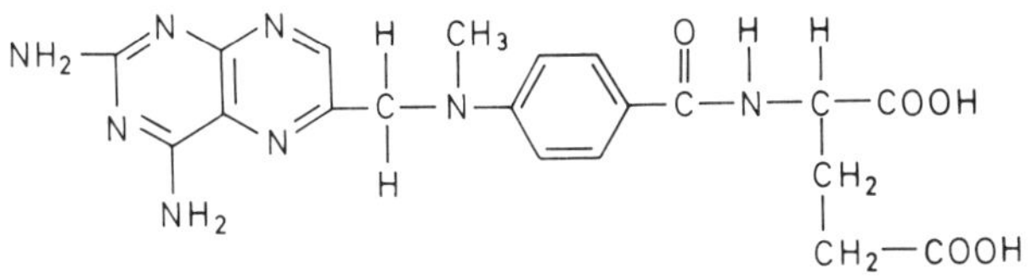

Figure 9.12. Methotrexate

The pyrimidine pathway is affected by the analogue fluorouracil (and iodoxuridine—used in antiviral therapy) causing synthesis of false metabolites.

Folic acid antagonists inhibit leukaemia. Methotrexate (*Figure 9.12*) blocks the enzyme dihydrofolate reductase.

Other methods include the use of anti-hormones for breast and prostatic cancers which seem to be hormone dependent; radioactive isotopes may destroy rapidly proliferating cells in which they become concentrated, and some antibiotics block nucleic acid synthesis.

Summary

The basic principle of chemotherapy is 'selective toxicity'. Drugs may damage bacteria for example without damaging adjacent tissue. Sulphonamides and antibiotics have been studied in great detail. Other categories considered here are antimalarials, antivirals and cancer chemotherapy agents.

Further reading

CARTER, S. K. and STAVIK, M. *Ann. Rev. Pharmacol.*, **14**. 157 (1974)
  Chemotherapy of cancer.
D'ARCY, P. F. and SCOTT, E. M. *Progress in Drug Research*, **22**, 93 (1978)
  Antifungal agents.
GILMAN, A. G., GOODMAN, L. S. and GILMAN, A. *The Pharmacological Basis of Therapeutics*, 6th edn, Macmillan, London (1980)
  Sections XII and XIII.
SALTON, M. R. and TOMASZ, A. *Annals. New York Acad. Sci.*, **235**, 1 (1974)
  Mode of action of antibiotics on microbial cell walls and membranes.
SMITH, R. A., SIDWELL, R. W. and ROBINS, R. K. *Ann. Rev. Pharmacol. and Toxicol.*, **20**, 259 (1980)
  Antiviral mechanisms.

Chapter 10

Other areas

This book is intended to provide a very condensed view of molecular pharmacology for the benefit of chemists who want to use their techniques in this area, and a convenient summary or introduction to students. It is clearly impossible to cover the whole field in depth and a very selective view has been presented in the previous chapters. Attention has been focused on neuro-transmission, both because this is the area where practising quantum pharmacologists have been most active and because the biochemistry of the transmission process is better understood than some other topics.

It would be very wrong indeed, however, if the impression were created that neuro-transmission was the only topic of molecular pharmacology or even that it was pre-eminent. In a balanced treatment the important research done in such areas as hormones or anti-inflammatory drugs, for example, would receive equal coverage. Some of these fields account for pharmaceutical sales running into billions of dollars.

On the other hand, in order to keep this introduction concise, these important topics are collected here in a single chapter and treated in a somewhat cursory fashion not because of their minor importance but rather because they are not, at the present time, frequently treated by quantum pharmacologists. They are the topics which ought to be tackled, so this chapter gives the briefest of introductions and some guide to the original literature.

Kinins

We have already encountered amines and polypeptides in neuro-transmission, but other polypeptides, the kinins, have effects somewhat similar to histamine on vascular smooth muscle, capillary permeability, and bronchial and intestinal smooth muscle. The best known kinins are bradykinins and kallidin which are found in plasma.

Bradykinin is a nona-peptide which can be synthesized and degraded very rapidly and is thought to play a role in the inflammatory process.

On a molar basis the kinins are the most powerful vasodilators known.

Prostaglandins

The prostaglandins are widely distributed acidic lipids but owe their name to the fact that they were first isolated from seminal fluid. They are thought generally to have a regulatory function related to adenyl cyclase. The wide-spread role of prostaglandins in both normal and disease processes is a major topic of current research. Prostaglandins are involved, *inter alia*, in the control of fertility, gastric secretion, inflammation, the blood clotting sequence and bronchoconstriction and relaxation. Their role in reproductive physiology has led to their use in the induction of abortion and synthetic analogues are used to regulate oestrus in cattle. A number of anti-inflammatory drugs, including aspirin, appear to act through inhibition of the enzyme prosta-glandin synthetase.

Anti-inflammatory drugs

Salicylates were originally extracted from the bark of the willow tree and were found to be effective in relieving aching pain. Derivatives have been found to have a spectrum of antipyretic (lowering fever), analgesic and anti-inflammatory properties (see *Table 10.1*).

The basis of the actions of these drugs is inhibition of the synthesis of prostaglandins. The variations in the activity of the different drugs may be

TABLE 10.1. Antipyretic analgesic drugs

	Analgesic	*Anti-inflammatory*	*Antipyretic*
Aspirin	∗∗∗	∗∗	∗∗
Phenacetin	∗∗∗	(∗)	∗∗
Indomethacin	∗	∗∗∗	∗

due to differential actions on tissues in various body areas and in the pathways involved.

Hormones

Hormones are involved in longer lasting control mechanisms than the nervous system. They are produced by glands and promote effect by interaction with receptors.

A key regulator of the metabolic processes is insulin, which is involved not only with carbohydrate metabolism. Deficiency results in many serious metabolic consequences. The hormone glucagon has some actions that are opposed to those of insulin and the ratio of the two hormones may determine their overall effect; both are small proteins.

The adrenal glands produce steroid hormones and, following the discovery that cortisone was beneficial to a patient suffering from rheumatoid arthritis, adrenal steroids and synthetic corticosteroids have become widely used in medicine.

The glucocorticoids, cortisol and corticosterone, are the principal glucocorticoids of the adrenal cortex. The rate of secretion shows a marked temporal rhythm. They affect the metabolism of carbohydrates, proteins, and fats. The clinical uses depend on inhibition of the inflammatory process. They also have anti-allergic effects which may be a manifestion of their non-

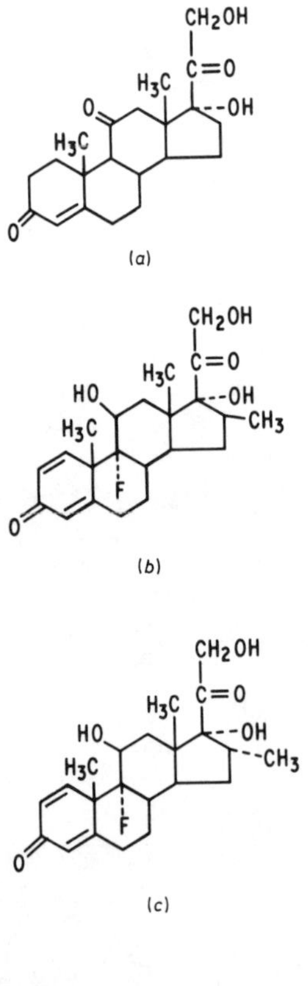

(a)

(b)

(c)

Figure 10.1 (a) Cortisone. (b) Betamethasone. (c) Dexamethasone

specific anti-inflammatory action. Cortisone and cortisol are beneficial in a large number of diseases but prolonged treatment does have disadvantages.

There are many synthetic corticosteroid compounds which have a spectrum of activity ranging from a pure glucocorticoid such as betamethasone and dexamethasone (*Figure 10.1*) to mainly mineralocorticoid such as fluoro-cortisone. The mineralocorticoid action resembles that of aldosterone which is secreted by the adrenal medulla and promotes reabsorption of sodium ions from the kidney.

The thyroid gland produces thyroxine (*Figure 10.2*) and triiodothyronine. These hormones are involved in regulating oxygen consumption, cardio-vascular function, cholesterol metabolism, neuromuscular activity and cerebral function. Deficient production of thyroid hormones also affects growth and development. The activities of the thyroid gland itself are greatly influenced by the thyrotropic hormone of the anterior lobe of the pituitary. Anti-thyroid drugs may act in a number of ways, for instance by inhibiting thyroxine synthesis or iodine trapping or, in the case of radioactive iodine, by the destruction of thyroid tissue.

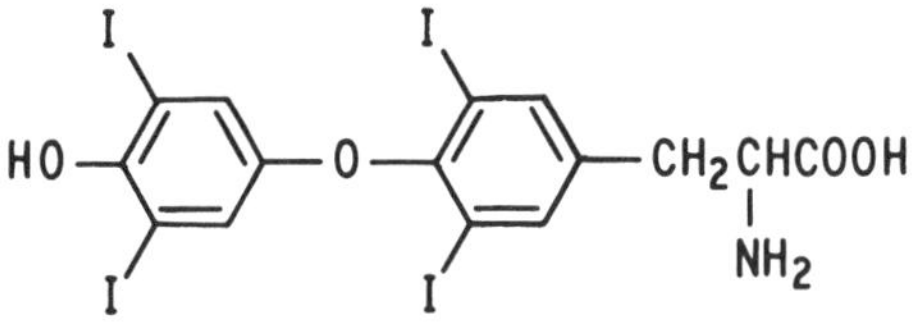

Figure 10.2. Thyroxine

Hormonal activity of the parathyroid gland determines plasma calcium levels and the intake of various forms of vitamin D. The plasma calcium level depends on the equilibrium between calcium salts in the blood and in bones and also the dietary intake and urinary secretion. Parathyroid hormone and calcitonin from the C cells of the thyroid are mutually antagonistic poly-peptides and these together with vitamin D regulate calcium homeostasis.

The posterior pituitary hormones vasopressin and oxytocin are both octa-peptides. There are two significant effects of the former. One is on the kidney where it has an antidiuretic function and the other is on the cardiovascular system where it increases blood pressure. Oxytocin, which is known to be related to the reproductive function in women, is used to induce labour and is involved in milk ejection. Since it is also found in males it presumably has other functions.

The anterior pituitary consists of several different types of cell which can produce their characteristic hormones independently. The secretion of these hormones is in turn controlled by hypothalamic releasing factors, themselves hormones, and is under the influence of various neuro-transmitters such as dopamine and serotonin.

The hormones of the anterior lobe of the pituitary include growth hormone, which stimulates growth, and prolactin, which has a large number of roles including control of mammary development, as well as two other hormones, follicle stimulating hormone and luteinizing hormone, which regulate the reproductive function in males and females and stimulate the secretion of

(a)

(b)

(c)

steroid sex hormones. These sex hormones control, for example, the ovulatory cycle. Oestrogens are used clinically to relieve menopausal disturbances and also, of course, in oral contraceptives.

Vitamins

Vitamins are organic constituents of diet which exert a large influence for small concentrations and which are indispensable for certain bodily processes. Some examples are given in *Figure 10.3*. Vitamins are administered to provide daily requirements or to correct a deficiency. In a few instances excessive

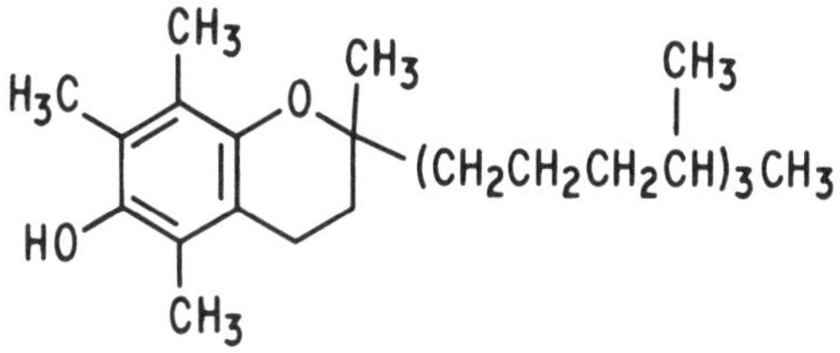

(*d*)

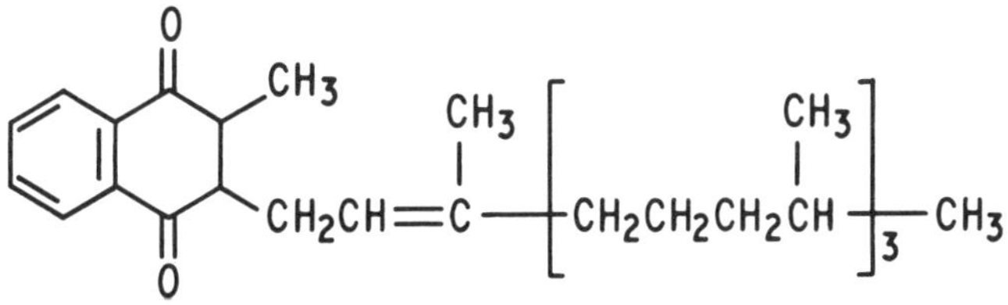

(*e*)

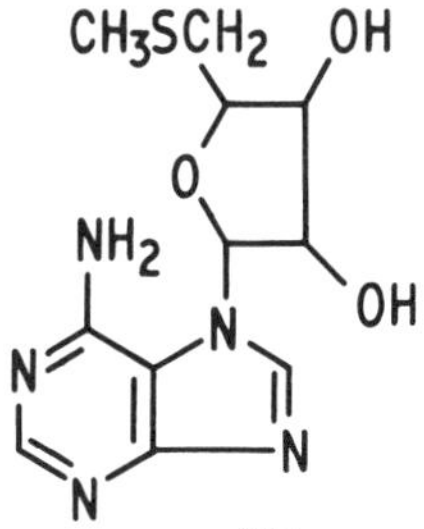

(*f*)

Figure 10.3. (a) Vitamin A. (b) Vitamin B_{12}. (c) Vitamin D_2. (d) Vitamin E. (e) Vitamin K_1. (f) Vitamin L

amounts are used therapeutically, such as vitamin D for parathyroid deficiency or vitamin K to antagonize anticoagulants. Overdosing can sometimes produce toxic effects.

Some water-soluble vitamins are precursors of coenzymes. Two such examples from the vitamin B complex are thiamine, a deficiency of which produces beri-beri, and nicotinic acid or niacin, a deficiency in this case causing pellagra. Vitamin C is an anti-oxidant.

Fat-soluble vitamins include vitamin A, a deficiency giving night blindness amongst other symptoms; the vitamin D group which are sterols; vitamin E which may be an anti-oxidant and vitamin K which is essential for pro-thrombin production by the liver.

Summary

Without being exhaustive this chapter has attempted to indicate some of the other areas of molecular pharmacology which are of current interest.

In every instance the original literature is replete with data for structure–activity studies, and in some cases clearly defined receptors are involved. Understanding in molecular terms is increasingly common.

Further reading

BRUNE, K., GLATT. M and GRAF, P. *General Pharmacology*, **7**, 27 (1976)
    Mechanisms of action of anti-inflammatory drugs.
DIPALMA, J. R. and RITCHIE, D. M. *Ann. Rev. Pharmacology*, **17**, 133 (1977)
    Vitamin toxicity.
GILMAN, A. G., GOODMAN, L. S. and GILMAN, A. *The Pharmacological Basis of Thera-peutics*, 6th edn, Macmillan, London (1980)
        Chapters: 27—Polypeptides
                  28—Prostaglandins
                  29—Analgesics, antipyretics and anti-inflammatory agents
        Sections: XV—Hormones and hormone agonists
                  XVI—The vitamins.
GORSKI, J. and GANNON, F. *Ann. Rev. Physiol.*, **38**, 425 (1976)
    Current modes of steroid action; a critique.
VANE, J. R. and FERREIRA, S. H. (eds) *Antinflammatory Drugs. Handbook of Experimental Pharmacology*, 50/11, Springer Verlag, Berlin, Heidelberg and New York (1979)

Part II

Molecular quantum mechanics

Chapter 11

Wave functions and orbitals

Wave functions

The Schrödinger equation lies at the heart of much of modern science. In its barest form it states

$$H\psi = E\psi$$

Here H is the short-hand notation for an operator which operates on a mathematical function, the wave function ψ, and E is the energy of the system. This notation disguises the fact that this equation is a differential equation, or rather a set of equations, with a function ψ_n corresponding to each allowed energy E_n.

In the case of the simple hydrogen atom system with a single electron outside a positively charged nucleus, the equation may be solved exactly providing the wave function, ψ, obeys a set of reasonable restrictions on its behaviour.

It must be emphasized that ψ is just a normal mathematical function. It has no supernatural properties. Plotting a function $f(x)$ against a coordinate x is a familiar procedure (*Figure 11.1*). In molecular quantum mechanics, since the problems concern three-dimensional molecular systems then the wave function also varies in these coordinates. Because of the essentially spherical nature of atoms, polar coordinates (r, θ and ϕ) are generally preferred over cartesian, x, y, z, coordinates (*Figure 11.2*).

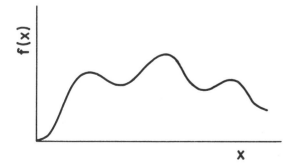

Figure 11.1. Graph of the function f(x) against the variable x

117

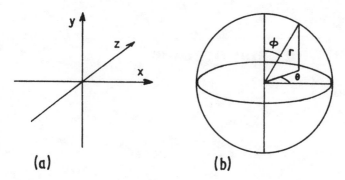

Figure 11.2. (a) Cartesian, x, y and z, coordinates. (b) Polar, r, θ and ϕ, coordinates

For the hydrogen atom the allowed wave functions or eigenfunctions are well known and an attempt to represent the three-dimensional functions in the two dimensions of the printed page is given in *Figure 11.3*.

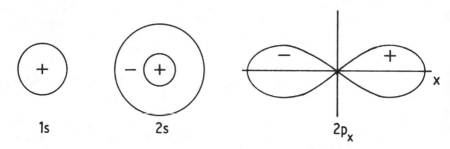

Figure 11.3. Allowed wave functions for the hydrogen atom

It can be seen in the figure that these resulting functions, one for each allowed energy or eigenstate, do satisfy the postulates of quantum mechanics in that they are 'well-behaved' functions. They go to zero at infinity and change smoothly, never doubling back on themselves, having discontinuities or even violent changes in curvature.

Once the wave function is known for a particular state of a system then any physical observable may in principle be determined using the prescription

$$\text{observable} = \frac{\int \psi^*(\text{operator})\psi\,d\tau}{\int \psi^*\psi\,d\tau}.$$

Integration over the element $d\tau$ means over all space and ψ^* is the complex conjugate of ψ; ($\psi^* \psi$) being the modulus of the square of the wave function. There is an appropriate operator for each different observable, be it energy when the hamiltonian operator, H, is the one to use, or another for the charge density, dipole moment or hyperfine coupling constant.

Orbitals

The wave functions which satisfy the Schrödinger equation for the hydrogen atom are sometimes called *orbitals*. A hydrogenic atomic orbital is thus merely a three-dimensional mathematical function from which one can calculate the energy or other properties of the single electron system.

In polyatomic atoms we adopt the so-called *orbital approximation*. This involves treating each electron separately, each with its own one electron wave function or orbital. This mathematical approximation is nothing more than the fundamental basis of the universal procedure of describing atoms by means of orbital configurations. Thus to write atomic electron configurations such as

Li : $1s^2 2s$

or

C : $1s^2 2s^2 2p^2$

is actually a mathematical approximation which treats each electron separately. In lithium two electrons have functions associated with them which are of the $1s$ shape and one with $2s$ form.

An orbital is thus merely a synonym for a one electron wave function. Each is a three-dimensional mathematical function which describes the behaviour of a single electron.

Generalizing this, with some formal notation, we may write for a poly-electronic atomic system, the total wave function for an atom, ψ, is a product of one electron atomic wave functions (χ_i), one for each electron, i.e.

$$\psi = \chi_1 \chi_2 \chi_3 \cdots \chi_n.$$

Spin-orbitals and antisymmetry

When we write the electronic structure of beryllium as $1s^2 2s^2$ we understand this as being a shortened form of

$1s^\alpha\ 1s^\beta\ 2s^\alpha\ 2s^\beta$

where α and β represent the two opposite directions of electron spin.

If we include the spin in our atomic orbitals writing either χ^α or χ^β or the equivalent shorthand, χ for an orbital associated with α spin and $\bar{\chi}$ for one with β spin, then our wave function for the whole atom is a product of *spin-orbitals*, for example:

He: $1s(1)\ 1\bar{s}(2)$,

and

Be: $1s(1)\ 1\bar{s}(2)\ 2s(3)\ 2\bar{s}(4)$.

In this expanded form of the common shorthand the numbers in parentheses indicate which electron is associated with each spin-orbital.

The expanded form of the notation enables us to see that we will need to make things a little more complicated before simplifying once more by means of a convenient notation.

Let us consider the case of the helium atom. If we write

$$\psi_{He} = \chi_{1s}\alpha(1)\chi_{1s}\beta(2)$$

or alternatively and equivalently

$$\psi_{He} = 1s(1)\, 1\bar{s}(2)$$

we can see that we are not satisfying the Pauli principle. In its fundamental form this states that the wave function for the system (ψ) must change sign if we interchange any pair of electrons, since electrons are identical fermion particles.

We have written our wave function as a simple product of orbitals when this is not sufficient, since

$$\psi = 1s(1)\, 1\bar{s}(2)$$

but on changing we get

$$\psi' = 1s(2)\, 1\bar{s}(1)$$

and ψ is not the negative of ψ'.

To overcome this we can write the wave function for the atom in the orbital approximation as

$$\Psi = \frac{1}{\sqrt{2}}\left[1s(1)\, 1\bar{s}(2) - 1s(2)\, 1\bar{s}(1)\right]$$

Now if we make the interchange, Pauli's principle will be satisfied (and the $1/\sqrt{2}$ retains the normalizing condition, $\int \psi^*\psi\, d\tau = 1$). Conventionally we write a volume element in three dimensions as dv, but if spin is also included the element is written as $d\tau$.

For beryllium, however, we must allow for any possible interchanges between four electrons so then

$$\psi = 1s(1)\, 1\bar{s}(2)\, 2s(3)\, 2\bar{s}(4)$$

has to be expanded to

$$\psi = 1s(1)\, 1\bar{s}(2)\, 2s(3)\, 2\bar{s}(4) - 1\bar{s}(1)\, 1s(2)\, 2s(3)\, 2\bar{s}(4) + 2s(1)\, 1\bar{s}(2)\, 1\bar{s}(3)\, 2s(4)$$
$$- 2\bar{s}(1)\, 1s(2)\, 1\bar{s}(3)\, 2s(4) + \ldots \text{ etc.}$$
$$\text{in all 24 such products.}$$

Fortunately notation can help us. All these products are simply the expanded form of determinants.

For He

$$1s(1)\, 1\bar{s}(2) - 1s(2)\, 1\bar{s}(1)$$

is the expansion of

$$\begin{vmatrix} 1s(1) & 1s(2) \\ 1\bar{s}(1) & 1\bar{s}(2) \end{vmatrix}$$

which is scarcely shorter. But for Be our long expansion above can be summarized as

$$\Psi = \frac{1}{\sqrt{4!}} \begin{vmatrix} 1s(1) & 1s(2) & 1s(3) & 1s(4) \\ 1\bar{s}(1) & 1\bar{s}(2) & 1\bar{s}(3) & 1\bar{s}(4) \\ 2s(1) & 2s(2) & 2s(3) & 2s(4) \\ 2\bar{s}(1) & 2\bar{s}(2) & 2\bar{s}(3) & 2\bar{s}(4) \end{vmatrix}$$

Since the diagonals of these determinants are sufficient to define them and because the value of the normalization constant is obvious ($1/\sqrt{n!}$ where n is the number of electrons), these expanded spin orbital wave functions are usually written as simple products

$$\Psi_{He} = 1s1\bar{s} \text{ or even } \Psi_{He} = 1s^2$$

$$\Psi_{Li} = 1s^2 2s$$

$$\Psi_{Be} = 1s^2 2s^2$$

The fact that these expressions are shorthand notation for determinantal wave functions is hidden in the notation.

When we want the wave function of an atom, Ψ, we write it in the form

$$\Psi = \chi_1 \, \chi_2 \, \chi_3 \cdots \chi_n$$

remembering that this is not a simple product.

The problem then becomes one of finding χ_1 etc. Each of these is a one electron function in coordinates r, θ and ϕ multiplied by a spin factor α or β. The individual χ_i can be taken as being hydrogen-like analytical functions but with different exponents appropriate to the particular atom or alternatively expressed (as any function can be) as a numerical value for each point defined by the three coordinates. This latter type of atomic orbital is called a numerical function.

Hartree produced some extremely accurate atomic functions of this numerical type which were later fitted to analytic forms by Slater and are called Slater atomic wave functions. They have the form

$$\chi_i = \text{Normalization constant} \times \text{(exponential function of } r)$$
$$\times \text{(spherical harmonic in terms of } \theta \text{ and } \phi)$$

The spherical harmonic part is identical to the shape variation found for hydrogen atom wave functions and the differences from atom to atom are found only in the r-dependent, or radial, part of the orbital. The quality of a wave function may be tested by using it to compute the energy of the system and using the well-known Variation Principle which states that the better the wave function the lower will be the resulting energy.

The atomic orbitals, χ_i, for all atoms encountered in pharmacological systems are well known and need only be taken from the literature.

A useful property of orbital functions of a given atom is that they may be made orthonormal. This means

$$\int \chi_i^2 \, d\tau = 1$$

integrating over space and spin coordinates, but

$$\int \chi_i \chi_j \, d\tau = 0 \text{ if } i \neq j.$$

Generally we use wave functions which are normalized but not orthogonal, i.e.

$$\int \chi_i \chi_j \, d\tau = S_{ij}.$$

This is the definition of the overlap integral S_{ij}.

Molecular orbitals

The wave function for a molecule is not in principle any different from that for an atom. We may use the symbol Ψ, to represent the molecular wave function and, as in the atomic case, we can make the orbital approximation,

$$\Psi = \phi_1 \, \phi_2 \, \phi_3 \, \ldots \, \phi_n$$

where each function ϕ_i will be a three-dimensional function which determines the properties of an individual electron in the molecule. We may include spin so that the wave function is a product of spin-orbitals. We must also remember that the wave function has to be antisymmetric with respect to electron interchange, or renumbering the electrons, with the result that the product as written represents the diagonal of a determinant.

The goal of most quantum molecular calculations is the production of a molecular wave function Ψ. This will be achieved if we know all the constituent molecular orbitals ϕ_i. In most of the methods currently applied to molecular questions the problem is broken down one stage further. We expand each of the unknown molecular orbitals ϕ_i as a linear combination of the known atomic orbital functions.

Thus

$$\phi_i = \sum_k c_{ik} \chi_k.$$

Each of the χ_k will be function of the form

$\chi_k = $ Constant $\times$ (function of r)

$\times$ (spherical harmonic function in terms of θ and ϕ)

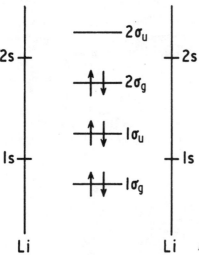

Figure 11.4. Molecular orbitals for diatomic Li$_2$

Here i is an index which labels the particular molecular orbital and k is a running index $1, 2, 3 \ldots$ whose range will depend on just how big an expansion is taken. Our problem in finding the wave function for the molecule, which means calculating the molecular orbitals ϕ, now reduces to finding the expansion coefficients c_{ik}.

For the simple case of a diatomic molecule like Li_2 this process can be illustrated pictorially by means of a molecular orbital diagram (*Figure 11.4*), in which we represent each molecular orbital as a sum of two lithium atomic orbitals. The molecular orbitals are labelled $1\sigma_g$, $1\sigma_u$ and $2\sigma_g$ for reasons of symmetry.

The molecular wave function for the ground state of Li_2 where the lowest (most tightly bound) molecular orbitals are each doubly filled will thus be

$$\Psi \ (Li_2; \text{ground state}) = \phi_{1\sigma_g} \bar{\phi}_{1\sigma_g} \ \phi_{1\sigma_u} \bar{\phi}_{1\sigma_u} \ \phi_{2\sigma_g} \bar{\phi}_{2\sigma_g}$$

with

$$\phi_{1\sigma_g} = c_{11} \ \chi_1 S_{Li} + c_{12} \ \chi_1 S_{Li}$$

and

$$c_{11} = c_{12} \text{ by symmetry}$$

$$\phi_{1\sigma_u} = c_{21} \ \chi_1 S_{Li} + c_{22} \ \chi_1 S_{Li}$$

and

$$c_{21} = -c_{22}.$$

The use of symmetry is convenient in small symmetrical molecules but plays very little part in molecules of biological interest which only rarely have symmetry.

An important principle in quantum mechanics, the Variation Principle, states that the more flexible the wave function the lower the energy and by implication the better the wave function. Zero on the energy scale has all particles separated at infinity. Calculated energies are thus negative numbers, the bigger the number the 'lower' the energy.

In the Li_2 example we can get a 'better' or 'lower' energy by using a more flexible wave function, perhaps extending our molecular orbital expansion

$$\phi_i = c_{i1} \ \chi_{1s_{Li}} + c_{i2} \ \chi_{2s_{Li}} + c_{i3} \ \chi_{2p_{Li}}$$

However lengthy our expansion the problem will remain the same: to obtain the molecular wave function, Ψ, we find the molecular orbital ϕ in terms of known functions multiplied by coefficients which have to be determined. This is done by the solution of the secular equations.

Secular equations

We have met the shorthand form of the Schrödinger equation

$$H\psi_n = E_n\psi_n$$

A similar equation may be written for each of the molecular orbitals

$$H\phi_i = \varepsilon_i\phi_i$$

but now H is a one electron hamiltonian, whose specific nature we will discuss later, and ε_i is the orbital energy or energy of one particular electron in orbital i. However we have seen that ϕ may be expanded as a linear combination of known atomic orbitals. Hence the one electron equations may be rewritten as

$$H\sum_k c_{ik}\,\chi_k = \varepsilon_i \sum_k c_{ik}\,\chi_k$$

Now we may multiply each side of the equation by χ_l (any one of the normalized set which includes χ_k) and integrate over all the electronic space coordinates (dv) giving the secular equations

$$\sum_k c_{ik}\left(\int \chi_l H \chi_k\,dv\right) = \varepsilon_i \sum_k \left(c_{ik}\int \chi_l \chi_k\,dv\right)$$

Conventional notation writes

$$H_{lk} \equiv \int \chi_l H \chi_k\,dv$$

and

$$S_{lk} \equiv \int \chi_l \chi_k\,dv$$

By this means the equations may be tidied up into the form

$$\sum_k c_{ik}\left(H_{lk} - \varepsilon_i S_{lk}\right) = 0.$$

Such a set of equations will only have a non-trivial solution if the following condition holds

$$\det\left|H_{lk} - \varepsilon S_{lk}\right| = 0.$$

This simple determinantal equation is the basis of all molecular orbital methods. In general the methods go directly to the secular determinant. All the terms (or matrix elements) H_{lk} and S_{lk} are computed. If the determinant were multiplied out this would yield a polynomial in ε, solutions of which would give the allowed molecular eigenenergies or orbital energies. Each ε_i in turn is then put into the secular equations and hence the desired coefficients are found.

Example

Let us consider a rather formal example which will illustrate the principles involved in calculating molecular orbital coefficients and is closely related to some genuine applications.

Suppose we are expanding the molecular orbitals in terms of three atomic orbitals,

$$\phi_i = c_{i1}\,\chi_1 + c_{i2}\,\chi_2 + c_{i3}\,\chi_3$$

The one electron equation is

$$H\phi_i = \varepsilon\phi_i$$

so that we have three such equations and can determine three molecular orbitals. We now multiply both sides of the equation successively by χ_1, χ_2 and χ_3 and integrate, giving three secular equations

$$c_{11} (H_{11} - \varepsilon S_{11}) + c_{12} (H_{12} - \varepsilon S_{12}) + c_{13} (H_{13} - \varepsilon S_{13}) = 0$$

$$c_{21} (H_{21} - \varepsilon S_{21}) + c_{22} (H_{22} - \varepsilon S_{22}) + c_{23} (H_{23} - \varepsilon S_{23}) = 0$$

$$c_{31} (H_{31} - \varepsilon S_{31}) + c_{32} (H_{32} - \varepsilon S_{32}) + c_{33} (H_{33} - \varepsilon S_{33}) = 0$$

For solution we must solve the determinantal equation

$$\det \begin{vmatrix} H_{11} - \varepsilon S_{11} & H_{12} - \varepsilon S_{12} & H_{13} - \varepsilon S_{13} \\ H_{21} - \varepsilon S_{21} & H_{22} - \varepsilon S_{22} & H_{23} - \varepsilon S_{23} \\ H_{31} - \varepsilon S_{31} & H_{32} - \varepsilon S_{32} & H_{33} - \varepsilon S_{33} \end{vmatrix} = 0$$

In this case we have a cubic equation in ε which has three roots.

Since more usually our expansions go well beyond three terms a more convenient method of solution of the determinantal equation is employed which makes use of the strength of computers.

Rows and columns of determinants may be added and subtracted or factors divided out without altering the value of the determinant. If by such adjustments we could rearrange the determinant into the form

$$\begin{vmatrix} (x - \varepsilon) & 0 & 0 \\ 0 & (y - \varepsilon) & 0 \\ 0 & 0 & (z - \varepsilon) \end{vmatrix} = 0.$$

where x, y, and z are numbers and all the rest of the determinant is zero, on multiplying out we should have the simple equation

$$(x - \varepsilon)(y - \varepsilon)(z - \varepsilon) = 0.$$

Computational methods for doing this or nearly equivalent simplifications are standard procedures. As a result there is no difficulty in solving the determinantal equation and hence finding the molecular orbital coefficients, no matter how extensive the expansion. The actual computer programs are invariably based on matrix diagonalization techniques which are equivalent to the above description, but particularly suitable for computers.

Matrix elements

Going directly to the secular determinant and thence to the secular equations to obtain molecular orbitals poses no serious problem providing all the 'matrix elements' H_{lk} and S_{lk} are easily found.

The matrix elements S_{lk} are called overlap integrals as they represent the overlap between the two three-dimensional functions χ_l and χ_k,

$$S_{lk} = \int \chi_l \chi_k \, dv$$

These integrals are reasonably easy to evaluate and again standard computer programs are available.

The matrix elements H_{lk} or

$$\int \chi_l \, H \, \chi_k \, dv$$

on the other hand include the one electron operator H. So far the precise nature of H has not been specified and indeed it is in the definition, or lack of it, that most of the molecular orbital methods differ. In the more sophisticated methods H is precisely defined. In the less precise approximations it is never defined and all H_{lk} matrix elements are replaced by parameters.

Self-consistent molecular orbitals

The most clearly defined molecular orbital calculations are based on the Hartree–Fock method. A hamiltonian operator contains terms for the kinetic and potential energy of the system. A suitable choice of units makes the equations look rather tidier than standard units. If we choose to take the electronic charge, e, and mass, m_e, each as unity and the unit of length as the Bohr radius then the Schrödinger equation for the hydrogen atom becomes

$$\left(-\frac{1}{2}\nabla^2 - \frac{1}{r} \right)\psi = E\psi$$

$$\underbrace{\phantom{-\frac{1}{2}\nabla^2}}_{\text{K.E.}} \underbrace{\phantom{-\frac{1}{r}}}_{\text{P.E.}}$$

where the kinetic energy is represented by the $-\frac{1}{2}\nabla_i^2$ term (∇^2 is shorthand for $\partial^2/\partial x^2 + \partial^2/\partial y^2 + \partial^2/\partial z^2$) and potential energy by the electron–nuclear attaction, $1/r$.

For the hydrogen molecule there are two electrons and the Schrödinger equation for the molecular wave function Ψ is

$$\left\{ -\frac{1}{2}\nabla_1^2 - \frac{1}{2}\nabla_2^2 - \frac{1}{r_{1A}} - \frac{1}{r_{1B}} - \frac{1}{r_{2A}} - \frac{1}{r_{2B}} + \frac{1}{r_{12}} \right\} \Psi = E_{el}\,\Psi$$

To this electronic energy E_{el} has to be added the nuclear–nuclear repulsion, $E_{nuclear} = 1/R$, where R is the separation of the nuclei A and B.

It may be seen that this equation represents the sum of two separate hydrogen molecule ion wave equations with the additional term, $1/r_{12}$, representing the repulsion between the two electrons.

When we come to one electron equations we want to include in the hamiltonian terms for all the energy contributions of that one electron. These will be kinetic energy, nuclear attraction and electron–electron repulsion. The kinetic energy term in the operator is $-\frac{1}{2}\nabla_i^2$ and the various nuclear attraction terms are

$$\sum_{\nu} Z_\nu/r_{i\nu},$$

where the nuclei are labelled by ν and the particular electron we are considering is electron i. These two parts can be grouped together and designated as H^N. If there were no other electrons in the molecule this would be a sufficient hamiltonian and the one electron energy would be the full molecular electronic energy which we could call ε_i^N.

When, as is usually the case, there are many electrons in the molecule a major part of the potential energy which must be represented in the hamiltonian is electron–electron repulsion. Now if we have two electrons with orbitals ϕ_i and ϕ_j, separated by a distance r_{12}, then the repulsion between them is given by

$$\int \phi_i^2(1)\frac{1}{r_{12}}\phi_j^2(2)\,dv_1\,dv_2,$$

since

$$\int \phi_i^2(1)\,dv_1$$

is the charge distribution of electron (1) (assuming ϕ_i is real). If ϕ is complex this should be replaced by

$$\int \phi_i^*(1)\phi_i(1)\,dv_1$$

The expression

$$\int \phi_j^2(2)\,dv_2$$

is the charge distribution for electron (2).

Thus we must include terms of this type in the one electron hamiltonian, suggesting that an expanded form of

$$H\phi = \varepsilon\phi$$

might be

$$\left\{ -\frac{1}{2}\nabla^2 - \sum_v \frac{Z_v}{r_{iv}} + \sum_{j=1}^{n} \phi_j^2(2)\frac{1}{r_{12}}dv_2 \right\}\phi_i(1) = \varepsilon_i\phi_i(1).$$

This equation due to Hartree would be correct if our orbital wave function were a simple product and not a determinant. To account for the determinantal form of Ψ the full self-consistent field equations or Hartree–Fock equations are

$$H^{SCF}\,\phi_i = \varepsilon_i\,\phi_i$$

where

$$H^{SCF} = \left\{ H^N + \sum_j J_j - \sum_j{}' K_j \right\}$$

and the shorthand notation used is defined by

$$J_j\phi_i(1) = \left(\int \phi_j^2(2)\frac{1}{r_{12}}dv_2 \right)\phi_i(1)$$

and

$$K_j \phi_i(1) = \left(\int \phi_j(2) \phi_i(2) \frac{1}{r_{12}} dv_2 \right) \phi_j(1)$$

with a prime on a summation indicating summing only over pairs of electrons of the same spin.

The Hartree–Fock equations contain the K_j or exchange terms in addition to the obvious coulombic interelectron interactions allowed for in the Hartree equations. These exchange terms arise as a result of the Pauli principle which leads to determinantal wave functions rather than products and exchange integrals between various cross-products of the expanded determinant.

This specification of H in the one electron equation leads to a lot of terms, but that is not a particularly difficult problem if we are using a computer.

More seriously the hamiltonian in $H\phi = \varepsilon\phi$ itself contains the various ϕ which we are trying to determine. That is to say the coefficients in

$$\phi_i = \sum_k c_{ik} \chi_k$$

must be known before we start. This is the origin of the term 'self-consistent' field. Starting values of c_{ik} are given from educated guesses or from the results of simple calculations. The determinantal equation,

$$\det \left| H_{lk}^{SCF} - \varepsilon S_{lk} \right| = 0$$

is solved after calculating all the integrals involved in H_{lk} and S_{lk}. Solution yields values of ε which are substituted in the secular equations to give new values of the various c_{ik}. The process may then be repeated until the c_{ik} resulting from one cycle are identical within prescribed limits with those used in the previous cycle. The results are then self-consistent.

The various simplified methods of calculating molecular orbitals are essentially approximations of a greater or less drastic nature which result in a reduction of the number of integrals necessary to build the matrix element H_{lk} and S_{lk} in the determinantal equation.

Configuration interaction

We have already met the variation principle which tells us that the more flexible a wave function the better it will be in terms of the energy which results. One way of improving the wave functions which we have as a result of self-consistent field or approximate calculation is to allow the interaction of configurations.

Formally this means allowing a further linear mixing to give an improved wave function,

$$\Psi_{\text{improved}} = a\Psi_0 + b\Psi_1 + c\Psi_2 + \dots$$

In this expression Ψ_0 is the wave function we first find and Ψ_1, Ψ_2 etc. are wave functions which would be appropriate for excited configurations of the same symmetry. The coefficients a, b, c etc. are mixing coefficients whose values are chosen so that energy improvement is maximized.

The problem with configuration interaction is knowing when to stop. Every extra configuration helps the energy a little. Although configurations closest in energy to the ground state may have an obvious influence others which are highly excited may also be significant.

In pharmacology most of the molecules of interest have closed electronic shells with no unpaired electrons and are not free radicals. There is a simple theorem due to Brillouin which proves that for such molecular species, excited states where only one electron is excited do not contribute directly to configuration interaction wave functions. In consequence configuration interaction is only of minor importance in applications to pharmacological problems.

Summary

The aim of molecular quantum mechanics is to produce a wave function Ψ, for the molecule of interest. The wave function Ψ is expressed in terms of one electron wave functions or orbitals ϕ_i, there being one such function for each electron in the molecule.

The individual ϕ_i are themselves expressed as coefficients multiplying known atomic functions χ_k,

$$\phi_i = \sum_k c_{ik} \, \chi_{ik}$$

The coefficients and hence ϕ_i and Ψ are determined by firstly solving the determinantal equation,

$$\det \left| H_{lk} - \varepsilon S_{lk} \right| = 0$$

after specifying H_{lk} and S_{lk}, yielding a set of orbital energies ε_i. Each of these on substitution into the secular equations,

$$\sum_k c_{ik} \left(H_{lk} - \varepsilon_i S_{lk} \right) = 0,$$

provides the coefficients.

The various molecular orbital techniques all use this method but differ in the manner of calculating or defining H_{lk} and S_{lk}.

All the methods produce a set of orbital energies ε_i each associated with a function ϕ_i expressed as coefficients c_{ik} multiplying a known set, or basis, of functions χ_k.

Further reading

ATKINS, P. W. *Molecular Quantum Mechanics*, 2nd edn, Clarendon Press, Oxford (1983)
DAUDEL, R., LEFEBVRE, R. and MOSER, C. *Quantum Chemistry; Methods and Applications.* Interscience, New York (1959)
PARR, R. G. *Quantum Theory of Molecular Electronic Structure*, Benjamin, New York (1963)
PILAR, F. *Elementary Quantum Chemistry*. McGraw-Hill, New York (1968)

These are all good basic texts which give a rather fuller account of the topics covered in this chapter.

Chapter 12

Approximate wave functions

All molecular wave functions are approximate; some are just more approximate than others. We can solve the Schrödinger equation exactly for the hydrogen atom but not even, despite what many textbooks say, for the hydrogen molecule ion, H_2^+. For H_2^+ we make the Born–Oppenheimer approximation which separates electronic and nuclear motion, and calculate the electronic energy of the ion with a given fixed internuclear distance and then obtain the total energy by adding the nuclear–nuclear repulsion term.

Molecular wave functions for molecules of chemical and biological interest are virtually all of the molecular orbital type. All the methods start with the determinantal equation and proceed in the manner described in the last chapter. In discussing various approximations used to build the terms necessary for this determinant, either of two sequences is possible. We can start with the more sophisticated methods and gradually whittle away difficulties by increasingly daring approximations, or we can start with the very simplest approximation and gradually make it more realistic and more complicated. It is probably simpler to follow the second path which mirrors the development of the subject. However, this course tends to make the reader feel that when half-way through the hierarchy of methods he has done sufficient as things have become complicated enough. For this reason we will adopt the former approach, starting with the more well-defined and lengthy methods, in part to underline just how horrendous are the approximations which we will adopt to avoid lengthy computations.

Computer programs for all the methods are freely available. It is not impossible to run molecular orbital calculations using any single one of the methods without knowing in detail how the computer program handles such necessary steps as performing integrals or diagonalizing matrices. On the other hand, the better the understanding of the methods the more wisely they are likely to be used and the less the likelihood of erroneous applications.

Ab initio methods

The term *ab initio* is perhaps unfortunate since it gives a spurious idea of quality, but it is universally used for calculations of orbital wave functions where the full Hartree–Fock self-consistent field operator is used in

$$\det \left| H_{lk} - \varepsilon S_{lk} \right| = 0,$$

$$H = \left[H^N + \sum_j J_j - \sum_j' K_j \right]$$

and all the integrals implied in H_{lk} and S_{lk} are computed.

Each molecular orbital will be in the form

$$\phi_i = \sum_k c_{ik} \chi_k.$$

If the expansion is infinite then we would achieve the most flexible wave function within the constraints of the self-consistent field hamiltonian which we have defined. The resulting energy would be the 'best' or biggest negative number we could obtain and is the Hartree–Fock limiting energy. In practice, if an expansion of thirty or forty terms is used for ϕ, then little further improvement in energy results and we can safely assume that we are close to the limit.

The larger the expansion in terms of atomic orbitals, the more integrals have to be computed and the more expensive computer time required. Thus for large molecules rather short expansions are used so that the resulting energy may be far from the best possible limit, and the wave function even though of *ab initio* origin is approximate even within the constraints of the method.

The most obvious set of atomic orbitals, χ_k, to use in the expansion are Slater-type atomic orbitals which were found by fitting analytical exponential functions to numerical atomic wave functions. If we use one such function for each atomic orbital which is filled, e.g. for C employing $1s$, $2s$ and $2p$ atomic orbitals, then the set of atomic functions or *basis set* is referred to as a *minimal basis*. If we use double that number, the basis set is of '*double zeta*' quality. Each of the atomic orbitals is of the form

$$\chi_k = C e^{-\zeta r} Y_{lm}$$

Here C is a normalizing constant; Y_{lm} is the angular part of the function (a spherical harmonic), and ζ is called the orbital exponent, zeta. The Y_{lm} are well known for $1s$, $2s$, $2p$ etc. so that a basis set may be specified by listing the exponents for each type of orbital used. Suitable basis sets are available in the literature.

To overcome some of the problems in doing integrals with exponential (or Slater-type) wave functions, the more tractable gaussian form of orbital dependence is often employed. The gaussian radial dependence has the less appropriate, e^{-ar^2}, form. To combine the suitability of exponential basis functions and the simplicity of calculating with gaussians, the obvious step of fitting gaussian shapes to an exponential has been taken. Thus one frequently sees in the literature expressions such as '. . . calculations performed with an STO-3G basis'. This indicates that a minimal basis set of Slater exponentials has been used but for the integrals each exponential function was fitted by three gaussian functions. An STO-4G calculation is likely to be closer to a true minimal basis calculation but even that would be some way from the limit of the method in terms of energy.

When running an *ab initio* calculation the starting point is a particular molecular geometry, the nature and coordinates of each atom being defined. Depending on which atoms are in the molecule a basis set of atomic orbitals is then decided upon, although the choice may be built into the computer program. The program will then compute all the integrals required in building up H_{lk} and S_{lk} using guessed trial coefficients, build and diagonalize the determinant and produce a set of orbital energies and first improved coefficients. As described earlier this process is repeated until self-consistency is achieved, when the program will print out a set of molecular orbitals ϕ_i in the form of the coefficients, and associated with each an orbital energy ε_i.

It is important to realize that even if we can afford to have long expansions of molecular orbitals and even reach the Hartree–Fock limit, there are still defects in the wave functions which arise from approximations in the actual Hartree–Fock equations.

There are two sources of error in the starting equations. The first comes about because the whole theory is based on the Schrödinger equation which is not relativistically correct. Fast moving inner electrons may move with speeds which are not negligible by comparison with the velocity of light and relativistic effects thus contribute; mass is not constant. Since most chemical and biological transformations of molecules do not involve core electrons this error is normally a constant and causes no serious difficulty.

The second error is more serious and is called the correlation energy error.

Correlation energy

Any defect in our wave functions will result in the calculated energy being less than the true energy. The correlation energy can be defined as

$$E_{\text{correlation}} = E_{\text{true}} - E_{\text{Hartree-Fock}} - E_{\text{relativistic}}$$

and represents the remaining energy error between the limiting Hartree–Fock energy and true total energy taking into account the relativistic effect. Correlation energy errors arise because of an unjustified approximation in the self-consistent field hamiltonian. This we write as

$$H = H^N + \sum_j J_j - \sum_j{}' K_j.$$

Involved in J and K are terms of the type

$$\int \phi_j{}^2(2) \frac{1}{r_{12}} dv_2$$

These are included to account for the interaction of one electron with another, the second electron being represented as a smoothed-out averaged electron density. Thus if we are considering the helium atom, each of the $1s$ electrons, as far as the calculation is concerned, would interact with the other as if the second electron was spherically distributed. In reality, of course, the two electrons will have their positions correlated, there being a higher probability of the two electrons being on opposite sides of the nucleus than there is of them being both on the same side, as self-consistent field theory allows.

The correlation energy error results from electron pair effects and is reasonably constant as molecular geometry changes providing the electron pairings in the molecule do not change. It is not a constant as bonds are stretched to the point of dissociation (*Figure 12.1*). Errors are thus quite serious in calculations of dissociation energies, and also in the estimations of ionization potentials or even pK_a values. On the other hand, if we merely change conformation and leave the electron pairings essentially unaltered, then the error may be constant (*Figure 12.2*).

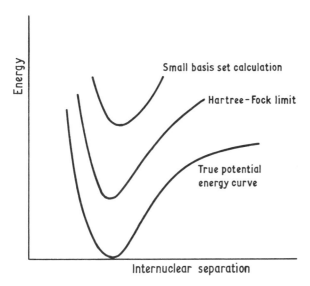

Figure 12.1. Errors in molecular orbital calculations for a diatomic molecule as a function of internuclear separation

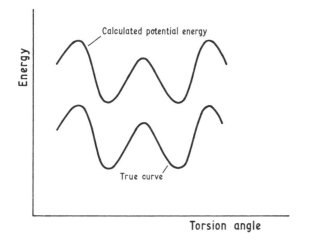

Figure 12.2. Errors in molecular orbital calculations as a function of conformational change

Semi-empirical calculations

Ab initio calculations are themselves not always perfectly successful in reproducing experimental observations. In addition the number of integrals required increases roughly as the fourth power of the number of basis functions in the molecule and for even quite small molecules many millions may be required. In consequence a great deal of effort has been expended devising so-called semi-empirical molecular orbital methods. These all start with the determinantal equation but make a variety of approximations to reduce the amount of computer time required.

All the commonly used techniques are valence electron calculations; that is they neglect $1s$ electrons since these play little part in chemical or bio-chemical behaviour. The $1s$ electrons are defined as part of the 'core' for first-row atoms and both K and L shell electrons for heavier atoms. The self-consistent field hamiltonian thus becomes

$$H = H^{core} + \sum_j J_j - \sum_j{}' K_j$$

and H^{core} incorporates kinetic energy and attraction to a core rather than to a bare nucleus. Integrals (or synonymously matrix elements) involving H^{core} are usually replaced by empirical or calculated parameters.

Particularly in instances where molecules of interest contain a heavy atom (such as a metal in an enzyme-binding site) an approximation at this level is introduced by incorporating a pseudopotential or effective potential into the hamiltonian. The resulting computed properties are not significantly different from those of full *ab initio* calculations in the cases of electron density or orbital energies. Savings of computer time by 50 per cent or more are however common.

There are two broad philosophies about the use of parameters in molecular orbital calculations. One school of thought takes the view that as *ab initio* calculations themselves are far from perfect, empirical parameters should be introduced so as to ensure agreement with experiment. In some ill-defined way this means that the parameterization includes correlation effects. Unfortunately correlation energy cannot be treated in this simple way in a universal fashion. Thus as long as the parameterization is related to experimental data which are closely related to those which one is trying to calculate, then this approach works perfectly. In the limit, of course, if you put some experimental data into the calculation you should at very least be able to get them out again. Generally semi-empirical methods using this philosophy give good agreement with experiment providing the experiment and the source of parameterization are related.

Alternatively there are methods which use parameters based on *ab initio* calculations and attempt to reproduce what a more costly rigorous calculation would have produced. This approach has the advantage of being clearly defined and it is not essentially biased in its parameterization towards one type of experiment or another. On the other hand the results can never be better than *ab initio* calculations.

The actual choice of method to be used in any pharmacological research project will depend on the computer time available, the number of calculations required and above all on the agreement of test calculations of properties which are related to the problem with physical measurements.

Neglect of differential overlap

The matrix elements H_{lk} in the secular determinant involve a large number of integrals over atomic orbital functions χ of the type

$$\int \chi_m(1)\chi_n(1)\frac{1}{r_{12}}\chi_l(2)\chi_s(2)\,d\tau_1\,d\tau_2$$

which are often written in the shorthand form $(mn|ls)$. These integrals are particularly difficult to evaluate if the atomic functions, χ_m etc. are centred on different atoms. In particular those integrals involving three or four centres are time consuming, perhaps prohibitively so, even using a computer.

An approximation which will surmount this problem at a stroke is to assume

$$(mn|ls) = \delta_{mn}\,\delta_{ls}\,(mm|ll)$$

with δ_{mn} and δ_{ls} being Kronecker deltas which are equal to zero unless the subscripts are equal. In this way, neglecting differential overlap of functions based on different centres, we eliminate not only all three and four centre integrals but most two and one centre integrals where different atomic orbitals are involved for either of the two electrons.

The study of *ab initio* results where these neglected integrals are computed confirms that they are significantly smaller than the integrals which remain but they may be by no means negligible. Consequently further approximations and parameterizations are normally added to counteract the omissions.

In the CNDO, or complete neglect of differential overlap method, this approximation is fully applied for the valence electrons with $1s$ electrons being treated as part of a nuclear 'core'. Integrals which remain are further approximated. The electron repulsion integral

$$(mm|ll)$$

is supposed to depend only on the atoms A and B on which χ_m and χ_l are situated and set equal to the parameter γ_{AB} which may be found from an actual calculation for a simple example such as $(2s_A\,2s_A|2s_B\,2s_B)$ or by the use of empirical data. Matrix elements of H^{core} are also parameterized and in particular atomic ionization potentials are frequently used to replace integrals which approximately represent the energy with which an electron is held by an atom. There are a number of alternative parameterizations, details of which can be found in the references.

Slightly less dramatic in the application of the neglect of differential overlap are intermediate neglect of differential overlap (INDO) schemes. these counter a defect in CNDO which results in there being no distinction between singlet and triplet electronic states. These have respectively two electrons paired in one case and of parallel spin in the other. Their energy difference is related to an exchange integral, K. Integrals of the form $(ms|ms)$ are not now neglected if χ_m and χ_s are centred on the same atom.

In the form of INDO used by Pople and co-workers the philosophy of keeping close to *ab initio* calculations is favoured. The more empirical line is followed by Dewar whose variant is given the acronym MINDO. The most recent parameterization of the latter, MINDO/3, does appear to give very satisfactory results when compared with a range of experimental observables. As yet, however, it has not been applied to many experiments akin to pharmacological problems. If it does prove as satisfactory as the most enthusiastic predictions then it could have a wide and reliable set of applications to biological problems.

The use of localized orbitals

In the realm of pharmacological problems one of the most widely applied molecular orbital methods and indeed the one which was designed with conformational problems largely in mind is the so-called perturbation configuration interaction using localized orbitals (PCILO) approximation.

This method is based on the expansion of the molecular orbitals, not as linear combinations of atomic orbitals but in terms of localized bond orbitals, which are constructed from hybrid orbitals taken in pairs. A set of localized antibonding orbitals are used to form excited configurations which are used in limited configuration interaction. The energy and wave functions are produced by perturbation theory, avoiding the necessity of matrix diagonalization. A series of terms just has to be summed to give contributions to the energy up to third order. The main approximations of the CNDO method are retained to compute the energy contribution terms, so that the method in its original form is roughly of comparable stature, although PCILO succeeds where CNDO fails and, occasionally, vice versa.

Since it is based on bonds there are some slight difficulties when dealing with non-classical structures and care has to be exercised in defining the bonds in the molecule. The great virtue of the method is its speed, permitting the calculation of many points on a potential energy surface even for a complex unsymmetrical molecule like a neuro-transmitter.

Use of an undefined hamiltonian operator

The methods considered so far are all in the spirit of self-consistent field calculations and use a formulation with a clearly defined one electron hamiltonian operator H. Variations are concerned with different ways of reducing the amount of calculation.

Very great increases in speed and hence range of accessible molecules may be gained if we drop the clearly defined nature of H and leave it totally undefined, hoping that multitudes of sins will be expurgated by means of wise parameterization.

Still we start with the determinantal equation,

$$\det|H_{lk} - \varepsilon S_{lk}| = 0$$

but since H no longer explicitly contains the functions and coefficients we are trying to find, the solution will be a once and for all diagonalization not a repetitive cycle. We use the valence electron approximation and have a basis set of $1s$ Slater functions for hydrogen and $2s$ and $2p$ Slater functions for first row atoms like carbon or nitrogen. The easy integrals, S_{lk}, i.e.

$$\int \chi_l \chi_k \, dv$$

are all computed.

Matrix elements H_{ll} are taken as measures of the electron attracting power of an atom and replaced by valence state ionization potentials. Off-diagonal elements of H are approximated as follows

$$H_{lk} = 0.5K \, (H_{ll} + H_{kk}) S_{lk}$$

with K being an empirical parameter.

This simple approach is called extended Hückel theory (EHT). Although very crude it is far from worthless if used with care and with experimental justification kept clearly in mind.

A slightly more realistic variant is iterative extended Hückel theory (IEHT) where the elements H_{ll} are weighted to allow for the fact that, for example, the electron density at all carbon atoms in a molecule will not be identical and hence the use of a universal ionization potential for H_{ll} may be inappropriate. Once a straightforward EHT calculation has been run the resulting coefficients may be used to estimate the charge density distribution (Chapter 13), this in turn being used to weight the ionization potentials preparatory to a second calculation. This procedure may be repeated until the results are consistent from cycle to cycle.

Computer programs for molecular orbital calculations

The brief details of the essentials of each of the most commonly applied molecular orbital methods presented above are amplified in the references cited, for those who want to know in more detail precisely what is going on when a particular method is used. The details given show how it is a relatively straightforward task to produce a computer program to perform the calculations providing one is supplied with routines for computing the integrals over atomic orbitals and for diagonalizing matrices.

It is not, however, necessary to write programs in order to conduct research in this area. The admirable Quantum Chemistry Program Exchange (QCPE) run from the Department of Chemistry at the University of Indiana has available tested programs with sample data and documentation for all the approximate methods and several variants of *ab initio* calculation.

It is more important to have a feeling for the reliability, the strengths and weaknesses, of the various methods than it is to be able to follow every line of FORTRAN in the program.

Summary

Figure 12.3 summarizes the hierarchy of molecular orbital methods. All are approximate and all are normally applied to the isolated molecule. Choice

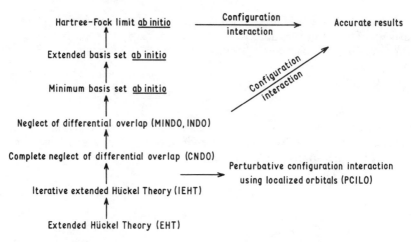

Figure 12.3. Summary of the various approximate molecular orbital methods. Accuracy improves both as going up the hierarchy of methods and from left to right as more configurations are added in configuration interaction

of a method will depend on the amount of computer time available and careful comparison of relevant experimental observations with calculated values.

For all of the methods computer programs are freely available. The programs usually contain the basis functions or parameters which will be employed so that the user will in general only have to specify the nature of the constituent atoms in the molecule and the precise molecular geometry for which the calculation is to be run.

For each specified geometry the result of a molecular orbital calculation will be a set of orbitals of the form,

$$\phi_i = \sum_k c_{ik} \chi_k$$

printed as a list of coefficients which multiply the known atomic basis functions χ_k. The coefficients are given both for the occupied and the unoccupied or 'virtual' orbitals. In addition an orbital energy ε_i is given for each molecular orbital and the total energy of the molecule.

The applications of the molecular orbitals involve the use of the coefficients and the orbital energies to calculate a number of useful properties.

Further reading

DEWAR, M. J. S., *The Molecular Orbital Theory of Organic Chemistry*, McGraw-Hill, New York (1969)

DEWAR, M. J. S. *Chem. in Britain*, **11**, (1975)

DUKE, B. 'Electronic calculations on large molecules', *Chem. Soc. Specialist Periodical Report – Theoretical Chemistry*, **2**, 159 (1975)

HOYLAND, J. R. 'Semi-empirical MO theories, A. Critique and a review of progress', in L. B. Kier (ed.), *Molecular Orbital Studies in Chemical Pharmacology*, Springer Verlag, Berlin (1970)

POPLE, J. A. and BEVERIDGE, D. L. *Approximate Molecular Orbital Theory*, McGraw-Hill, New York (1970)

RICHARDS, W. G. and COOPER, D. L. *Ab initio Molecular Orbital Calculations for Chemists*, 2nd edn, Clarendon Press, Oxford (1983)

SCHAEFER, H. F. III, *The Electronic Structure of Atoms and Molecules*, Addison-Wesley, Reading, Mass. (1972)

SCHAEFER, H. F. III (ed) *Methods of Electronic Structure Theory*, Plenum Press, New York (1977)

SCHAEFER, H. F. III (ed) *Applications of Electronic Structure Theory*, Plenum Press, New York (1977)

Chapter 13

Calculated molecular properties

Every physical observable has associated with it a quantum mechanical operator, O. The value of an observable or eigenvalue, ω, can in principle, be found by using the eigenvalue equation in which the operator operates on the wave function appropriate to the state and condition of the molecule in which we are interested,

$$O\Psi = \omega\Psi$$

Mean values of ω may be extracted from such equations using the formula

$$\omega = \frac{\int \Psi^* O \Psi \, d\tau}{\int \Psi^* \Psi \, d\tau}$$

In the neater and powerful notation of Dirac this equation is written in the form

$$\omega = \frac{<\Psi|O|\Psi>}{<\Psi|\Psi>}$$

In fact, apart from the case of energy, where O is the hamiltonian operator, H, this pure approach is rarely used and calculated properties are generally based on the orbital energies ε_i and the expansion coefficients of the molecular orbitals in terms of atomic orbitals, c_{ik}.

Energies

Molecular energies are particularly important as so many other properties may be inferred from a study of the variation of energy with some molecular parameter such as bond length or angle.

A calculation is run for a particular defined geometrical arrangement of the constituent atoms yielding molecular orbitals and their orbital energies. From these we may calculate the electronic energy, E_{el}. To this must be added the nuclear–nuclear repulsion terms

$$\sum_{\mu,\nu} Z_\mu Z_\nu / R_{\mu\nu}$$

where Z_μ and Z_v are the charges on the nuclei μ and v, and $R_{\mu v}$ their separation. The total energy E_{total} is thus a smaller negative number than E_{el}.

The electronic energy, E_{el}, can be expressed in terms of integrals involving the molecular orbitals, ϕ_i.

$$E_{el} = \sum_i \varepsilon_i^N + \sum_{i>j} J_{ij} - \sum_{i>j}' K_{ij}.$$

Here

$$\varepsilon_i^N = \int \phi_i^* \, H^N \, \phi_i \, d\tau$$

and represents the energy an electron in orbital ϕ_i would have were it the only electron in the molecule, i.e. its kinetic plus nuclear attraction terms;

$$J_{ij} = \int\int \phi_i^*(1)\phi_i(1)\left(\frac{1}{r_{12}}\right)\phi_j^*(2)\phi_j(2)\,d\tau_1\,d\tau_2$$

$$K_{ij} = \int\int \phi_i^*(1)\phi_j(1)\left(\frac{1}{r_{12}}\right)\phi_i(2)\phi_j^*(2)\,d\tau_1\,d\tau_2$$

Exchange terms, K, only occur between electrons of the same spin, indicated by the prime on the summation.

Now orbital energies ε_i are also related to the three terms ε_i^N, J_{ij} and K_{ij}, leading to the convenient result for closed-shell molecules which have no unpaired electrons,

$$E_{el} = \sum_i \left(\varepsilon_i^N + \varepsilon_i \right).$$

This rigorous formulation is used in *ab initio* methods, the ε^N being computed from the orbitals ϕ_i.

For many of the semi-empirical methods the approximation is made that

$$E_{el} = \sum \varepsilon_i.$$

Such an assumption may appear gross but it does seem to produce numbers which vary sensibly with other molecular parameters.

Every type of molecular orbital computer program incorporates the calculation of E_{el} and E_{total} within its own framework and this is invariably printed out. It must be remembered however that only the *ab initio* energies have any absolute meaning, being related to a zero of energy where all particles are removed to infinity. Semi-empirical calculations all use ionization potentials as parameters and consequently energies cannot be compared between one type of calculation and another. Within one method and for different arrangements of the nuclei in one molecule the energies may be compared.

Molecular geometry

If we take the simple example of the water molecule, we may run a molecular orbital calculation for any number of relative positions of the atoms H and

O. The minimum energy geometry found in all types of calculation is similar to the experimental geometry with an angle between the two OH bonds.

In principle this procedure can be followed for a molecule with any number of constituent atoms but the number of calculations required would soon become prohibitive. In practice the starting values of bond lengths and angles are usually taken from known data from spectroscopy or crystal structures, or from values known for similar species. Small variations are then investigated.

Some examples of predicted bond angles in small molecules are given in *Table 13.1.*

TABLE 13.1.
Bond angles predicted by molecular orbital calculations

Molecule	Experiment	Ab initio	INDO	CNDO	EHT
H_2O	104.5	110		107.1	150
CH_2	103.2		106.0	108.6	
NH_3	106.6	106.6	106.4	106.7	
MeOH	(HCH) 109.5		108.2		
	(HCO) 109.5		110.7		
	(COH) 105.9		107.3		
C_2H_6	(HCH) 108.8		106.6		
	(HCC) 110.1		112.2		

Just how well the geometry of isolated molecules can be predicted by calculation may be illustrated by the typical case of NH_3.

Molecular geometries are more often used to confirm the validity of calculations than calculations are used to determine geometries, since there is an abundance of experimental techniques available for investigating molecular geometry. The principles may, however, be carried over to determine other molecular energy variations which are less amenable to experiment.

One such example is the case of vibration frequencies. The energy of a molecule may be calculated as a function of stretching a bond or bending an angle. If the resulting potential curve is then fitted to a suitable expression (even a simple quadratic expansion will do in many cases) then rough estimates of vibration frequencies may be found. Such quantities are on the other hand more of interest to spectroscopists than to medicinal chemists.

An important aspect of the calculation of accurate geometries for small molecules is the current interest in optimizing programs. Such programs calculate an *ab initio* molecular wave function and then optimize the geometry using the gradient of the energy with respect to the 3N nuclear coordinates (N being the number of atoms). A particular computer program which is available from the Quantum Chemistry Program Exchange named 'HONDO' is widely used, especially by those who have access to super-computers which have associated parallel and vector processors. [HONDO, rather than an acronym, is the name of a basket-ball player!] As yet, however, questions of molecular geometry, as opposed to conformation, have not seemed critical in molecular pharmacology.

Conformation

The molecular energy property which is of most interest to researchers interested in small biologically active molecules is conformation. As we have seen in Part I, the majority of the interesting molecules are conformationally flexible. Questions about molecular geometry can be answered with the aid of molecular models, but these leave open a whole range of conformations because of free rotation about single bonds. This is one area where calculations can be of real value to medicinal chemists.

Experimental techniques such as crystallography and nuclear magnetic resonance spectroscopy cannot give more than a small portion of the whole conformational picture.

Quantum chemical calculations may treat conformation exactly like geometry. A calculation is performed for a series of positions of one part of a molecule with respect to another and the energies for each position compared.

If there is only one bond about which rotation can occur then the results may be presented in the form of a curve of energy against angle (*Figure 13.1*).

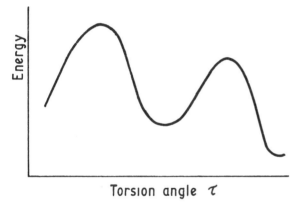

Torsion angle τ

Figure 13.1. Variation of conformational potential energy with one variable torsion angle

For pharmacological species it is frequently the case (e.g. acetylcholine, catecholamines, histamine, dipeptides) that two rotational angles are required to specify conformations. In this case it is sensible to present the required three-dimensional diagram (energy, torsion angles τ_1 and τ_2) as contour diagrams as in *Figure 13.2*. On these energy maps, minima indicate stable conformational structures with the relative depths being indicative of relative stability or enthalpy. The maps also give the heights and shapes of barriers between conformational isomers from which it is possible to calculate rates of interconversion.

As with geometries, the normal computational practice is to start with the bond lengths and angles found for the molecule in the crystal structure and then to hold everything constant except the rotations which are being

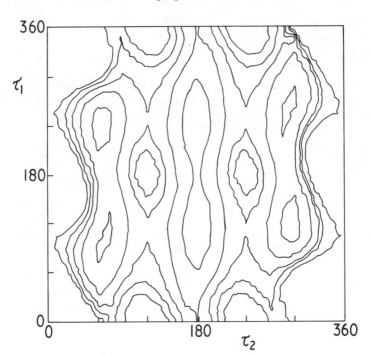

Figure 13.2. Variation of conformational potential energy with two variable torsion angles presented as equal energy contours

investigated. This procedure is not ideal. Given unlimited facilities the logical procedure would be to do *ab initio* calculations, optimizing both the basis set and the geometry for each point on the potential surface. Thus, in a calculation on the conformation of ethane we would allow for the fact that in an eclipsed conformation the H–C–H angles would differ from those in a staggered conformation.

Fortunately as *Table 13.2* shows, barriers to internal rotation found without optimizing geometries at each point on the conformational surface are nonetheless quite close to experimental values.

TABLE 13.2.
Barriers to internal rotation

| Molecule | Barrier (kJ mol^{-1}) | |
	Calculated	Experiment
C_2H_6	12.83	12.25
CH_3NH_2	8.44	8.28
CH_3OH	4.43	4.47
$NH_2–CHO$	90.71	84.44

The experimental values in *Table 13.2* are from gas phase measurements of microwave spectra. The pharmacologist is interested in conformation in a biological environment. However the agreement of careful calculations with measurements in the gas phase does give some encouragement to the hope that the calculated conformational maps where only torsional angle variation has been considered will contain the essential details of conformational preference and hindrance. As ever, however, it will be safest to use experimental data to support the calculations and to eliminate environmental effects by comparing conformational potential surfaces for similar compounds rather than looking at single molecular species.

Conformational free energies

The advent of conformational energy maps, largely owing to increasingly rapid molecular orbital calculations, underlines an obvious point of thermodynamics that is often ignored. If there are several minima on a surface then the relative populations depend on free energy differences and not on the calculated energy differences which are internal energies. Entropy effects will frequently be very important. The relative populations of two dips in a potential surface will depend both on how difficult it is to get out of a valley and the ease with which molecules can enter the holes owing to varying widths.

In *Figure 13.3* the case of a wide shallow depression and a narrow deep one are contrasted for both the one-dimensional and two-dimensional conformational diagrams. In both cases the population of molecules with the conformation labelled *A* with a broad shallow depression of the surface might be more abundant than the internal energy favoured *B* with a deep narrow hole in the potential surface but with a low probability.

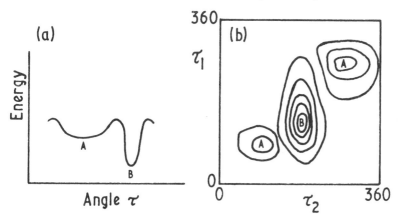

Figure 13.3. Variations of potential energy with conformation showing hollow minima (A) and deep minimum (B) for (a) one variable angle and (b) two variable angles

The diagrams also highlight a semantic difficulty in deciding just what area of the map can be referred to as 'conformation' *A* or *B*. The boundaries are essentially arbitrary. This point is of relevance to experimental work as well as theoretical calculations since it would remain true even with perfect, real potential surfaces. For this reason many published solution conformation population ratios derived from n.m.r. coupling constant measurements are not very accurate numbers.

If we use some statistical ideas it is possible to compute conformational free energies from the energy maps and hence genuine equilibrium constants. It is reasonable to assume that altering conformation has only a minimal effect on volume so that the maps may be considered as enthalpy, ΔH, surfaces, ΔH being equal to $\Delta E + P\Delta V$. For each region which we define as a conformation, a Boltzmann partition function may be calculated. The partition function Z is a number which indicates how the molecules are spread amongst available energy levels. For the single angle case this would be defined as

$$Z_{\text{conformational}} = \sum_{\tau} \exp\left[- E(\tau)/kT\right]$$

and in the two variable angle instance

$$Z_{\text{conformational}} = \sum_{\tau_1 \tau_2} \exp\left[- E(\tau_1, \tau_2)/kT\right]$$

where $E(\tau)$ or $E(\tau_1, \tau_2)$ is the calculated energy for a conformation defined by τ or (τ_1, τ_2), k is the Boltzmann constant, and T is the temperature (normally 37°C). The summations have to be taken over a regular grid of points, fine enough to reflect the shape of the surface appropriate for a given conformer. Effectively we are using a numerical form of integration, assuming that the torsional energy levels are very close together. The appropriate portion of the surface can be defined by taking a local minimum point and defining as a conformer all space within a contour set at $2kT$ above the minimum. Then

$$\Delta G^{\circ} = -kT\ln\left(\frac{Z_{\text{conformational}}A}{Z_{\text{conformational}}B}\right).$$

There is a further important application of the use of conformational partition functions which is of particular value when we wish to compare the conformational flexibility of a series of similar molecules. We may be interested in knowing for a series of similar, conformationally flexible, compounds, just how flexible they are and what range of conformations is likely at body temperature for each molecule.

This information is contained in the potential energy map but there is so much detail that comparisons are far from obvious. As in computing free energies we can associate with each point on the energy surface a probability

$$Z_{\tau_1 \tau_2} = \exp\left[- E(\tau_1 \tau_2)/kT\right].$$

The probability function can then be integrated numerically over the total surface using Simpson's rule to yield Z and normalized by correcting the points using

$$Z^{\text{new}}_{\tau_1 \tau_2} = Z^{\text{old}}_{\tau_1 \tau_2}/Z$$

so that the function integrates to unity.

We can now generate probability maps, single contoured diagrams with the same axes, say τ_1 and τ_2, where the contour will contain within it an indication of a given percentage of molecules for a chosen temperature. If we consider the two-torsion angle case which is appropriate for all the transmitter substances, clearly the square defined by the axes contains 100

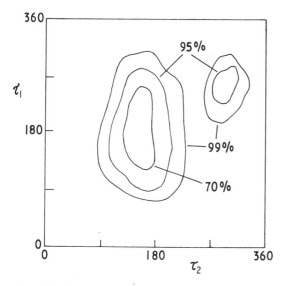

Figure 13.4. Population map with contours defining the region of conformational space containing defined percentages of molecules for a given temperature

per cent of molecules but, as we become more restrictive, we can emphasize just how flexible a molecule is, as in *Figure 13.4.*

With these 'population maps' it is possible to see at a glance just how flexible a molecule may be and which regions of conformational space are favoured. Even more usefully we can compare many members of a series by taking, for example, the 99 per cent contour diagram for each compound and ask the question whether, if biological data are available, there is any indication of conformational requirement for activity.

Ionization potentials and electron affinities

The ionization potential and electron affinity of a molecule should, in principle, be simple to calculate. All that seems necessary is to do a calculation for the neutral molecule in its ground state geometry and conformation and similar calculations for the positive and negative ions, then by difference we will obtain the desired energies. In practice this obvious path is rarely followed.

One reason why it is not popular is that such a procedure would only be expected to yield values in accord with experiment if the correlation energy error, the relativistic error and the discrepancy from the Hartree–Fock limiting energy were identical for the calculations on the molecule and on the ions. Unfortunately the correlation energy error, being dependent to a first approximation on the number of electron pairs in the molecule or ion will certainly differ in the two situations even though the other two errors may cancel.

A further problem when considering electron affinities but not ionization potentials is that self-consistent field calculations frequently do not converge for negative ions.

In consequence a much more drastic but simply applied approximation is often employed. This equates the ionization potential of an electron with the orbital energy ε_i associated with that electron. This is known as Koopmans' theorem. It implies that not only are relativistic and correlation energies the same in the molecule and in the ion but also that there is no reorganization of electronic structure or distribution on ionization. Clearly such approximations are not valid. Once again, however, when considering differences between ionization potentials for a series of similar molecules many of the errors are constant and an acceptable indication of trends in values on chemical modification can be obtained. The energy of the highest occupied molecular orbital which approximates to the ionization potential is often given the acronym HOMO and used as a parameter in correlations with measured biological activities.

For electron affinities the energy of the lowest unoccupied molecular orbital, ε_i for the first virtual orbital, may give an indication of the ease with which the molecule may accept an electron. In addition to the assumptions involved in Koopmans' theorem this approximation is made even less acceptable since there is no definite physical meaning for the virtual orbitals. If an *ab initio* computation is run, the virtual orbitals are very variable as a function of the size of the basis set, the only mathematical constraint upon them being one of orthogonality between themselves and with occupied orbitals. The energy of the lowest unoccupied molecular orbital is frequently referred to as LUMO and again is used in statistical correlations.

Electron affinities then are not well calculated although the simple equation of ionization potential with orbital energy is satisfactory for comparative purposes. Absolute calculation requires a lot of work.

Charge distribution

Possibly more important than nuclear conformation are the details of electronic charge distribution or potential revealed by calculations. The pharmacological receptor, when it experiences the influence of a transmitter molecule, or a drug, must do so by the interaction of electron densities on the two partners. Thus charge distribution is of central importance in any application of quantum mechanics to pharmacology, especially as the theoretical methods should be capable of yielding details of charge distribution within the molecule, unobtainable from experiment.

Ever since the earliest days of quantum mechanics the square of a wave function at a point in space has been interpreted as a probability. If we have an electronic wave function, Ψ, and integrate this function squared over a volume $dv = dx \times dy \times dz$ then the result will be a sum of the probabilities of finding the electrons in this volume element or an electron density ρ, with

$$\rho = \int \Psi^* \Psi \, dv.$$

This direct head-on calculation of the charge within a defined volume in a molecule has only recently been used to produce charge distribution data.

The problem which hindered the use of the direct approach was the difficulty of doing the integrals for volumes of space which bear an awkward relationship to the coordinate system being used for the molecular calculation.

The recent progress has been based on the realization that it is easy to integrate Ψ^2 (or $\Psi^*\Psi$ if Ψ be complex) over a spherical volume if the sphere is centred at the coordinate origin. In these circumstances the charge within a sphere of radius r centred at the origin of the coordinate scheme being used for the problem will be

$$q = \int_0^{2\pi} \int_0^{\pi} \int_0^{r} \Psi^*\Psi r^2 \sin\theta \, dr \, d\theta \, d\phi.$$

Because wave functions may now be computed very quickly it has been realized that we may use the direct approach and calculate the charge within any sphere merely by putting the sphere at the coordinate origin. Thus if we want to know the charge within a sphere of covalent radii centred on each of the atoms of a molecule we can run several molecular orbital calculations, putting each atom in turn at the origin. A convenient matrix transformation in fact exists to transform results, so that in practice only a single molecular orbital calculation is necessary.

The result of such calculations will give clearly defined measures of the charge within each sphere. In principle any volume may be used, not just spheres and, for example, for lone-pair electrons we may be more interested in the charge density away from an atomic centre. The choice of the radius of spheres or dimension of volume considered is arbitrary, but the covalent radius is one obvious simple choice which is related to the rather woolly concept frequently employed by chemists who speak of the charge 'on' an atom (in reality its nuclear charge) when they are more concerned with the charge near an atom. What is meant by 'near' may vary for a given nucleus depending on its environment, with consequent chemical implications.

The results found for the total electronic charge found within a sphere of defined size highlight one of the main difficulties of all approaches to calculating reactivity or binding possibilities by consideration of a single isolated molecule. Consider the charge density in a sphere sited where one expects to find the 'lone pair' on the nitrogen atom of ammonia. A calculation reveals no large concentration of charge corresponding to a 'lone pair' of electrons. Although at first sight this is a puzzling revelation, further thought leads to the conclusion that *isolated* ammonia will not have a 'lone pair'; electrons after all repel each other. However if a proton, or indeed any electrophile, approaches then ammonia reacts as if it had two electrons ready to form a bond. In isolation, however, the 'lone pair' will be smoothed out in a diffuse manner in the region away from the bonds.

An attractive way of using the direct integration approach to charge distribution is to plot contours of charge density. This is full of information but has the disadvantage of difficulty of presentation when a molecule has little symmetry as is the case with most pharmacological species.

This problem of presentation of computed data for molecules which lack obvious symmetry elements has hampered the use of computed properties in molecular pharmacology. In Part III of this book we shall see that computer graphics, particularly those employing colour, are likely to transform this situation.

The pure approach to charge distribution has, as yet, scarcely been applied to pharmacological problems, although it promises to yield much interesting information. Instead a computationally convenient approximation is almost universally made.

Mulliken population analysis

A conveniently programmed way of gaining an idea of charge distribution in molecules comes from the so-called Mulliken population analysis. In one line of computer program we can produce figures to be associated with each atom in a molecule, the figure being the number of electrons 'associated' with the particular atom. In this way all the electrons in the molecule are assigned to nuclei, even though they may not spend much time very close to the particular nucleus. Thus the meaning in physical terms is imprecise although mathematically Mulliken population analyses are clearly defined.

If we are dealing with molecular orbital wave functions,

$$\phi_i = \sum_k c_{ik}\, \chi_k$$

then the net atomic population of a given atomic orbital, χ_k is defined as

$$P_k = 2\sum_i c_{ik}^2$$

Here the subscript i labels the molecular orbital and k refers to the atomic basis function, χ_k. In this we use the concept of the square of a wave function representing a charge density and the atomic basis functions are assumed to be normalized,

$$\int \chi_k^2\, d\tau = 1.$$

The overlap population—the population shared by atomic orbitals k and l—is further defined as

$$O_{kl} = 2\sum_i c_{ik}\, c_{il}\, S_{kl}$$

with

$$S_{kl} = \int \chi_k\, \chi_l\, d\tau.$$

Since $P_k = O_{kk}$ we can write the gross population of atomic orbital χ_k as

$$P_k = \sum_l O_{kl}.$$

The total population at any nucleus can be found by adding all the values of P_j for orbitals χ_j which are centred on atom n.

Most molecular orbital programs incorporate the facility of computing Mulliken population analyses. The numbers so generated are then frequently used in applications to biological problems. It is therefore necessary to add a few cautionary words.

To state the obvious, the only charge on an atomic nucleus is its nuclear charge. This will not change with the environment of the nucleus in a molecule. We are more interested in the charge near to a nucleus but 'near to' has to be defined. In population analyses all the charge is associated with nuclei. The charge between two nuclei is divided equally between the two, even if the atoms have very different electronegatives.

A more worrying feature of population analyses emerges if *ab initio* molecular orbital functions are used. The resulting populations are not invariant to the basis set. In particular if the basis set is gradually increased in size the results may become bizarre. It is even possible to produce negative populations since S_{ij} integrals can be both positive and negative. Experience has shown that the picture of charge distribution derived from minimal basis set computation is frequently more realistic in terms of accord with experiment than when an extended basis set is employed.

These observations are included to urge caution when using population analyses. They are not useless by any means, but their meaning is not quite as clear cut as is often inferred from the presentation of a diagrammatic molecule together with a number (the net charge) associated with each atom.

Despite its weaknesses the rough pattern of charge distribution is indicated by a population analysis. Plots of population analyses against rigorously computed charge densities are linear. Above all when comparing charge distributions of similar molecules the analysis is valuable in indicating trends. Differences are more meaningful than the absolute values.

Molecular potential fields

In some ways more revealing than even an accurate picture of the charge distribution in a molecule would be an indication of the molecular potential field, particularly if drug–receptor interactions are largely electrostatic in nature.

The electrostatic molecular potential is taken as the interaction energy between a unit positive charge and the unperturbed molecular charge distribution. The latter is due to negative electrons and positive nuclei, so that the electrostatic molecular potential $V(k)$ at a point in space labelled k is

$$V(k) = -\int \rho(1)\frac{1}{r_{1k}}dv_1 + \sum_\alpha \frac{Z_\alpha}{R_{\alpha k}}$$

where Z_α is the nuclear charge of nucleus α.

The first order electron density $\rho(1)$ may be derived from an *ab initio* calculation by taking the occupied molecular orbitals and squaring them, i.e.

$$\rho(1) = \sum_{\substack{\text{occupied} \\ \text{mo}}} n_i\, \phi_i^*(1)\phi_i(1).$$

A full calculation of this nature can provide what is sometimes referred to as an 'exact' potential. However, more frequently, further approximations are introduced. Often semi-empirical wave functions are used and the electronic distribution replaced by a set of point charges computed from the wave function, perhaps by the use of population analyses.

For very large molecules the electronic distribution may be based on transferable bond orbitals. Náray-Szabo has produced a computer program which will consider a system of up to six hundred atoms.

Because of the speed with which potential field computations may be carried out using gaussian basis functions it becomes possible to treat large molecules of pharmacological interest and to present the results in the form of isopotential maps. An example is shown in *Figure 13.5*. The potential maps represent contours connecting points at which the energy of interaction of the unperturbed molecule with a proton is identical or 'isopotential'. The main features revealed by this diagram are a positive region extending round the cationic head and two regions of negative attractive energy near the two oxygen atoms. In the figure and in the calculations a hypothetical negative NH_2^- group has been included to simulate an anionic binding site.

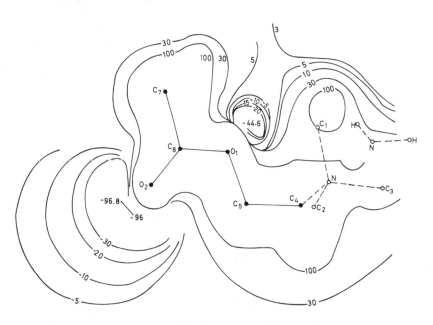

Figure 13.5. Molecular potential field [reproduced with permission from H. Weinstein *et al.*, *Molec. Pharmac.*, 9, 820 (1973)]

Electrostatic molecular potential field calculations have established themselves as a major technique in quantum pharmacology. To an extent their value rests upon the fact that like charge distribution, good results can be obtained from relatively unsophisticated wave functions. This is due to the fact that charge density depending on the square of the wave function is not hypersensitive to the sign of the function at any point. Numerous studies have shown, particularly in areas where differences in otherwise similar molecules are being considered, that useful potential maps can be derived from small basis set calculations and from calculations using pseudo-potentials and even more approximate semi-empirical approaches.

As with charge-density contours a major disadvantage is the presentation of the results for molecules without obvious symmetry. The potential maps look complicated to the uninitiated. As with charge-density pictures the solution to this problem lies in the use of computer graphics, particularly if colour can be used to distinguish regions of positive and negative potential. With such support, the electrostatic potential method can be utilized by experimental chemists and not remain the province of full-time computational chemists.

Frontier electron density

The frontier electron theory was originally developed to explain the difference in reactivity at each position in an aromatic hydrocarbon. It is based on the intuitive idea that the reaction should occur at the position of the largest density of the electrons in the frontier orbitals, which are defined according to the type of reaction:

(1) In an electrophilic reaction, the highest occupied molecular orbital (HOMO).
(2) In a nucleophilic reaction, the lowest unoccupied molecular orbital (LUMO).
(3) In a radical reaction, both of these.

This theory was later given a sound theoretical basis by Fukui, Yonezawa and Shingu who then introduced the concept of superdelocalizability. Denoting the occupied molecular orbitals by $1, 2, \ldots m$, and the unoccupied levels by $m + 1, m + 2, \ldots N$ the superdelocalizability, S_r, is given for the three types of reaction by:
(a) for an electrophilic reaction

$$S_r^{(E)} = 2 \sum_{j=1}^{m} \frac{c_{rj}^2}{\lambda_j}$$

(b) for a nucleophilic reaction

$$S_r^{(N)} = 2 \sum_{j=m+1}^{N} \frac{c_{rj}^2}{\lambda_j}$$

(c) for a radical reaction

$$S_r^{(R)} = \sum_{j=1}^{m} \frac{c_{rj}^2}{\lambda_j} + \sum_{j=m+1}^{N} \frac{c_{rj}^2}{-\lambda_j}$$

where c_{rj} is the coefficient of the rth atomic orbital in the jth molecular orbital, and λ_j is the coefficient in the orbital energy, which is given as $\varepsilon_j = \alpha + \lambda_j \beta$ (α is an ionization potential and β an empirical energy parameter used in simple π-electron Hückel theory).

The orbital which mainly determines the value of S_r in each type of reaction is the same as the frontier orbital previously considered.

There are problems in the use of both frontier electron density and super-delocalization. The latter concept was originally put forward considering the π-electron part of the molecule only, with the energies of the orbitals being given in units of the resonance integral of a C–C bond in benzene, β. This means that in a series of molecules there would be a common zero of energy. Using all-valence molecular methods, the energies are obtained in absolute terms, so that the zero of energy is in the unoccupied orbitals. This is obviously not constant in a series of molecules.

The frontier electron density strictly permits only a comparison of re-activities at different positions within the same molecule. In order to extend this concept for use over a series of molecules, a further quantity, F, may be considered:

$$F = f_r/\varepsilon$$

where f_r is the frontier electron density, ε is the energy of the appropriate frontier orbital.

F may be thought of as a weighted frontier electron density, in the sense that ease of removal of the particular electron is also considered.

Frontier orbital theory may be made more rigorous if *ab initio* sphere charges which have been described above are used to provide the charge in specified regions of particular orbitals. Particularly for comparative purposes it is simple using freely available programs to calculate the charge in a sphere of defined radius on an atom, in a bond or indeed at any suitable point in space. This charge may be broken down into orbital contributions by giving an occupation number (the number of electrons in the orbital) equal to zero for all molecular orbitals other than the one of interest. The orbital of interest is likely to be the HOMO if the molecule is thought to be donating charge but LUMO if it is postulated to be acting as an electron acceptor.

Frontier rate factors can be produced by weighting the sphere charge density by the orbital energies, analogously to the definition of super-delocalizability. *Figure 13.6* gives an example of a correlation produced by

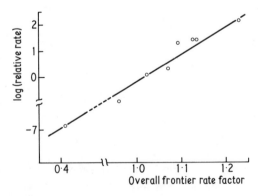

Figure 13.6. Logarithm of overall rate vs. frontier rate factor for nitration of some aromatics

plotting the relative rates of nitration of some aromatic molecules against frontier rate factors.

Static indices

The use of charges, frontier electron densities and other static indices derived from calculations on an unperturbed molecule as a guide to its reactivity is very dangerous. Reactivity is dependent on transition states and not on the unreacted starting materials as illustrated in *Figure 13.7*. All that the calculations on an isolated species may indicate which is of any relevance to the reactivity is the initial slope of the curve shown above.

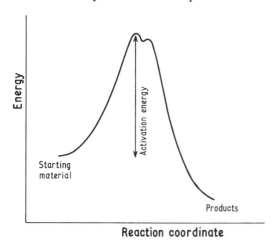

Figure 13.7. Profile of energy of a chemical reaction. Static indices usually refer to the starting materials not the more relevant transition state

As far as pharmacological binding to the receptor is concerned the use of static indices may be less dangerous. If the binding is not covalent but rather based on electrostatic and dispersion forces then the binding free energy may be small. Thus the initial slope of the reactivity curve may give a good indication of the height of the maximum since it is not very far from the unperturbed case. Particularly for comparative purposes static indices then may be useful but the inherent dangers should always be kept in mind.

Summary

Wave functions and energies can be computed for molecules for any set of nuclear coordinates. By changing the atomic positions systematically an energy surface as a function of conformation or geometry can be obtained. The potential energy surface may indicate which conformations are stable, the relative free energies of conformers and equilibrium constants between them. The barriers between conformers can in principle yield rates of inter-conversion.

Charge distributions can be derived from the square of the wave function at a point in space and integrated over defined volumes. Indications of charge distribution come very simply from population analyses. Electrostatic potentials displayed as contour diagrams are among the most useful calculated properties.

The calculations are almost invariably run for isolated molecular species so that conclusions from theoretical calculations are more significant when applied to biological situations if attention is focused more on differences between molecular systems than on individual molecular species.

Further reading

ELLIOTT, R. J., SACKWILD, V. and RICHARDS, W. G. *J. molec. Struc.*, **86**, 301 (1982)
  Quantitative frontier orbital theory.
FARNELL, L., RICHARDS, W. G. and GANELLIN, C. R. *J. theoret. Biol.*, **43**, 389 (1974)
  The calculation of conformational free energies.
HINCHLIFFE, A. and DOBSON, J. C. *Chem. Soc. Rev.*, **5**, 79 (1976)
  Charge-density calculations.
NÁRAY-SZABO, G. *Int. J. Quantum Chem.*, **16**, 265 (1979)
  Electrostatic isopotentials for large biomolecules.
POLITZER, P. and TRUHLAR, D. G. (eds) *Chemical Applications of Atomic and Molecular Electrostatic Potentials*, Plenum Press, New York (1981)
RICHARDS, W. G. *Int. J. Mass Spec. and Ion Phys.*, **2**, 419 (1969)
  The use of Koopmans' theorem.
RICHARDS, W. G., WALKER, T. E. H. and HINKLEY, R. K. *A Bibliography of Ab Initio Molecular Wave Functions*, Clarendon Press, Oxford (1970), Supplement for 1970–73, Supplement for 1974–77, Supplement for 1978–80
SCROCCO, E. and TOMASI, J. *Topic. Curr. Chem.*, **42**, 95 (1973)
  Review of isopotential calculations.

Chapter 14

Running a calculation

This chapter will have something of the flavour of a cookery book, but such advice is essential for anyone who wants to follow the suggestions of earlier parts of this book and apply the quantum mechanical techniques to pharmacological problems. This is the way in which the best work is likely to be done, by experimental research workers who use the theoretical methods as a tool when it seems appropriate to do so, rather than by professional theoreticians who seek problems on which to apply their techniques. The direction of research should be given by the problems to which answers are sought and not by the answers seeking the problems.

The intention of this chapter is to answer the questions which might arise when an experimentalist tries to use molecular orbital calculations to answer his research problems.

Atomic coordinates

An experimentalist will be interested in a particular molecule, or preferably a series of chemically similar molecules, if he wants to rationalize structure–activity differences. In order to run a molecular orbital computer program the input data required will be cartesian coordinates for each of the atomic nuclei in the molecule. Any one of the atoms can be chosen as the origin of a cartesian coordinate system. To produce coordinates of the other nuclei the normal source will be data on bond lengths and angles from which the rectilinear coordinates may be calculated using standard trigonometry. This last phrase covers a nasty calculation if performed by hand, but short computer programs which convert from bond lengths and angles to coordinates are widely available. A routine to transform the data may also be an option at the start of a molecular orbital program.

Bond lengths and angle data may be of two types. It may be that the crystal structure of the interesting molecule is known or alternatively standard values may be used.

Crystal data are preferable but must be used with a little caution. Molecules may not have precisely similar shapes in a crystal and in solution or in an active environment. Crystal structures of ions may vary depending on the nature of counter-ions. The crystal bond lengths and bond angles may be only appropriate for an energy minimum and distortions will occur when groups are rotated or twisted away from equilibrium values.

When crystallographic information is not available, it may be possible to use X-ray data for similar molecules. Failing this, resort has to be made to so-called standard values. There are tables (see list of reading at the end of this chapter) which give the bond lengths and bond angles of known compounds. Average values may then be taken from molecules as similar as possible to the molecule of interest. This practice is frequently taken to what may seem dangerous lengths. In calculations on molecules containing a substituted aromatic ring, all the bond lengths and angles may be assumed to be benzenoid (*Figure 14.1*). If the problem under consideration is, for example, a conformation of a side chain where the aromatic ring is a constant feature then this approximation may not be influential. On the other hand, if the charge distribution in the ring is the point at issue then more care must be taken about the geometry.

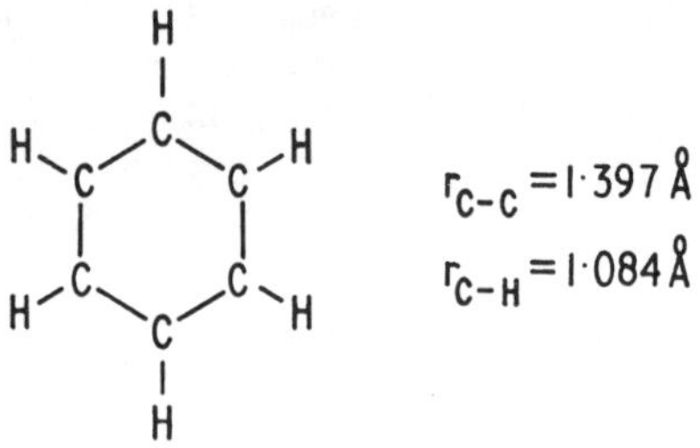

$$r_{C-C} = 1.397 \text{ Å}$$
$$r_{C-H} = 1.084 \text{ Å}$$

Figure 14.1. Geometrical data for a calculation on benzene

Molecular models

Even before deciding upon the nuclear coordinates for a calculation it is sensible to study a molecular model of the system upon which calculations are to be run. This is particularly important if molecular conformation is a crucial point. Preferably both bond models, such as Dreiding models, should be used and space-filling models of the Corey–Pauling–Kolthun (CPK) type (*Figure 14.2*). The models will indicate which molecular conformations are quite impossible within reasonable energies, and about which bonds 'free' rotation is possible and ought to be investigated.

Careful study of the model may also indicate in advance reasons why

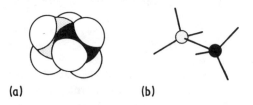

(a)   (b)

Figure 14.2. Molecular models of methyl ammonium $CH_3NH_3^+$. (a) CPK (Corey–Pauling–Kolthun) type of space filling model. (b) Dreiding molecular skeleton models

calculations in a particular case may yield seemingly spurious results. This is above all true if the model indicates the possibility of intramolecular hydrogen bonds. If they can be formed in a model without distortion, good calculations may indicate (quite rightly) that such bonds would be formed if the molecule were to exist in an isolated form. This knowledge should forewarn the investigator to be suspicious of the results if applied unquestioningly to solution or a polar medium. It may be necessary to take action to prevent unrealistic distortion by perhaps including a molecule of water in the calculation or just ignoring the results of a particular computation on the basis of knowledge available prior to seeing the results.

Atom–atom potential calculations: molecular mechanics

A great deal of nonsense has been spoken and written about atom–atom potential calculations or the methods of molecular mechanics, so let us state quite clearly that these calculations are useful, they are inexpensive to perform, but they are not complete alternatives to quantum mechanical calculations except for a narrow range of questions.

If it were possible to write the potential energy, U, between two atoms in a molecule just as if the atoms were like atoms in a rare gas we could write

$$U = \frac{A}{r^6} + B \exp(-Cr)$$

a van der Waals' attraction and an exponential repulsion term. If the constants A, B and C are known for every atom pair in the molecule the total energy would merely be a sum of such terms for all pairs. For a computer this is a trivial problem and there exist many variants in this simple theme.

In general, particularly when there are very few different atoms in a molecule or polymer, very sensible indications of preferred conformations are given. What then are the objections to the use of potential functions? The answer is 'none', so long as it is realized that the status of such a calculation is only an extension of the use of molecular space-filling models.

The mere incorporation of interatomic attraction and repulsion is insufficient to provide valuable indications of molecular conformational energy. Torsion potentials are very important; but these too may be included in an appropriate functional form. The end result is a molecular mechanics computer program which may contain tens of adjustable parameters, each with very little physical meaning. However, so many years of development and refinement of these programs have now taken place that the current versions (available from the Quantum Chemistry Program Exchange) are both highly sophisticated and quite accurate. *Table 14.1*, for example, gives some examples of barriers to internal rotation calculated with a molecular mechanics program and compared with values from *ab initio* molecular orbital calculations.

The agreement is very satisfactory and it must be emphasized that the molecular mechanics demands only a small fraction of the computing time required for a quantum mechanical calculation. For many applications to

TABLE 14.1.
Comparison of *ab initio* and molecular mechanics calculations of rotational barriers or energy differences

Molecule	Barrier (V) or energy difference (ΔE)	Observed†	Energy difference/ kJ mol^{-1}	
			Ab initio	Molecular mechanics
CH_3–NH_2	V (Me)	8.27	9.15	7.90
CH_3–OH	V (Me)	4.48	6.48	3.09
CH_3–CH_2F	V (Me)	13.83	11.65	13.64
CH_3–CHF_2	V (Me)	13.31	9.12	15.58
CH_3–CF_3	V (Me)	13.60	7.27	17.43
CH_3–CH_2Cl	V (Me)	15.42	12.76	15.42
CH_3–$CHCl_2$	V (Me)	19.91	14.70	18.45
CH_3–CCl_3	V (Me)	27.57	16.72	20.92
CH_3–CH_2NH_2	V (Me)	15.65	13.96	11.40
CH_3CH_2–NH_2	ΔE (t–g)*	1.24 (ir)	1.47	0.13
CH_3CH_2–NH_2	V (g–g)	6.40 (ir)	9.32	7.07
CH_3CH_2–NH_2	V (g–t)	9.53 (ir)	10.74	6.83
CH_3–CH_2OH	V (Me)	13.93	11.46	11.46
CH_3CH_2–OH	V (g–g)	5.05	6.28	4.31
CH_3CH_2–OH	V (t–g)	5.60	8.02	3.45
$(CH_3)_2$–CHOH	V (Me)	14.20 (t)	16.21	12.75
$(CH_3)_2CH$–OH	V (t–g)	7.03	7.59	4.11
$(CH_3)_2CH$–OH	ΔE (t–g)	1.17	1.60	2.07
CH_3–CHO	V (Me)	4.89	4.91	4.50
$(CH_3)_2$–CO	V (Me)	3.26	5.13	2.90
CH_3–CH_2CHO	V (Me)	9.54	12.32	15.19
CH_3CH_2–CHO	ΔE (g–c)*	3.76	3.64	3.48
CH_3–COC_2H_5	V (Me)	2.17	4.71	2.93
CH_3–CO_2H	V (Me)	2.02	1.88	1.77
$H(CO)O CH_3$	V (Me)	4.98	3.66	7.87
$H(CO)O$–C_2H_5	ΔE (g–t)	0.78	3.82	0.41
$H(CO)O$–C_2H_5	V (t–g)	4.60	4.88	2.77
CH_3–CO_2CH_3	V (Me)	1.25	1.86	1.82
CH_3–OCH_3	V (Me)	11.38	12.58	10.23
CH_3–SCH_3	V (Me)	8.92	5.49	8.03
CH_3–SH	V (Me)	5.31	5.33	4.41

* t = *trans*; g = *gauche*; c = *cis*.
† All barriers measured by microwave spectroscopy except those indicated: ir = infrared; t = thermodynamic.

Neither set of calculations involved geometry optimization.

questions of conformation of large molecules, molecular mechanics has become the method of choice.

In a CPK model the atoms have a square-edged potential (*Figure 14.3* for two H atoms in a –C–H group). The atom–atom potential adds a soft edge to the potential and is clearly more realistic. Thus using an atom–atom potential program is a sensible extension of the use of molecular models, being even more realistic. This may be sufficient to answer some questions.

However, the potentials are only devices to produce potentials of roughly the correct softness of approach of atoms. They do not have any real significance; a whole range of consistent potentials may be used, each giving the same indication of conformation.

Exponential, r^{-6}, potentials are not very satisfactory for the gaseous argon–argon case. In intermolecular force work on gases it is clear that the total energies are not 'pair-wise additive'; three body interactions are significant. The r^{-6} van der Waals' term is only appropriate for spherical charge distributions. (It is not widely appreciated that the dispersion force between two identical atoms, one in an S state and one in a P state is of the form r^{-3} and is repulsive!)

Atom–atom potentials may take no account of variations in delocalization as molecular geometry changes.

The chief distinction between the methods of molecular mechanics and quantum mechanical calculations, apart from practical considerations about computer time, is that the former methods yield energies while the latter give both energies and wave functions. The uses of the wave function, such as revelations about electron distributions, are restricted to molecular orbital methods.

If in the past there was something akin to rivalry, even enmity, between practitioners of the two approaches, this is no longer the case. Each has seen the merits in the techniques of the other and theoretical workers in drug design use both. Molecular mechanics is a good way to answer questions of shape: quantum mechanics for electronic properties.

Choice of the molecular orbital method

An experimentalist may be prejudiced as to the method or technique to be used on a problem by what is available. No such constraint need govern theoretical calculations. Apart from the program writers who may display understandable preferences, the general user can use objective criteria for choice.

Programs for all the molecular orbital approximations discussed in this book and methods of molecular mechanics are available at low cost from the Quantum Chemistry Program Exchange run from the Chemistry Department of the University of Indiana. The programs are all available in FORTRAN so that transcription for almost any computer is not a very difficult task. How then is a research worker to choose which method to try?

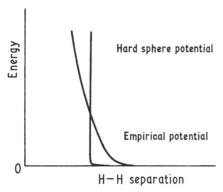

Figure 14.3. Atom–atom potentials for H–H non-bonded interactions

As a general rule the higher up the hierarchy of sophistication the more computer time and storage space is required. This may provide some limitation.

For accurate work on small gas-phase species the more high level the method the better, in general, are the answers. In biological applications this may not be true. The safest approach is to adopt an experimental criterion. If the calculations are being used to illuminate a conformational problem then the calculations should be tested against known facts about the molecule concerned or about similar ones. The crystal structure and n.m.r.-derived conformational preferences should be consistent with the calculation. Barriers to internal rotation should be in reasonable accord with those derived for suitable model systems for which gas-phase microwave data are available. If agreement is satisfactory then the calculations can add considerably to the experimental information since the latter is restricted to equilibrium forms of the molecule.

For calculations which set out to investigate charge distribution on a sub-molecular scale the computed results must be in harmony with bulk measures of charge distribution such as dipole moment.

When the energies of excitation or removal of electrons are the focus of attention then reasonable correlation with data from ultraviolet spectra of photo-electron spectroscopy is an essential prerequisite for confidence in the calculations.

When supported in this manner it is often not the most expensive calculation which is required. Even though extended Hückel theory may be derided for its lamentable failures in many respects, it does nonetheless frequently give good indications of aliphatic conformation; it should do so as the method was parameterized with this in mind.

This final observation suggests an approach which can be adopted if calculations are to be used in a major project such as a structure–activity relationship involving many compounds. It is possible to reparameterize one of the semi-empirical methods to ensure agreement with experiment for some members of the molecular series. The quantum mechanical formulae will then be almost interpolation formulae, relating one molecule to another. However, although this idea may be superficially attractive it should not be undertaken lightly as the problem is a multivariational one since the various empirical parameters may not be varied independently.

Basis sets

Ab initio molecular orbital calculations require a basis of atomic orbitals χ_k. Some of the available computer programs of this type (for example Gaussian '70) have this built into the program so that the user does not have to specify the orbital exponents, ζ, to be used in the equation

$$\chi_k = C \, e^{-\zeta r} \, Y_{lm}$$

for Slater-type orbital, or a in the gaussian

$$G_k = C \, e^{-ar^2} \, Y_{lm}$$

(C represents a normalization constant, r distance from the atomic nucleus and Y_{lm} the angular part of the atomic orbital in terms of angles θ and ϕ).

The *ab initio* programs which allow a choice of basis set (e.g. POLYATOM, IBMOL or ATMOL) may require the size and details of the basis set to be included in the data for running the program. The basis set must be equally 'good' in energy terms for each type of atom in the molecule, otherwise we may encourage much of the charge to be concentrated on one atom for purely spurious reasons. Fortunately tables of atomic basis functions are available (*see* reading list) providing bases of a variety of numbers of terms and consequent energies. An example is given in *Table 14.2*. Programs with built-in bases normally only employ a minimal basis set.

TABLE 14.2
Basis sets of atomic orbitals for the carbon atom

	Orbital	Exponent	
1. A minimal basis set			
	1s	5.673	
	2s	1.608	
	2p	1.568	Total energy of atom -37.62239 au
2. An extended basis set			
	1s	9.153	
	1s	5.832	
	2s	1.428	
	3s	3.076	
	2p	5.152	
	2p	2.177	
	2p	1.150	Total energy of atom -37.68855 au
3. An accurate basis set			
	1s	9.055	
	1s	5.025	
	2s	2.141	
	2s	1.354	
	3s	6.081	
	2p	6.827	
	2p	2.779	
	2p	1.625	
	2p	1.054	Total energy of atom -37.68862 au

Semi-empirical molecular orbital programs do not require basis functions as data, but are also normally constructed with an implied minimal basis.

Configuration interaction

In Chapter 11 the possibility of improving a calculation by configuration interaction was introduced. This facility is an option in some published computer programs.

For pharmacological applications the molecules or ions will normally be closed-shell cases with no unpaired electrons. In this case the Brillouin theorem applies and only excited states with two electrons excited interact directly with the ground state. Such excited states are so highly excited that the effects will not be very significant and configuration interaction is unlikely to be of value.

In the case of free radicals with doublet electronic ground states, monoexcited states which are close in energy may influence the ground state quite profoundly. If configuration interaction is included in the calculation the user will have to decide just how many excited states he must include in the computation. As stated earlier the results do not converge very quickly so the best criterion is probably an experimental test. A suitable set of data are coupling constants which are readily measured and should be proportional to charge densities at the appropriate atoms. For example if we calculate molecular orbital wave functions for the allyl radical, the lone π-electron will have a node at the central carbon (*Figure 14.4*). However the coupling constants are in the ratio $14:4:14$ indicating that the electron does spend a portion of its time in the vicinity of C_2. Configuration interaction will add wave functions which allow this and probably two or three excited states will usually be sufficient for biological problems. However, there is no good answer to the question of when to stop configuration interaction.

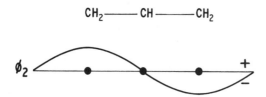

Figure 14.4. Schematic illustration of the molecular orbital ϕ_2 of the unpaired electron in the allyl radical, showing the node at the central carbon atom

Computed properties

Any molecular orbital calculation will yield the total energy of the molecule for a given geometrical arrangement of the atoms and normally in addition the various orbital energies and molecular orbitals in a form of the list of the coefficients which multiply the known basis set. Other properties are computed only if asked for in the data.

The amount of computer time required to compute properties such as population analyses from wave functions is marginal by comparison with the original calculation so that it is sensible to include these properties routinely even though they may not be of immediate interest.

An example of a calculation: methylamine

The geometry of the molecule, obtained from Sutton's Tables, is as follows

Bond length, C–N = 1.474 Å
Bond length, N–H = 1.014 Å

Bond length, C–H = 1.093 Å
Angle, H–N–H   = 105.8°
Dihedral angle = 112.2°
Angle H–C–H   = 109.471°

Input

The initial data for a molecular orbital calculation are likely to indicate the nature of the calculation: closed or open shell; minimal or extended basis; and number of gaussians to be fitted to each Slater orbital. A title may be given and an indication as to whether the species is charged and its spectroscopic multiplicity.

The atomic centres are numbered, equivalent atoms having the same number, and for each the geometrical data are provided, beginning with the atomic number of the atom which we will call X. This is followed by atom A, the length XA; atom B, angle XAB. Next atom C is given followed by the dihedral angle $XABC$ (positive in a clockwise direction round the bond AB looking towards C) if zero or blank follow; or alternatively this second angle is XAC if followed by ±1 ($+$ indicating above the plane XAB and $-$ indicating that the atom is below). Thus in our example:

Atomic number of atom:	X	Atom A	XA	Atom B	XAB	Atom C	XAC	a
The origin is at N_1;	7							
	6	1	1.474					
	1	2	1.093	1	109.471			
	1	1	1.014	2	112.2	3	300.5411	
	1	1	1.014	2	112.2	3	59.4789	
	1	2	1.093	1	109.471	3	109.471	$+1$
	1	2	1.093	1	109.471	3	109.471	-1

In column a, blank indicates angle in column XAC is dihedral $XABC$; $\pm$ indicates above and below plane XAB.

Output

The output usually starts with a presentation of the input data including the cartesian coordinates of each separate atom. These are useful for checking that no errors have been made in the preparation of the data. Details of the basis set chosen are also often produced and a matrix giving the distances between all pairs of atoms.

The molecular orbitals are also printed in matrix form. In our example, if we are running a minimum basis set calculation there will be 15 basis functions; $1s$, $2s$ and $2p$ on N and C with $1s$ on each hydrogen. The matrix will thus be a 15×15 matrix, each column of which will be the 15 coefficients of the basis function for a particular molecular orbital. The orbital energy of each molecular orbital is also given. For example, the first column might contain the following information (*see* table overleaf).

Not surprisingly the most tightly bound molecular orbital is almost entirely a nitrogen $1s$ atomic orbital as indicated by its large coefficient. Similar columns are given for all the fifteen molecular orbitals. Since the molecule has 18 electrons the first 9 molecular orbitals have negative orbital energies; that is, they are bound. The remaining 6 are the virtual orbitals.

Molecular orbital 1

Index	Atom	Basis function	Coefficient
1	N	$1s$	-0.99338
2	N	$2s$	-0.03161
3	N	$2p_x$	-0.00422
4	N	$2p_y$	0.00000
5	N	$2p_z$	-0.00088
6	C	$1s$	-0.00049
7	C	$2s$	0.00515
8	C	$2p_x$	0.00020
9	C	$2p_y$	0.00000
10	C	$2p_z$	-0.00428
11	H	$1s$	-0.00035
12	H	$1s$	0.00672
13	H	$1s$	0.00672
14	H	$1s$	-0.00025
15	H	$1s$	-0.00025

orbital energy -15.30029 au

If requested further output is usually given such as the density matrix used in calculating molecular properties and a Mulliken population analysis.

Computers

The more rigorous theoretical methods generally demand the largest computers, whereas the simple approximations are not so stringent in their demands. Most of the readily available computer programs run without trouble on standard mainframe machines such as the IBM 360 series or CDC 7600.

More recently the explosion in the number of minicomputers available has resulted in the standard programs being rewritten and made available for use on minicomputers such as the VAX 11/780. This has brought the application of the techniques discussed in this book within the range of cost typical for a major laboratory experimental tool and escaped the expense of a dedicated professional computer service. Array and vector processors can also greatly speed calculations. The most recently released microcomputers seem equally capable of performing many of the molecular orbital calculations, bringing down the expense even further and extending the likely range of users. Coupled with this, as has been mentioned several times, are the developments in graphics systems which permit the presentation of computed results in a form which is helpful to a practical chemist who is not a full-time theoretician.

It is not possible to present a rigorous guide to the relative speeds of various machines, but a rough guide is provided by *Table 14.3*. In this table, based on benchmark programs for single precision FORTRAN, performance

TABLE 14.3.
Relative computing speeds

Computing system	Speed relative to IBM 360/195
IBM 360/195	1
IBM 4331–1	0.03
IBM 4341–1	0.20
IBM 3033U	1.1
Amdahl 470/V8	1.5
Burroughs B 7750	0.16
CDC Cyber 170–20	0.18
CDC 7600	2.0
CDC Cyber 205 (2 PIPE)	2.4 (Scalar)
	42 (Vector length 1000)
Cray 1	3.2 (Scalar)
	20 (Vector length 64+)
CTL Modular 1	0.008
Data General Eclipse S/200	0.10
DEC KL 10	0.24
DEC PDP 11/45 (FPP)	0.04
DEC VAX 11/780 (FPA)	0.24
GEC 4080	0.05
Harris S 500 (SAU)	0.16
H 3000–III	0.04
Honeywell 6/43 (SIP)	0.05
Honeywell 6080	0.16
ICL 1904S	0.04
ICL 2960 (VME/B)	0.08
ICL 2980 (FMDU)	0.72
ICL System 4/72	0.06
Modcomp Classic	0.19
Nord 50	0.11
Perkin Elmer 3220	0.11
Prime 750	0.20
SEL 32/77 (HW FL PT)	0.12
Siemens 7748	0.06
Univac 1108	0.16

is compared with that of an IBM 360/195 computer, but wide variation may be expected for specific applications.

The system of choice for many in the pharmaceutical industry as well as in academic departments would be a minicomputer plus interactive coloured graphics display.

Summary

Before running molecular orbital calculations it is sensible to study molecular models of the molecule concerned. An even more realistic notion of shape can be derived from an atom–atom potential calculation, useful for energies but giving no information about the electrons in a molecule. The type of approximate method to use is best decided upon by reference to relevant physical data.

The advent of minicomputers, microcomputers and graphics systems will enable more and more research groups to use theoretical calculations as research tools without being dependent on gigantic computing facilities or professional theoreticians.

Further reading

KENNARD, O. *et al. Molecular Structures and Dimensions*, International Union of Crystallography, Chester (1972)
SUTTON, L. E. (ed) *Tables of Interatomic Distances and Configurations in Molecules and Ions*, Special Publication of the Chemical Society, London, Vol. 11 (1958); Supplement, Vol. 18 (1965)
The sources for bond lengths and angles.

Basis sets of atomic orbitals may be found in the following references:

BASCH, H., HORNBACK, C. J. and MOSKOWITZ, J. W. *J. chem. Phys.*, **51**, 1311 (1969)
CLEMENTI, E. Tables of atomic functions, Supplement to paper in *I.B.M. J. Res. Develop.*, **9**, 2 (1965)
CLEMENTI, E., MATCHA, R. and VEILLARD, A. *J. chem. Phys.*, **47**, 1865 (1967)
VEILLARD, A. *Theoret. chim. Acta*, **12**, 405 (1968)
WACHTERS, A. J. H. *J. chem. Phys.*, **52**, 1033 (1970)

Details of the Quantum Chemistry Program Exchange which produces a regular newsletter from

QCPE,
Department of Chemistry, Indiana University,
Bloomington, Indiana 47401, USA

Part III

Applications of theory
to experiment

Chapter 15

Conformations

The results presented in Part I suggest that theoretical calculations can offer an important contribution to the understanding of the behaviour of nerve transmitters and their agonists and antagonists. All the transmitter substances are small flexible molecules which appear to interact with quite distinct receptors. One possibility is that separate conformations are involved for different receptors. If this is so, equilibrium structural studies such as crystallography or n.m.r. spectroscopy may not be capable of providing sufficient information. Active conformations may not be those stable in the solid or in solution and indeed may not be stable at all except in the receptor environment. Calculations of conformational potential energy should supplement the experimental data about conformation.

Before discussing the results and value of calculations of conformation one important and not merely semantic problem must be discussed. What is a conformation? When using models which give a good notion of shape, but no indication of the dynamical behaviour of the internal degrees of freedom of a molecule, the importance of this question may not be apparent. A $1:2$ disubstituted ethane molecule will have *gauche* (*syn*-clinal) and *trans* (*anti*-periplanar) forms, but where does one form change to the other and how far from an energy minimum can one stray before ceasing to be in a 'conformation' referred to by reference to the energy minimum?

Let us consider the general form of a transmitter substance as shown in *Figure 15.1* where τ_1 and τ_2 define the conformation.

A possible potential energy surface showing only the valleys corresponding to stable conformations is illustrated in *Figure 15.2*.

In the figure a conformation is described as *trans* (t) or *gauche* (g) (more properly *anti*-periplanar or *syn*-clinal) if it lies within a specified boundary

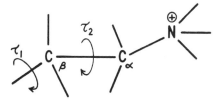

Figure 15.1. Twist angles defining the conformation of molecules with two variable torsion angles

171

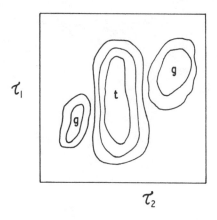

τ_1

τ_2

Figure 15.2. Conformational potential energy surface for a molecule with two variable angles. Only valleys, labelled t and g for the stable conformations, are shown

on the surface. The choice of this boundary is arbitrary. The point at which a molecule ceases to be in a *trans* or *gauche* conformation and should be considered as being in a transitional form is not obvious. An identical range of energy above each potential minimum may seem to be a sensible restriction. In the case illustrated however this may leave a problem as to whether the two minima in each *gauche* form should be treated independently since the barrier between these two forms may be much lower than that between *trans* and *gauche*. These arbitrary decisions may have serious repercussions in computing equilibrium constants between various conformational forms of a molecule.

Calculation procedure

Solution of a set of molecular orbital equations yields an energy and a wave function for a prescribed set of nuclear coordinates. Conformational work utilizes the energies, frequently displayed as above in a contour diagram. As no use is made of the wave function in conformational studies, the option of using the methods of molecular mechanics is open and is often followed, especially for very large time-consuming molecules. It is a sensible precaution to test the quality of a potential energy surface with some discrete *ab initio* molecular orbital calculations, especially for rotational barriers.

The procedure for calculating potential surfaces was covered in Part II, but a brief summary may be helpful. In molecular orbital methods, the bond lengths and bond angles of the molecule other than those involved in conformational rotations are taken from crystal data or standard values. They are not usually changed or optimized during a conformational change. Although this might seemingly lead to calculated torsional barriers being higher than reality, it does not seem to produce serious anomalies.

Molecular mechanics calculation may incorporate optimization of bond length and angle with conformational change, but in this case the difficulty may be the choice of parameters for molecules containing a variety of hetero-atoms or structural units.

Notation and presentation of results

There is an accepted convention for the description of the conformation of molecules in terms of torsion angles. The eclipsed conformation of A–X–Y–B which is configurationally described as *cis* has a torsion angle of 0°. The extended *anti*-planar conformation which is configurationally called *trans* has a torsion angle of 180°. When looking from X towards Y, the convention defines the clockwise movements of B relative to A as positive. The conformational terms used to describe special values of torsion angles are as follows: 0° is *syn*-periplanar or *syn*-planar; ±60° is ±*syn*-clinal; ±120° is *anti*-clinal and 180° is *anti*-periplanar or *anti*-planar.

Nonetheless some papers do use the main convention reversed with the *syn*-planar conformation called 180° and extended periplanar called 0°. This can be confusing and care is necessary in interpreting conformational potential energy maps. The use of molecular models is almost essential.

Even in the presentation of conformational potential energy surfaces there is no uniformity of practice. If we restrict consideration to the case which is of major importance in the pharmacology of the nervous system, with conformation described by two twist angles, then the same diagram may have the axes running from 0° to 360° or from −180° to +180°, restricting ourselves to the most obvious possibilities. The former convention is aesthetically the more pleasing since the valleys representing stable conformations usually appear in the body of the figure while in the latter they are frequently on the axes and interpretation requires more mental agility. The second convention on the other hand is in closer accord with the Ramachandran diagrams used in the dipeptide model for proteins.

In the case of the results presented in this chapter all the work will be transformed into the 0–360° convention as these maps are easier to visualize. Most of the figures represent recalculations of original work referenced in the bibliography.

As well as presenting energy surfaces for a number of key molecules we will also on occasion give percentage or population maps. These are even easier to interpret and bear a closer relationship to experiment since they incorporate entropy considerations as explained in Chapter 13.

Results for isolated molecular species

Calculations performed on a single isolated molecule are perhaps surprisingly in general agreement with shapes found from X-ray crystallographic determinations. This is particularly surprising when it is recalled that even the solid state structures may vary as a function of the counter-ion used, the solvent or the preparation of the crystal. The agreement must imply that the essential features responsible for conformation are intramolecular but it is also fair to point out that the experimental crystal data are often incorporated into the calculation in the form of bond lengths and bond angles other than the conformational torsion angles.

The following sections give some sample results for molecules of major importance and details of the many calculations to be found in the literature can be taken from the bibliography.

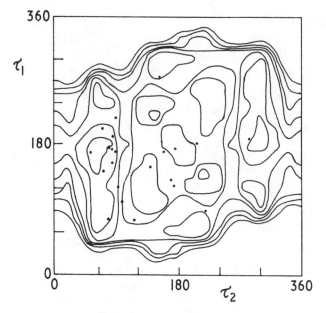

Figure 15.3. Conformational potential energy surface for acetylcholine calculated using the PCILO approximation. The points which cluster round the minima refer to measured X-ray crystal structures

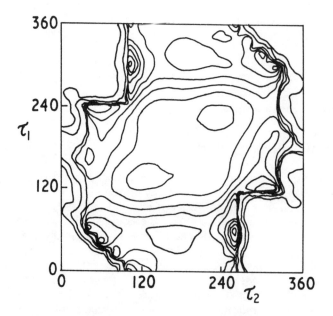

Figure 15.4. Conformational potential energy surface for acetylcholine calculated in the INDO approximation

Acetylcholine

Figure 15.3 is a conformational energy map for acetylcholine computed in the PCILO approximation with relevant crystallographic data also indicated.

For comparison in *Figure 15.4* a similar diagram for acetylcholine calculated in the INDO approximation is presented. It may be seen that the overall results are very similar.

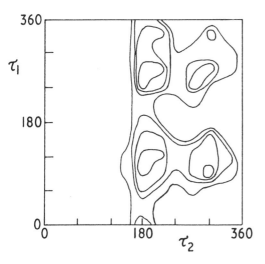

Figure 15.5. Conformational potential energy surface for noradrenaline computed using the PCILO approximation

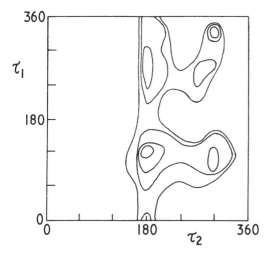

Figure 15.6. Conformational potential energy surface for adrenaline computed using the PCILO approximation

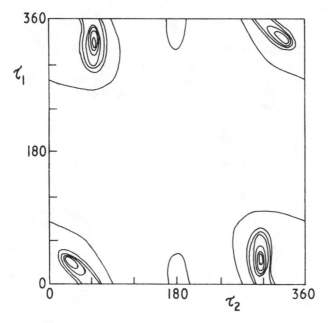

Figure 15.7. Conformational potential energy surface for histamine computed using the PCILO approximation

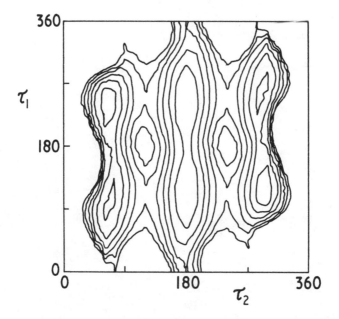

Figure 15.8. Conformational potential energy surface for histamine computed using the EHT approximation

Catecholamines

Figures 15.5 and *15.6* show PCILO calculations for isolated noradrenaline and adrenaline.

Histamine

Histamine has proved a more troublesome problem than the other small flexible amines largely because solvation effects seem to be more important than for some of the transmitters.

Figures 15.7 and *15.8* compare the PCILO and extended Hückel conformational potential surfaces.

It may be seen that the surfaces are strikingly different indicating certain defects in the simple Hückel approximation even though owing to a cancellation of errors the surface so calculated is capable of reproducing results from solution experiments.

5-Hydroxytryptamine

Finally the PCILO surface for conformational variation in 5-hydroxytryptamine is given in *Figure 15.9*.

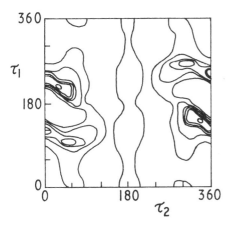

Figure 15.9. Conformational potential energy surface for 5-hydroxytryptamine computed using the PCILO approximation

The details of many more calculations on the conformational potential surfaces of isolated molecules may be found in the bibliography, together with further details of those presented here and sufficient data to recompute any particular case.

Limitations of isolated molecule calculations

The selection of results given above is quite typical of the sort of accord found between calculation and experiment. Such agreement is of only limited value however. It is more an encouragement to the theoretical chemist than an incentive to the medicinal chemist. The results lend confidence in the ability of the methods to reproduce experimental findings, but calculations on single molecules in the isolated environment cannot provide the basis of any structural explanation of the interaction between a small active molecule and its macromolecular receptor.

The effect of water as solvent on a molecule will be considered in a later chapter, but before tackling that complicated problem we can consider one way in which isolated molecule or solvated molecule calculations can lead to definition of conformation essential for biological activity.

The Venn diagram approach

The starting point for this approach is the realization that the environment of the small molecule when it fulfils its biological role is totally unknown. It is by no means clear what the pH of the medium is, even if such a concept has meaning at a microscopic molecular level; we do not know what ions will be in close proximity to the molecule; we are unsure whether a lipid or aqueous phase is the more appropriate environment; we know nothing of the cell surface where the receptor is frequently to be found. Under these circumstances the only recourse is to look at the varying biological effects of a series of chemically and physically similar compounds in the hope that environmental perturbations will be constant for the whole series.

Calculations may then be performed on the set of compounds, each being treated either as an isolated molecule or perhaps, more realistically, solvated.

In principle either a series of agonists or a series of antagonists may be chosen. The former have the advantage of no ambiguity as regards the site of action but the disadvantage of having a biological activity dependent both on the affinity of the small molecule to the receptor and the efficacy of such binding. Antagonists have only affinity but the difficulty now becomes one of being certain that each member of the series produces its effects in the same manner by binding very strongly into the site designed to accept the natural compound, or at least into the same site for the whole series. It is also possible that different agonists or antagonists bind to a given receptor in somewhat different conformations, trading off conformational energy for close fit to different extents. A possible example is the binding of methotrexate to dihydrofolate reductase.

'Lock and key' as a model for the interaction between small biologically active molecules and their receptors served from the time of Erlich for several decades. It has been replaced by a more exact analogy, that of a 'hand and glove'. The newer model includes the notion of an intimate fitting between the macromolecule receptor and the small molecule, but in addition the possibility of flexibility in both partners is incorporated. There is abundant evidence of conformational change in proteins when small molecules are bound into specific sites (including oxygen binding to haemoglobin). Enzyme substrates are frequently bound in conformations which differ from those of the unbound form. A change of conformation of the small partner on attachment seems particularly probable in the case of neuro-transmitters and there is some strongly suggestive evidence that this does take place. Most of the putative neuro-transmitters bind to more than one quite distinct type of receptor, this being certain for acetylcholine, noradrenaline, dopamine, histamine and GABA. In all these instances there could be a variety of reasons for the use by nature of a single small molecule to bind to distinguishable receptor sites. The use of different ionic forms or different sides of the same molecule are possibilities. More likely seems to be the use of different conformers of the flexible ligand. These conformers need not be stable forms, the prerequisite is merely that the required shape is not too far energetically from a minimum on the energy surface. It is this possibility which leads to the use of theoretical methods. If the required shapes are non-equilibrium conformations then they are not amenable to study by X-ray crystallography or n.m.r.

Calculations, since they are equally valid for unstable as well as stable shapes, permit the answering of the question, 'Is there a particular conformation of a neuro-transmitter which is essential for binding to a given receptor?'

In outline, the procedure for answering questions about essential conformations for particular receptors which will be illustrated below is as follows. We need to be able to calculate those shapes of a molecule which can be adopted and then to compare the available conformations for active agonists to set up hypotheses about shapes which are prerequisites for activity. These hypotheses can then be tested by additional molecules and the idea rejected or refined. In a sentence, the strategy is to produce Venn diagrams related to conformation which will lead to necessary but not sufficient criteria for reactivity (*Figure 15.10*).

The first stage in the implementation of this process is to produce a potential energy surface.

The energy map contains a great deal of information but it is not suitable

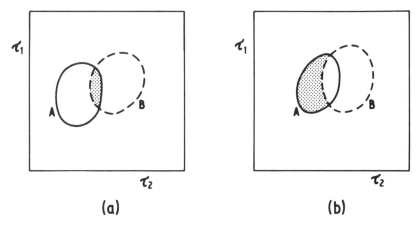

Figure 15.10. Venn diagrams showing conformations necessary but not sufficient for activity (shaded). (a) Molecules A and B both active. (b) Molecule A active but B inactive

to use in a Venn diagram. What is required is a simplified version which will reveal only an answer to the question of what range of shape is available to a molecule. The simplest manner to achieve this is to take some arbitrary contour above the global minimum on the surface. The defect of this solution is that it takes no account of the details of the surface shape. Wide shallow depressions will contain a bigger population of molecules than deep narrow holes: in other words entropy effects are important and we need free energy information rather than internal energy. This can be achieved by taking Boltzmann factors and plotting diagrams with a single contour which encompasses say 99 per cent of the molecules at physiological temperature; that is we use the population maps discussed in Chapter 13.

An old example which has withstood the test of time and many subsequent challenges from new compounds is that of the essential conformation for activity at the histamine H1 receptor. *Table 15.1* lists the series of compounds and their biological activities at H1 and H2 receptors.

TABLE 15.1.
Agonist activities of methylhistamines

Compound	H1 activity	H2 activity
histamine	100	100
2-methyl	16.5	4.4
3-methyl	0.42	<0.1
4-methyl	0.23	43.0
β-methyl	0.83	0.89
α-methyl	0.36	0.74
N-methyl	72.0	74.0
N,N, dimethyl	44.0	51.0
α, 4-dimethyl	0.08	2.96–7.4

The fact that the potential surfaces computed, even with the almost disreputable extended Hückel theory, are realistic is supported by the figures in *Table 15.2*.

TABLE 15.2.
Calculated (EHT) and observed (n.m.r.) percentages of anti-periplanar conformers of some methyl histamine dications

Compound	Anti-periplanar (per cent)	
	EHT	n.m.r.
3-methyl	65	57
4-methyl	65–75	57
N-methyl	65	59
N,N dimethyl	80	72
N,N,N trimethyl	>99	92

Figure 15.11 shows an example of the Venn diagram including three members of the series which leads to the suggestion of a fairly well-defined region which can be labelled as 'essential' for this type of activity. Ability to adopt this particular non-equilibrium conformation is a necessary but not sufficient condition for H1 agonist activity.

Much more recently a fascinating experimental result (see *Table 15.1*) has permitted a similar comparison to be made for the more exciting H2 activity. Histamine itself is, of course, active at both its receptors, while 4-methyl

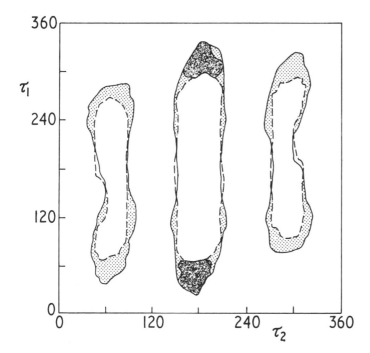

Figure 15.11. Comparison of conformational percentage maps. The dotted area indicates regions available to histamine but not to the 4-methyl compound. The dark area is within the 99 per cent contour for all H1 active agonists and represents the conformation 'essential' for this type of activity

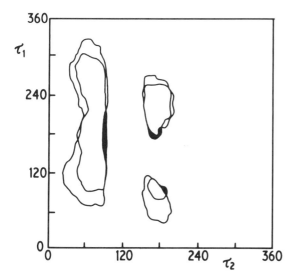

Figure 15.12. Population maps for α-methyl histamine and 4-methyl-α-methyl histamine with the shaded areas being possible essential conformations

histamine is barely active at H1 and about half as active as the natural compound at H2 (a fact used in the H1 essential conformation argument and incorporated into the very successful H2 antagonists). The α-methyl substituted histamine is scarcely active at either site. However the dimethylated compound, α-methyl 4-methyl histamine has greatly increased H2 activity. This is a rare example of an increase in activity on methylation, steric assistance rather than steric hindrance.

Figure 15.12 shows the associated Venn diagram which permits the hypothesis of the H2 essential conformation.

The defect in this work is the reliance on a crude potential energy calculation. Unfortunately, more sophisticated methods for this particular molecule lead to the indication of a very stable intramolecular hydrogen bond involving the lone pair on the imidazole ring nitrogen and the side chain ammonium group. Methods of incorporating solvent to preclude this are not sufficiently reliable to trust so that the problem remains somewhat inconclusive despite its tremendous importance.

Some conclusions of a similar nature can be drawn for dopamine acting at the D1 receptor, although a lack of experimental data precludes definitive statements. Dopamine and N-methyl dopamine are equipotent but α- and β-methyl dopamines while still active are less so. *Figure 15.13* shows population maps for these four compounds which conform with n.m.r. data.

The only conformational region which seems to show dopamine and the N-methyl analogue conformational flexibility to be similar and to discriminate α- and β-compounds is that with an anti-periplanar ($\tau_1 = 90°$ or $270°$; $\tau_2 = 180°$) shape. Some support for this suggestion is provided by the semi-

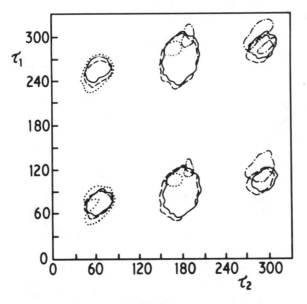

Figure 15.13. Population maps for dopamine and substituted dopamines. Dopamine and N-methyl dopamine are equipotent but α- and β-methyl compounds are less active. The only shape which appears to discriminate is the anti-periplanar conformation $\tau_1 = 90°$ or $270°$; $\tau_2 = 180°$)

rigid D1 agonist ADTN (2-amino 6,7 dihydroxytetranaphthalene). The oxygen–nitrogen atom separations in the equatorial form of ADTN are similar to this anti-periplanar form of dopamine. This is clearly a case where the testing of further simple agonist molecules would be helpful and would encourage further more sophisticated calculations.

Calculations on GABA are complicated by the fact that being a zwitterion, isolated molecule computations are dominated by the intramolecular charge–charge interaction. There is no totally satisfactory answer to this although solvated supermolecule calculations are probably realistic in predicting a variety of allowed stable conformers. It is possible to investigate the neutral non-ionic form assuming the biological environment will preclude the intramolecular interactions. Biologically the GABA recognition site seems to be part of a supermolecular complex consisting of a GABA receptor site, a receptor which will bind benzdiazepines and an ionophore. Agonists of GABA bind at the GABA sites to produce some pharmacological effects and also stimulate benzdiazepine binding. *Figure 15.14* shows a conformational percentage map for neutral GABA computed using *ab initio* methods.

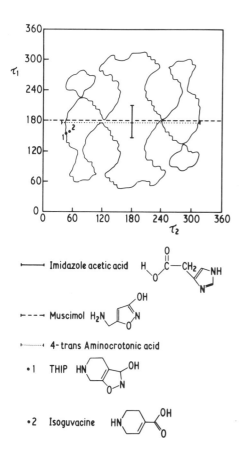

Figure 15.14. A population map for GABA with available conformations for some agonists

Superimposed lines show the flexibility of agonists with a single variable torsion angle and points indicate rigid agonists.

At least one molecule (imidazole acetic acid) does not fit in with the rest of the series, but otherwise the hypothesis of a form of GABA with approximate angles $\tau_1 = 180°$ and $\tau_2 = 60°$ as an essential conformation is suggested.

Again there are not enough experimental data to give firm conclusions and the theoretical methods are open to question, but nonetheless a working hypothesis can be derived and the calculations do suggest obvious further experiments which can test this hypothesis.

Even if the essential conformation is defined in this way we are left with the question as to what is the nature of the essentiality. The precisely defined conformation could either be a conformation through which a molecule must pass in order to gain access to the receptor or equally possibly it could reflect the precise conformation required for effective binding to the receptor from which receptor site characteristics could be inferred.

Although it may be tempting to hope that the second alternative is appropriate there are no compelling grounds for believing that this is so. All the transmitters and many drugs are flexible so it is possible that adaptation of shape to reach the most favoured binding position is common. Stepwise binding involving first the positive amino-nitrogen atom followed by the rest of the molecule seems an obvious possibility.

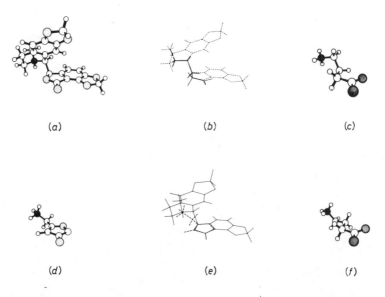

(a)   (b)   (c)

(d)   (e)   (f)

Figure 15.15. Structural similarities between GABA, bicuculline and muscimol.
(a) Bicuculline in a low energy form (H–C1–C9–H angle 90°). (b) GABA
fitted to this form of bicuculline. (c) GABA in the 'bicuculline conformation'.
(d) Muscimol conformation (N7–C6–C5–C4 torsion angle 39°) which affords
maximum overlap with bicuculline. (e) Overlay of muscimol on bicuculline.
(f) GABA in the 'muscimol conformation' which differs only in the position
of carbon atom 4 from the 'bicuculline conformation' [reproduced with
permission from P. R. Andrews and G. A. R. Johnston, *Biochem. Pharmac.*, **28**,
2697–2702 (1979)]

The use of computer graphics

In theoretical calculations of conformation the burgeoning use of computer graphics has already had a profound influence. At its lowest level a display of the geometry entered into a computer program will provide a rapid and simple test for errors in data. More usefully it is possible to test the superimposability of molecules graphically in a manner not possible with models.

A good example of this procedure is provided by the work of Andrews and Johnston on the GABA problem discussed above. Their figure (*Figure 15.15*) shows the structural similarities between GABA, muscimol and the rigid agonist bicuculline.

Series with several torsion angles

Although the Venn diagram approach, preferably coupled with the use of graphics systems, is powerful for cases where a two-dimensional population map summarizes all the flexibility data, things are more intractable when there are several variable angles. It is still possible however to use a Venn diagram logic but in a slightly different manner. Diagrams are produced for each member of the series of compounds with each entry on the diagram revealing the variation in specific conformational parameters.

A particularly interesting example is some work by Heritage who introduced this procedure, although similar ideas in terms of excluded volume have been exploited by Marshall. The study concerns the activities of some rather complicated pyrethroid molecules (*Figure 15.16*).

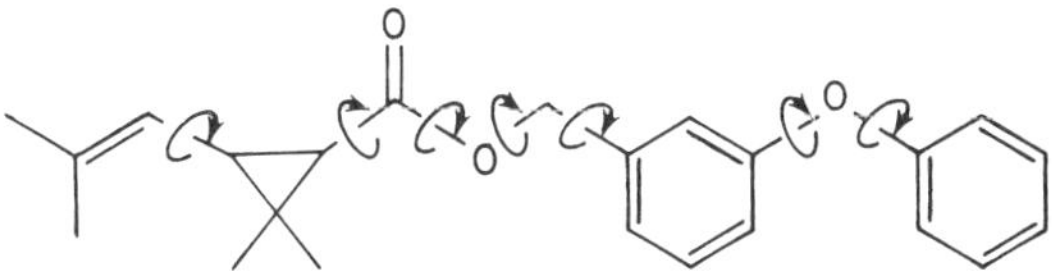

Figure 15.16. A synthetic pyrethroid showing the seven torsion angles

A synthetic compound with high intrinsic activity, bioresmethrin is shown in *Figure 15.17* together with two methyl analogues; 2-methyl substitution gives a small reduction in activity while α-substitution reduces potency by several orders of magnitude. The flexibility indicated in the accompanying maps suggests that we need τ_3 somewhere near $0°$.

The other five torsion angles are held at minimum energy values to give an extended conformation which acts as a sort of template. Variation in activity is seen as the outer aryl ring is altered in its manner of attachment (*Figure 15.18*).

It is then possible to produce a Venn diagram for each molecule rather than comparing several different molecules. On each diagram are three boundaries; one refers to conformational flexibility in terms of an energy contour or population; a second is provided by a distance between the

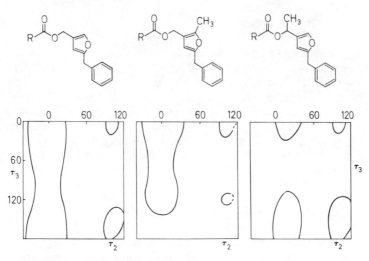

Figure 15.17. Bioresmethrin analogues and energy maps

conformationally variable outer ring and a fixed ring; the third is the angle between the two aryl rings, based on the supposition that they need to be parallel as well as close in space. *Figures 15.19* and *15.20* show such Venn diagrams for the two instances with the outer ring attached in meta- and para-positions. In the former case there is a wide range of overlap on a τ_4 against τ_5 diagram but very little common area in the para-instance where with a less good fit we get a less active isomer.

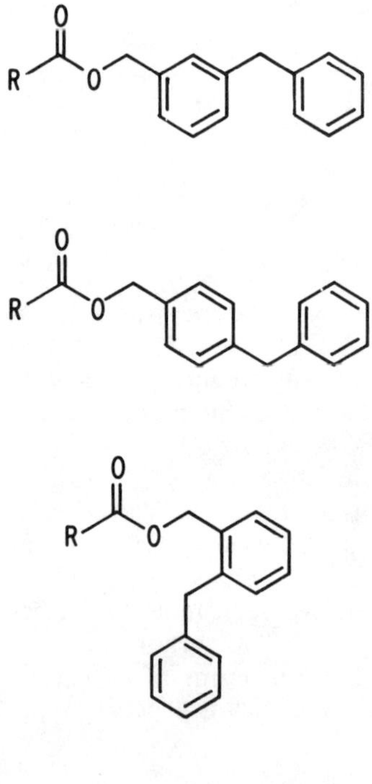

Figure 15.18. m-, p- and *o*-benzyl benzyl isomers

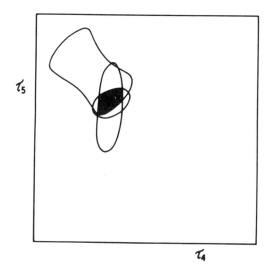

Figure 15.19. Venn diagram for the meta-isomer with good overlap

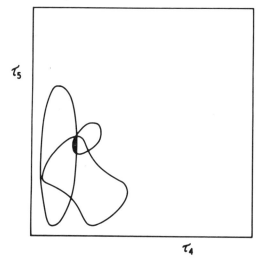

Figure 15.20. Venn diagram for the para-isomer with poor overlap

As a general technique this extension relies upon the use of a template molecule to which other active alternatives have to approximate in conformation to bind. The closeness of the approximate fit is indicated by maximum overlap of areas of conformational freedom on the Venn diagram.

Summary

Calculations of conformational internal energy surfaces for flexible pharmacological molecules which treat the molecule or ion as isolated in space produce results which are in good agreement with experimental data derived from crystallographic studies.

If a series of similar molecules with varying activities is studied from a conformational point of view, it may be possible to define the precise conformation of molecules which is essential for activity; calculations are helped by the use of computer graphics.

In molecules with several variable conformational features the adaptability to the conformation of a postulated template can be revealed by Venn diagrams.

Further reading

ANDREWS, P. R. and JOHNSTON, G. A. R. *Biochem. Pharmacol.*, **28**, 2697 (1979)

BERGMANN, E. D. and PULLMAN, B. (eds) 'Conformation of biological molecules and polymers', *Proc. 5th Jerusalem Symposium on Quantum Chemistry and Biochemistry*, Academic Press, New York (1973)

CHRISTOFFERSEN, R. E. in B. Pullman (ed) *Quantum Mechanics of Molecular Conformations*, John Wiley, London (1976)
    The article on 'Molecules of Pharmacological Interest' contains an excellent bibliography.

FARNELL, L., RICHARDS, W. G. and GANELLIN, C. R. *J. med. Chem.*, **18**, 662 (1975)
    The use of population maps.

KIER, L. B. *Molecular Orbital Theory in Drug Research*, Academic Press, New York (1971)
    A wide-ranging account of the use of extended Hückel theory in conformational problems.

PULLMAN, B. 'Conformational studies in quantum biochemistry', in R. Daudel and B. Pullman (eds), *The World of Quantum Chemistry*, D. Reidel, Dordrecht, Holland (1974)

RICHARDS, W. G., CLARKSON, R. and GANELLIN, C. R. *Phil. Trans. R. Soc. Lond. B.*, **272**, 75 (1975)

Chapter 16

Electronic charge distribution and potential

In many ways far more important than the energy derived from a molecular orbital calculation is the wave function. From the wave function it is possible to compute a wide variety of physical observables by using the appropriate operator. Amongst these possibilities the charge density is perhaps the simplest and most useful.

The utility of information on the distribution of electrons, or the potential field which this distribution creates, derives from the obvious fact that the chemistry, the affinity, the efficacy and the reactivity of a molecule are properties of electrons. When molecules encounter each other it is the electrons which interact. Shape is defined by the electrons in a molecule: the nuclei are merely inert positive centres, the skeleton on which the electrons provide the flesh.

It is fortunate that the quantum mechanical operator needed to compute charge is the particularly simple unit operator, or in other words, as has been known since Born's conjecture at the dawn of quantum mechanics, the square (Ψ^2 or $\Psi^*\Psi$ if Ψ be complex) of an electronic wave function at any point in space is a measure of the electron density or probability of finding an electron at that point. Since the wave function is squared, many of the subtle counter influences of positive and negative portions of the wave function are rendered unimportant in the case of charge distributions. Wave functions which are of insufficient accuracy to compute satisfactorily other molecular properties are good enough for charge distributions and many apparent liberties may be taken in the calculation of electrostatic molecular potentials without compromising the value of the work.

The wave function may be used to reveal charge distribution details in a variety of ways. Once again a major difficulty in an otherwise simple topic has been the manner of display of the information, particularly if it is to be used as a tool by a non-specialist. As in many such instances the escape from this impasse has been the introduction of computer graphics displays.

189

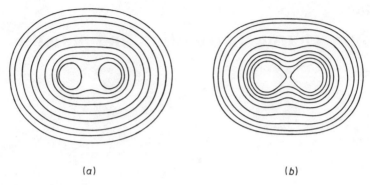

Figure 16.1. Molecular charge-density contours for C_2 (a) and O_2 (b)

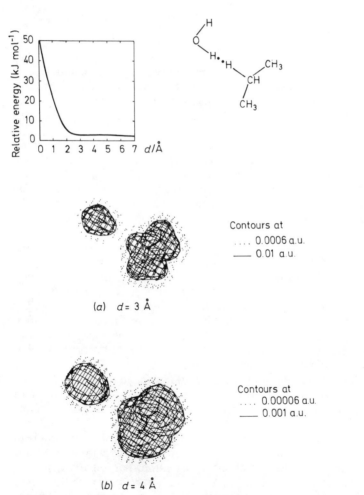

Contours at
.... 0.0006 a.u.
——— 0.01 a.u.

(a) $d = 3$ Å

Contours at
.... 0.00006 a.u.
——— 0.001 a.u.

(b) $d = 4$ Å

Figure 16.2. The $CH_3CH_2CH_3 \ldots H_2O$ system

Charge-density contours

In elementary chemistry texts it is common to find figures such as *Figure 16.1* which give the electron density in the form of contour diagrams. This full use of the information contained in a wave function is of value when introducing concepts about bonds and regions of high electron density. The drawback in the case of pharmacologically interesting molecules is twofold: the molecules are much more complex and the plane through which the contour diagram is drawn is arbitrary.

With the aid of current computer graphics technology it is possible to produce quasi-three-dimensional representations of charge density. The molecular skeleton in a form similar to a Dreiding model is displayed with depth-cueing to give an impression of three dimensionality. Surrounding the molecule, a net (preferably in a different colour) is drawn corresponding

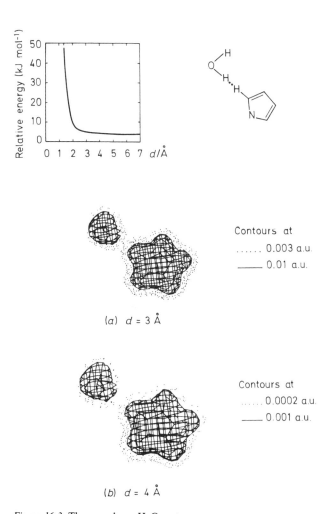

Figure 16.3. The pyrrole ... H_2O system

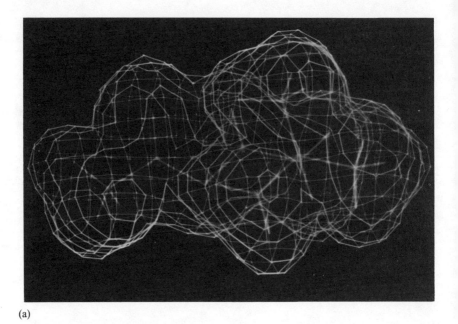

(a)

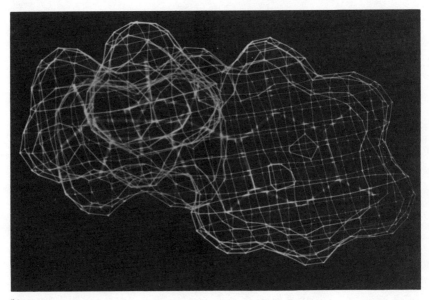

(b)
Figure 16.4. (a) Acetylcholine. (b) Nicotine

to a prescribed level of electron density. Crystallographers call the use of a net in this way a 'chicken-wire' representation of charge or shape.

The actual density for which the net is drawn is clearly arbitrary but for small molecules tests have shown that 0.002 atomic units of charge gives a definition which is in accord with the Van der Waals radii and also incorporates some 95 per cent of the total molecular charge [1 a.u. of charge density $= 67.49$ e/Å^3].

Another way of defining the most useful contour to take is to investigate the interaction of two molecules and to observe the position where they repel or appear 'hard'. *Figure 16.2* shows water interacting with propane and shows a choice of charge-density contours. The interaction between water and pyrrole is similarly shown in *Figure 16.3*.

From such studies, we have concluded that a net cast around the molecular framework at a density of 0.01 a.u. gives the most appropriate indication of molecular shape, albeit the hard shape. *Figure 16.4* compares the hard outline of acetylcholine and nicotine in this way although the coloured original, it must be stressed, is far more revealing than the black and white reproduction.

In instances where comparative studies are being made for a series of compounds it may be more useful to look at the electron density of individual orbitals rather than the total density, as illustrated by the example in *Figure 16.5*.

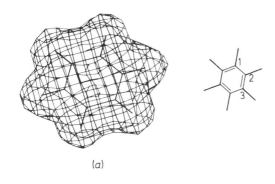

(a)

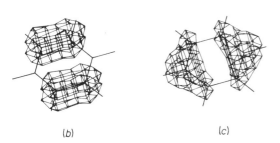

(b)   (c)

Figure 16.5. The total and orbital electron density maps of benzene. (a) Total electron density. (b) HOMO electron density. (c) NHOMO electron density (next highest molecular orbital)

Charge in spherical regions

Computer generated pictures of molecular shape in terms of a charge-density contour net can be used to compare molecules, but only in a qualitative way. If we want to be able to make a quantitative comparison we need numbers. For this reason and to provide a simple means of displaying the charge-density information, the method of calculating the electron density in a defined sphere was developed. In this technique a molecular wave function of the *ab initio* type is squared and summed over a sphere for which the radius and location are specified (the computer program is available from the Quantum Chemistry Program Exchange).

The charge Q in a sphere of radius R can be computed from the wave function as

$$Q(R) = \int_0^{2\pi} \int_0^{\pi} \int_0^R \Psi^*\Psi_r{}^2 \sin\theta \, dr \, d\theta d\phi.$$

If Ψ is a linear combination of atomic orbitals

$$Q(R) = \sum_j D_{jj} \int \chi_j^2 dv + \sum_{jk} D_{jk} \int \chi_j\chi_k dv$$

with D_{ij} being the density matrix

$$D_{ij} = \sum_k n_k c_{ik} \, c_{jk}$$

The results of such a calculation for ethane are shown in *Figure 16.6*. The numbers in the spheres, which may be placed at points centred on nuclei, in bonds or at any specified point, can then be used in a correlation.

Just as with charge-density contours, it may be more sensible to look at the charge in specific orbitals rather than the total amount in a particular

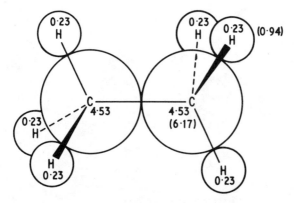

Figure 16.6. Numbers of electrons contained in spheres of covalent radius centred on the nuclei of ethane (Mulliken population analysis values in parentheses)

region. Reactivity will depend on the amount of charge available for donation or the amount which can be received, but also the strength with which the electrons are held. With this in mind it is possible to develop a form of frontier molecular orbital theory starting with a calculation of the charge within a defined sphere in a single orbital. Computationally this may be achieved by altering the occupation number n_k, which appears in the density matrix given above. If n_k is equated to zero for all orbitals but one, then the charge is given for that one molecular orbital. In particular the charge in the highest occupied and lowest unoccupied orbitals (HOMO and LUMO) are of most interest, with the next to highest occupied orbital also sometimes contributing.

As an example of a quantitative correlation we can consider aromatic substitution. The charge in the highest occupied orbital and the next highest weighted by the energy separation of the orbital does correlate with the rate of nitration of aromatic species as shown in *Figure 13.6* (p. 154).

We have also seen that a frontier rate factor defined as ($q_{HOMO}/\varepsilon_{HOMO} + q_{NHOMO}/\varepsilon_{NHOMO}$) also produces an excellent correlation with the pesticidal activity of a chlorosubstituted molecule where electrophilic substitution by an enzyme was believed to be responsible for activity. Some details of the results are given in *Table 16.1*. The activity is correctly ranked as $1 < 7 < 10 < 9 < 2 < 3 < 6 < 8 < 4 < 5$, and correlation statistics are impressive.

TABLE 16.1. Sphere charges (0.7Å) and electrophilic frontier rate factors for halosubstituted sites in some pesticides

Compound ref. no.	HOMO energy (a.u.)	NHOMO energy (a.u.)	HOMO charge (electrons)	NHOMO charge (a.u.)	F_r
1	−0.2671	−0.2733	0.1262	0.0003	0.4736
2	−0.2682	−0.2955	0.1377	0.0406	0.6508
3	−0.2540	−0.2807	0.1213	0.0525	0.6821
4	−0.2826	−0.3164	0.2006	0.0130	0.7509
5	−0.2680	−0.3086	0.2258	0.0022	0.8497
6	−0.2299	−0.2697	0.1288	0.0372	0.6982
7	−0.2626	−0.2946	0.1255	0.0108	0.5146
8	−0.2961	−0.3456	0.1838	0.0441	0.7483
9	−0.2390	−0.2974	0.1062	0.0595	0.6444
10	−0.2426	−0.2826	0.1128	0.0491	0.6387

The defects of sphere charges as input for correlations are firstly the arbitrary choice of sphere size and location, and more fundamentally the fact that although accurate in themselves, the numbers refer to the unperturbed reactant, not a transition state. The former objection may be overcome using the techniques being developed by Bader who uses catastrophe theory to define regions of electronic charge which should be associated with particular atoms.

Molecular electrostatic potentials

Charge density, either in the form of a contour diagram or simplified into spherical regions is, of course, a property of an isolated molecule. More interesting from a reactivity or pharmacological binding point of view is the effect of a molecule on its surroundings. A first step towards this is to convert the information contained in the wave function into an electrostatic molecular potential.

The electrostatic molecular potential $V(r)$ may be calculated from the molecular density distribution $\rho(r)$,

$$V(r) = \sum_{\substack{\text{all nuclei} \\ \mu}} \frac{Z_\mu}{R_\mu - r} - \int \frac{\rho(r')}{r' - r} \mathrm{d}r$$

and displayed in maps. The contours will indicate positions of equal interaction energy of the unperturbed molecule with a unit positive charge, a proton. The maps are thus the first stage towards an interaction picture. As such they have been proved to be one of the most significant tools in theoretical studies of pharmacological problems.

A number of objections and worries about the use of electrostatic potentials have been voiced, but most have been investigated and the validity of the approach is well documented. In part this again results from insensitivity to the quality of the wave function. Ideally a large basis set *ab initio* function will be calculated and the energy of interaction with the proton recomputed at every point on a grid covering the space surrounding the molecule. In practice it has been demonstrated that a simple charge distribution may be used without recomputing at each point; small basis sets or pseudo-potentials are adequate and even semi-empirical wave functions do not introduce serious errors. The strategy followed is generally the typical one in all such work. The best function obtainable at reasonable cost is employed. When dealing with general questions about a series of otherwise similar molecules errors tend to cancel and trends emerge. Only when small differences between reactive sites are in question are the results sensitive to such niceties as the basis set.

More fundamental doubts about the approach include the influence of surrounding molecules or ions on the calculated field and interactions other than electrostatic. These are valid causes for caution but once again the utility of the use of potentials has been in comparing species which act in otherwise similar surroundings. Caution is wise and appeal to experiment for justification reassuring when possible. The best support on the other hand comes from actual pharmacological studies using the potentials.

Much of the more notable work has been performed by Weinstein and his colleagues and in particular the detailed series of papers on the LSD/serotonin receptor stand out as models of care, and what is more, lead to a major level of understanding of the action at the receptor and the different properties of agonists.

The series studied by Weinstein and his collaborators include a number of 5-hydroxytryptamine congeners; tryptamine and hydroxylated molecules with the hydroxyl in several positions, which incorporate the high affinity

5-hydroxy, low affinity 6-hydroxy and intermediate 4- and 7-hydroxy-
tryptamines. The group of molecules also bear a strong structural resemblance to LSD (*see* page 80).

The first and most obvious use of the electrostatic potential maps is to
provide a pattern for the natural agonist which must be matched by other
agonists if they are to behave similarly towards the receptor. This reproduction of a similar electron pattern for the recognition process has been termed
'the interaction pharmacophore' but in essence merely states that in order
to act in a similar way molecules must look the same *at the electronic level.*

The electrostatic molecular potentials were computed for the free base
forms of the molecules rather than for the ionic form which abounds in
solution on the grounds that the cationic group is presumably neutralized
by binding to an anion group in the receptor as the first step in binding.
Supporting calculations show that interaction of the cations with free OH^-
do indeed lead to a potential pattern appropriate to free bases for the indole
portion of the molecules. It is believed that it is the neutralized form of
serotonin and other indoles which acts as electron donor in complexation
with electron acceptors.

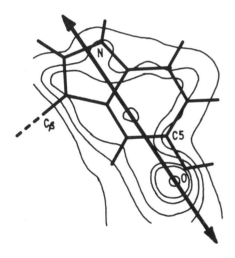

Figure 16.7. Molecular electrostatic potential
map for serotonin in a plane above the indole ring
with an indication of the direction of the
orientation vector

Figure 16.7 shows a molecular electrostatic potential map for serotonin
together with a vector connecting the minima through the areas of steepest
change in potential. These vectors are thought to serve as orientation vectors
which indicate the preferred alignment of a molecule towards a field
generated by positive charges placed above it. Similar maps for other members
of the series differ in the direction of the orientation vector, that for 6-
hydroxytryptamine being almost perpendicular to the one for 5-hydroxy-
tryptamine. The difference may be postulated as one reason for the differing

affinities. Further it is possible to set up an hypothesis concerning recognition at the serotonin receptor sites:

(1) The positively charged alkylamine side chain interacts with an anionic group, preparing the indole position of the molecule to form a stacking complex.
(2) The electrostatic molecular potential orientates the indole ring system.

Weinstein has further suggested that the other hydroxytryptamines anchor themselves in a similar manner but have to adjust their conformation to orientate the electrostatic vector. The measured difference between the affinity of 5-hydroxytryptamine and any other member of the series for the LSD–serotonin receptor results from the discrepancy between the orientations vectors.

Support for this hypothesized mechanism comes from model calculations on stacking complexes of serotonin and similar molecules with the imidazolium cation which apes the receptor. These calculations, performed for a variety of alignments and interplanar distances indicate that complex formation is dominated by electrostatic interactions.

The pattern of the serotonin electrostatic potential map is reproduced by LSD as is the direction of the orientation vector (*Figure 16.8*). The two molecules then should be recognized by the same receptor and indeed they are.

Superficially it might have been expected that LSD would be closer to the unsubstituted molecule tryptamine but in fact the C12–C13 double bond of LSD produces the effects of the OH in serotonin. This contention is supported by further work by Weinstein *et al.* on the compound hexanoic

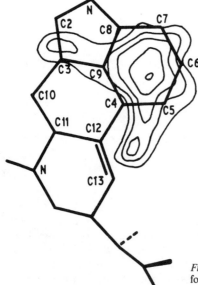

Figure 16.8. Molecular electrostatic potential for D–LSD in a plane above the indole rings

acid 4-aza-4,5-dimethyl-6-(3-indoyl)-N,N diethylamide (SKF 10856) which resembles LSD but lacks the double bond (*Figure 16.9*). The electronic properties now resemble unsubstituted tryptamine. The experimental findings support the hypothesis. SKF 10856 is not recognized like LSD on the LSD–serotonin binding sites, rather it resembles tryptamine. On the other hand it does antagonize histamine H2 sites in the central nervous system like LSD with which it shares structural similarities enabling it to block H2 agonists such as dimaprit (*see* page 63).

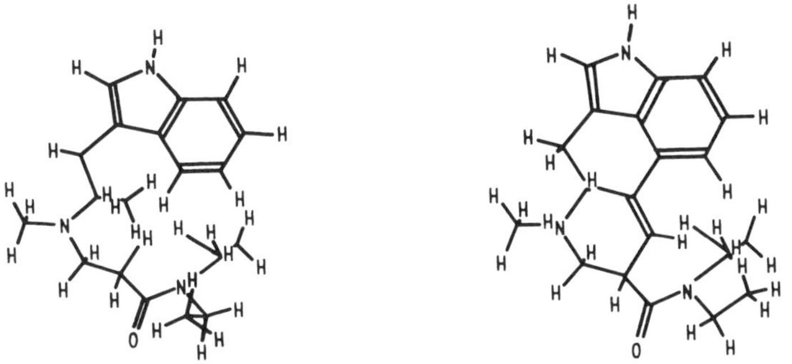

Figure 16.9. Molecular structure of SKF 10856 and D–LSD

Molecular electrostatic potentials of known receptors

Rather than calculate the electrostatic potential of the small molecule involved in the receptor binding process, it would be preferable to produce the potential for the receptor. Of course in general not enough is known about receptors at the present time for this to be feasible. However in a series of papers of almost heroic proportions the Pullmans and their collaborators have looked at the electrostatic molecular potentials of various DNA and RNA molecules. The work, which can be illustrated by giving just one single example, does offer the hope that when molecular details of receptor sites become known the electrostatic molecular potentials can be computed even if they involve hundreds of atoms and that these will lead to a better understanding of interaction and binding.

As an example of this work we may consider the calculation of the electro-static molecular potential of yeast tRNA. The potential was calculated at sites bridging the anionic oxygens of each of the 76 phosphates in the molecule using the known crystal structure. The influence of all 76 phosphates and the sugar and bases were incorporated. This amounts to 228 molecular subunits or some 2500 atoms. This large set of components is treated as a set of subunits for which point charges are computed from *ab initio* wave functions. Using a multipolar expansion the charges yield individual electro-static potentials which are then superimposed to provide the total potential of the macromolecule. With such an approximation the potential is probably realistic at points more than 2 Å from the constituent atoms but not closer to nuclei.

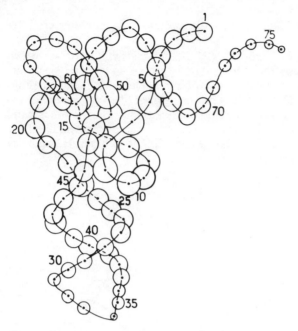

Figure 16.10. Schematic representation of the potentials at the phosphate bridge sites. The radii of the spheres about each phosphate are proportional to the corresponding bridge site potentials [reproduced with permission from R. Lavery, A. Pullman and B. Pullman, *Theoret. chim. Acta. (Berl.)*, **57**, 233–243 (1980)]

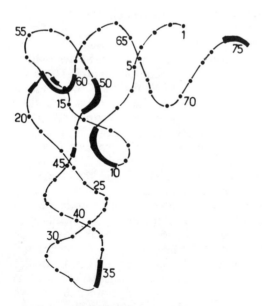

Figure 16.11. Representation of the phosphate groups having anionic oxygens with low accessible areas (————) [reproduced with permission from R. Lavery, A. Pullman and B. Pullman, *Theoret. chim. Acta. (Berl.)*, **57**, 233–243 (1980)]

For comparative purposes the position where a sodium ion might be expected to bind was considered for each phosphate group: potentials vary due to the folding of the molecule. *Figure 16.10* gives a schematic illustration of the potentials at the phosphate bridge sites.

When considering reactivity at these sites access is as important as a favourable potential. An attempt to quantify this was made by using a variant of the scheme frequently used to calculate accessibility of solvent. A van der Waals envelope for the macromolecule is calculated by placing spheres of appropriate radius at each atomic centre. Accessibility of a sodium ion to each of the anionic oxygens of the phosphates was then calculated by bringing the cationic sphere into van der Waals contact with the oxygen sphere and then moving the cation over the surface of the latter sphere, noting whether it intersected with any of the atomic spheres. By studying a large number of configurations for each anionic oxygen and taking the ratio of accessible conformations and total conformations a quantitative measure of relative accessibility emerges. *Figure 16.11* gives the gist of such calculations. This type of procedure could be extended to cover more complex substrates. The actual reactivity of a site will depend on both the potential at the site and the ease of access in possibly quite a complex manner.

From the point of view of quantum pharmacology the message from this work is that it ought to be possible to do something similar with a receptor site or enzyme-binding site with a variety of agonists, antagonists or substrates. The sheer size of the problem is not the limiting feature. Yet again in such a situation computer graphics would make the results of any such work both more intelligible and accessible to the medicinal chemist.

Displaying potential fields

The system of a net appropriate to a given contour described earlier for change-density pictures may also be applied with advantage to electrostatic molecular potentials. This is particularly true if the results are to be handled by a working medicinal chemist rather than a full-time computational expert. Inevitably also, colour is a great asset, permitting positive and negative regions of potential to be distinguished with ease. *Figure 16.12* shows a two-dimensional slice through the potential for ammonia.

Currently work is in progress to display electrostatic potentials in coded colour on a surface of molecules and enzyme binding sites.

Summary

Since molecules interact by virtue of their electronic clouds the wave function from a quantum mechanical calculation can be helpful in understanding the details of binding.

Electron density plots can highlight similarities in molecular shape which are not apparent from models. Charge located in precise regions of space can yield quantitative criteria to be used in a statistical study.

Electrostatic potential maps give a first approximation to the field experienced by a receptor due to an approaching molecule. The maps point out similarities in molecules and distinguish different orientations in

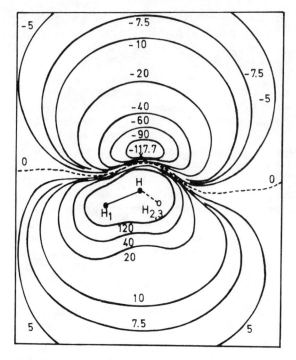

Figure 16.12. A slice through the electrostatic potential of ammonia

approach. Recent work suggests that there is no limit to the size of molecular system which can be considered in this way if we superimpose the potentials of constituent subunits.

Further reading

BADER, R. F. W. *J. chem. Phys.*, **73**, 2871 (1980)
  Molecular change distributions.
ELLIOTT, R. J., SACKWILD, V. and RICHARDS, W. G. *J. molec. Struct.*, **86**, 301 (1982)
  Use of charge in a sphere to indicate reactivity.
LAVERY, R., PULLMAN, A. and PULLMAN, B. *Theoret. chim. Acta*, **57**, 233 (1980)
  Electrostatic potential of RNA.
WEINSTEIN, H., OSMAN, R., GREEN, J. P. and TOPIOL, S. in P. Politzer and D. G.
  Truhlar (eds), *Chemical Applications of Atomic and Molecular Electrostatic Potentials*, Plenum
  . Press, New York (1981)

Chapter 17

Solvation

Logically it may seem that the way to take into account the effect of a solvent on a solute would be to start with a calculation on the isolated solute molecule and then to graft on the effects of the solvent. Such an approach is followed by the work discussed in this chapter. The two extreme methods consider the solvent as molecular in one case and as a continuum in the other. Both have scored notable successes in dealing with apparent anomalies in the deductions which might be drawn from isolated molecule calculations concerned with conformation. It is also only reasonable to point out that in the case of water as solvent, which is often assumed for pharmacological species, we are dealing with an exceptionally difficult problem. The structure and properties of water itself pose many serious questions and only very approximate methods can be used in theories of solvation.

As mentioned in the introduction, even a perfect understanding of the role of water as solvent would not suffice to explain the properties of drugs in active environments which will certainly bear little resemblance to pure water. The unknown biological environment can only be taken into account in theoretical studies by examining series of compounds which are likely to respond identically to that environment.

Nonetheless, so many physical experiments of relevance to pharmacology are performed in water that it is essential that there should be a good understanding of its role, particularly perhaps in modifying conformational preference.

The supermolecule approach

In essence the supermolecule approach is very simple. It concentrates on water molecules which are likely to be tightly bound by hydrogen bonds to the solute and then includes these extra atoms in the calculation of conformational energy maps of a larger, but still isolated, species.

The most favourable hydration sites and hydration geometries have been determined by *ab initio* or reliable semi-empirical calculations on model compounds. A calculation of the charge distribution of an isolated molecule, together with a little experience of chemistry, can indicate the atomic positions where hydration is most likely. The precise manner in which the water molecule attaches itself can then be determined by varying the position of the water molecule and looking for the most favourable situation from energy considerations. Alternatively, the charge distribution of solute and isolated water found from calculations can be used to estimate the dominant electrostatic contribution to the hydrogen bond energy using a multipole expansion for the charges. The results of such calculations have been reviewed

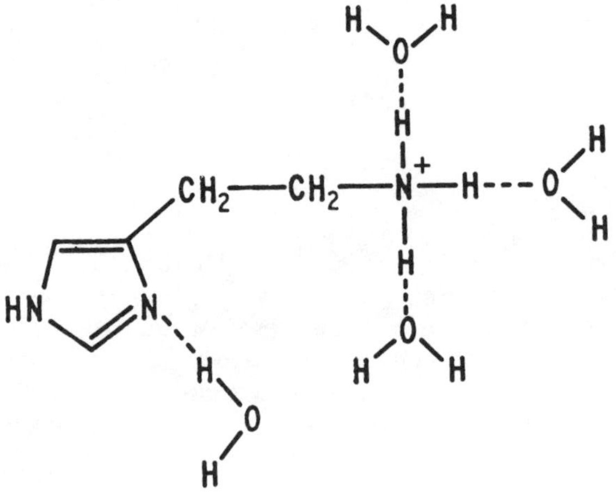

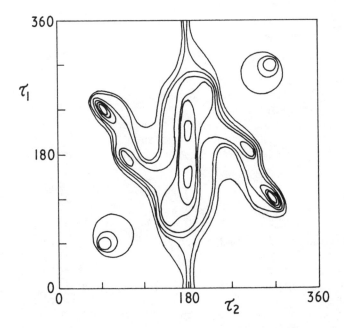

Figure 17.1. Hydration sites of histamine monocation

Figure 17.2. Conformational potential energy surface for the hydrated histamine molecule computed in the PCILO approximation

by the Pullmans, and seem eminently sensible although the actual estimates of hydrogen bond energies are generally far too high.

With the water molecules included, a new conformational map may be compiled. The case of histamine is illustrated in *Figures 17.1* and *17.2*; the former indicates the hydration sites. *Figure 17.2* shows the conformational energy map of the supermolecule which should be compared with the PCILO map for the isolated molecule given in *Figure 15.7*. Whereas the isolated molecule is shown as preferring a *gauche* conformation with the side chain positively charged nitrogen atom bound by a hydrogen bond to the unprotonated nitrogen in the ring, such intramolecular effects are precluded in the solvated supermolecule and the *trans* conformation found by n.m.r. in solution is favoured. The conformer population ratio is quantitatively correct as well as qualitatively.

When H_2O molecules are included in the supermolecule the conformational preference of acetylcholine has been shown to be the *gauche syn*-clinal form as is found by n.m.r. in solution and similar satisfactory results have been obtained for a number of indolealkylamines, phenethylamines and phenethanolamines. In most cases the solvent is predicted to increase the probability of *trans* forms over what would be expected in isolation.

Perhaps particularly interesting is the case of GABA (γ amino butyric acid). *Figure 17.3* shows PCILO conformational maps for isolated and solvated zwitterionic forms. The second figure predicts the coexistence of several conformers in solution and n.m.r. studies suggest that at least five conformational species are present in water.

The successes of this simple approach ought not to overwhelm us and it is important to realize that it represents only a first step which must contain a portion of the important contributions from the solvent. Since a major factor in increasing the indicated amount of *trans* form in monocations is merely bulk which precludes the side chain folding back to bind to the nitrogen-containing ring, it is possible that we are disguising the real effects. Any bulky substituent or even bound inert gas atoms would have the same effect. If we have merely constrained the calculations to give the right answer by making the conformations such as *gauche* very unstable by putting atoms in the way, we may not have a real physical effect. In the case of monocations we need to remember that in solution there probably exists a negatively charged ion in the vicinity of the cationic head to preserve local neutrality. Attempts to include a chloride or fluoride ion in the calculated supermolecule suggest that this too could alter conformational preference, but there is no obviously valid means of deciding upon its location.

The supermolecule approach is probably most useful when there exists very specific tight binding of water molecules. However, energetically good solvation sites may be of minor importance in thermodynamic properties because of their low statistical weight; an argument parallel to the difference between conformational energy and conformational free energy discussed in Chapter 13.

Extended Hückel calculations frequently give good indications of solution conformation preference, even when no water is included, for quite the wrong physical reasons; possibly the exaggerated charge distribution makes intramolecular hydrogen bonding insufficient to overcome the repulsion between electronegative atoms. The success of the supermolecule technique is on better

(a)

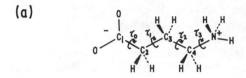

(b)

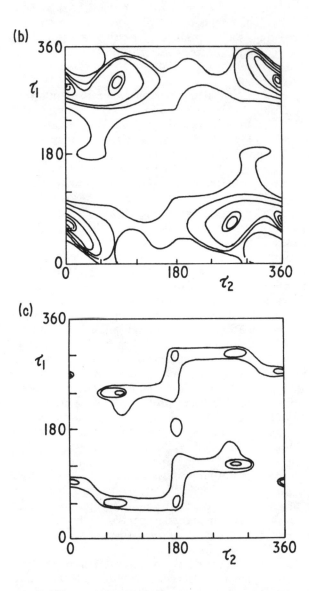

Figure 17.3. (a) GABA zwitterionic structure. (b) Isolated species conformational potential energy surface. (c) Solvated supermolecule conformational potential energy surface

grounds than this; water is included but it is by no means clear that the results are truly based on the physics of the situation.

The continuum model

The use of a continuum model to account for the influence of solvents on the conformational preferences of pharmacologically active compounds was pioneered by Beveridge. It is based on the classical electrostatic treatments of interacting systems by Born, Onsager and Kirkwood.

The total energy of a molecule or ion with a defined geometry and conformation can be written approximately as

$$E_{total} = E_{solute} + E_{solvation}$$

with E_{solute} being the energy found in an isolated molecule computation.

The solvation energy, $E_{solvation}$, is made up of three contributions,

$$E_{solvation} = E_{es} + E_{dis} + E_{cav}$$

E_{es} is the electrostatic solvent–solute binding energy arising from the interaction of permanent and induced electric moments; E_{dis} is the interaction energy resulting from dispersion forces; both are negative. E_{cav}, which is positive in sign, is the energy required to form a cavity in the solvent to accommodate the solute molecule. Each of these terms may depend parametrically on quantities which vary as functions of molecular conformation or geometry.

For the calculation of E_{es} the solute is treated as a point dipolar ion of charge Q and total dipole moment m at the centre of a sphere of effective radius α imbedded in the solvent. The solvent is represented as a polarizable dielectric continuum of dielectric constant ε. The solute induces a reaction field E_R in the solvent which then acts back on the solute system. If differences in the monopolar term as a function of conformational change are ignored, the following expression for E_{es} is given

$$E_{es} = -\frac{1}{2}m.\ E_R$$

with

$$E_R = \frac{2(\varepsilon - 1)\ m}{(2\varepsilon + 1)\alpha^3}.$$

Both m and α depend on conformation; m can be computed from the wave function and α is the molecular cavity radius defined by equating the molecular volume with the volume of a sphere,

$$\alpha = (3V/4\pi)^{1/3}.$$

The molecular volume is estimated from the cartesian coordinates of the atoms used in the isolated molecule calculation.

E_{dis} is estimated using the expression

$$E_{dis} = \frac{\rho}{2} \int_0^\infty v^{eff}(r)g^{(2)}(r)4\pi r^2\ dr$$

where ρ is the number density of the solvent, v^{eff} is the effective pairwise potential function for solute–solvent interaction and $g^{(2)}(r)$ is a radial distribution function. For simplicity $g^{(2)}(r)$ is taken as zero for $r < \alpha$ and unity for $r > \alpha$. The function v^{eff} may be a modified Kihara potential.

E_{cav} is estimated from the cavity area, A, and the solvent surface tension γ as

$$E_{\text{cav}} = f \cdot 4\pi\alpha^2\gamma$$

where f is a factor which relates macroscopic to microscopic dimensions.

Both E_{dis} and E_{cav} vary parametrically with conformation through the cavity size α.

The most striking feature of this summary of the continuum model is the fact that every attempt is made to treat the physics of the problem in an honest way, but that because of the complexities of the solvent species, so many very crude approximations have to be made. The parameters entering the calculations are based on physico-chemical properties of the solvent and are not designed to produce agreement with experiment.

Figure 17.4 shows INDO calculations on acetylcholine with water as solvent. The solvated acetylcholine molecule is indicated as having a *gauche* (*syn*-clinal, *anti*-periplanar) conformation as is found from the spin coupling analysis of n.m.r. spectra in D_2O. The major contributing factor is the electrostatic term.

The chief defects of the simple continuum scheme are the lack of explicit consideration of solute–solvent hydrogen bonding effects which are clearly important as indicated by supermolecule calculations and the lack of water–water interactions.

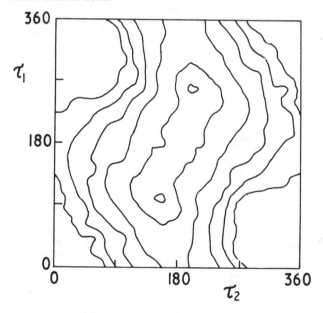

Figure 17.4. Conformational potential energy surface for acetylcholine in water, treated as a continuum using the INDO approximation

An obvious extension is to try to amalgamate the features of the two approaches. This again has been done by Beveridge.

The combined approach

Statistical thermodynamics provides both the basis for a combined approach and highlights the essential differences between the two extremes of simple first approximation just discussed.

From the point of view of statistical thermodynamics we can treat a dilute solution as an ensemble of systems consisting of a solute molecule surrounded by a large number of solvent molecules. All the thermodynamic properties will depend on a partition function, Z, the number which indicates the distribution of molecules over allowed energy states

$$Z = \int \exp(-E(Q)/kT)dQ$$

where Q represents the internal and external coordinates of all the molecules in the system, both solute and solvent.

The reduced partition function for the solvent molecule may be written as

$$Z(\tau_1) = \int \exp(-E(Q)/kT)dQ'$$

with Q' the same as Q except that it no longer includes the dihedral angles (τ_1) of the solute.

The continuum and supermolecule models can be regarded as alternative approximations for the calculation of $E(Q)$. The former approximation is based on

$$E(Q) \doteqdot E^{\text{eff}}(\tau_1) + E_{\text{solvent}}$$

with $E^{\text{eff}}(\tau_1)$ as an effective energy including all solute–solvent interactions by treating the solvent as a polarizable continuum.

The supermolecule makes the alternative approximation

$$E(Q) \doteqdot E(\tau_1, q_2, q_3 \ldots) + E_{\text{solvent}}$$

where τ_1 is the coordinate describing the conformation of the solute and q_2, q_3 etc. are the coordinates of the water molecules incorporated in the supermolecule.

The union of the two models could be achieved if the energy was approximated by

$$E(Q) \doteqdot E^{\text{eff}}(\tau_1, q_2, q_3 \ldots) + E_{\text{solvent}}$$

In qualitative terms this would mean using the supermolecule approach by including as part of the solute these water molecules which are tightly bound, but at the same time recognizing that the bulk water will have a major influence and incorporating in some manner factors which are revealed by the dielectric and surface tension of the liquid.

Simulation methods

The two approaches to solvation discussed above are self-evidently crude and designed to go some way towards treating the solvation problem in complicated real molecular problems. Simulation methods on the other hand attack the problem of solvation as a physicist would, taking model systems and avoiding crude approximations wherever possible. The techniques of computer simulation do not offer a realistic hope of being able to incorporate solvation into calculations in a routine fashion. Rather, the aim of such work is to understand principles which can then be applied qualitatively or semi-quantitatively.

Computer simulation includes both the methods described as 'molecular dynamics' and 'Monte Carlo' techniques. Both approaches have the advantage of including in consideration not only the solute but possibly several hundred water molecules so that the all-important water–water interactions are not ignored. Molecular dynamics considers a solute surrounded by water molecules and starts by computing the forces on the particles followed by their subsequent motion according to Newton's classical mechanics. A Monte Carlo calculation similarly considers a solute molecule in a box containing solvent molecules. Periodic boundary conditions ensure that if a molecule leaves the box through one wall it reappears through the opposite one, thus keeping the density a constant. The energy of the whole system of interacting particles is computed using appropriate intermolecular potentials and possibly intramolecular potentials as well. One particle is moved randomly and the energy recomputed. If the new energy is lower, this new position is accepted. On the other hand if the new energy indicates less stability, the result is multiplied by a random number between zero and unity and accepted or rejected on the basis of a predetermined threshold. In this manner (the Metropolis algorithm) the sampling of all positions of particles, weighted towards the more likely arrangements leads to computed partition functions.

Both molecular dynamics and Monte Carlo methods depend on the availability of inter- and intramolecular potentials in an energetic form suitable for rapid computation. Typically potentials are utilized in the form of Lennard-Jones ($Ar^{-6} + Br^{-12}$) potentials. This form is known to be less than perfect even for rare gas interactions and non-pairwise effects are ignored. Potentials become even more complex when they need also to reflect the orientational effects of real non-spherical molecules.

A variety of potentials are available for water–water interactions and some solute–water instances. For simulations of liquid water those of Stillinger and Rahman and of Matsuoka, Clementi and Yoshimine are often favoured. Pure water simulations have been very successful in describing some thermodynamic and structural properties, but less so for phenomena involving polarization.

Although potentials are available for some small ion–water interactions, and for formaldehyde and methane with water there are no published potentials for interactions of complicated solutes and water. Potentials can be found from *ab initio* molecular orbital calculations on important configurations of the solute–water dimer. The resulting energies are then fitted to suitable functional forms by least-squares. However the number of degrees of freedom becomes very large for molecules of the size of a neuro-transmitter, especially if conformational flexibility is incorporated.

The techniques have progressed to the point where a conformationally flexible dipeptide model has been studied, but there seems little prospect of simulations being routinely used to graft solvent influence on to free molecule molecular orbital calculations.

The question as to which of the alternative approaches, molecular dynamics or Monte Carlo calculations, is to be preferred is not fully resolved. There are proponents of both. Molecular dynamics calculations have the advantage that transport phenomena can be analysed. On the other hand, for large solutes there are few experimental data with which to compare this analysis. Monte Carlo computations have the advantage that the choice of thermo-dynamic ensemble is not a problem. Recently the distinctions between the alternatives have become somewhat blurred with both forces and statistical random walks being incorporated into both methods.

For either method a major stumbling block remains the lack of suitable intermolecular potentials. Even though these may be obtained in principle by fitting the results of *ab initio* molecular orbital calculations, such pre-parative work is both dull and very expensive in terms of computer time.

As in so many aspects of contemporary work a major influence and aid is, yet again, computer graphics. It is possible to observe the behaviour of water molecules surrounding a solute as the simulation progresses. Even the qualitative picture from computer graphics makes it abundantly plain that the solute influences the water structure for a considerable distance from the molecule. This emphasizes why it is so difficult to do anything accurately about solvation if one restricts consideration to tightly bound water, or treats water as a continuum, or indeed indulges in simulation which does not allow a very large solute–solute repeat distance containing very many water molecules.

Status and future of solvent effect calculations

Although both the supermolecule and dielectric continuum approaches do have some record of success in confirming the changes in conformation on going from an isolated or crystal phase into solution, neither can be accepted as satisfactory. The obvious improvements which are necessary seem exceed-ingly complicated to apply to situations as complex as those of relevance to pharmacology.

At the level of physical chemistry and simple model systems the picture is much brighter. The dynamical Monte Carlo calculations on pure water and other liquids represent a real advance in the understanding of the liquid state. The way is open for a similar enlightenment of solutions but the enthalpy and entropy effects involved in the solution of rare gases, metal ions, small hydrocarbons and inflexible organic solutes must be studied in detail before it is profitable to consider the additional complexities introduced by conformational freedom.

In the opinion of the present author such a situation lends strength to the notion of treating solvation effects semi-empirically. In order to have some data on which to base such a parameterization scheme the following information should be sought: small flexible molecules should have their conformational preferences studied in both the gas and solution phases. For gaseous systems a small amount of data may come from microwave spectroscopy or electron diffraction, but accurate Hartree–Fock calculations should provide essential detail for the gas phase conformational energy diagrams. In solution, high-resolution n.m.r. studies can give accurate population ratios. By comparing the conformer population ratios for the two environments it ought to be possible to devise an empirical scheme whereby isolated molecule calculations can be modified to incorporate solvation effects.

Summary

Although biologically active molecules do not bind to receptors in a simple aqueous medium the effects of water on conformation are of major importance in understanding the results of physical measurements made on solutions.

Specific solvent interactions may be incorporated into isolated molecule calculations by placing water molecules at the most likely hydration sites. In particular, water molecules on terminal charged nitrogens in side chains will not favour *gauche* conformations and lead to agreement with solution n.m.r. studies.

The water may also be treated as a dielectric continuum and its effects considered as a sum of solute–solvent interactions resulting from polarization and cavity formation.

The two approaches can be combined and in principle a rigorous molecular dynamics or Monte Carlo calculation could be used to study the effects of water if all the relevant solute–solvent potential functions were known for all possible solute conformations.

At present the complexities of water structure leave the problem of the influence of water on conformation incompletely solved.

Further reading

BEVERIDGE, D. L., KELLEY, M. M. and RADNA, R. J. *J. Am. chem. Soc.*, **96**, 3769 (1974)
A full account of the continuum method.
BEVERIDGE, D. L. and SCHNUELLE, G. W. *J. phys. Chem.*, **78**, 2064 (1974)
Supermolecule–continuum model.
EISENBERG, D. and KAUZMANN, W. *Structure and Properties of Water*, Oxford, London (1969)
A readable account of water structure.
FRANKS, F. (ed) *Water—A Comprehensive Treatise*, Vols 1–6, Plenum, London (1972–4)
Especially see article by Franks in Vol. 4 and by Wood in Vol. 6
HAGLER, A. T., OSGUTHORPE, D. J. and ROBSON, B. *Science, N.Y.*, **208**, 599 (1980)
Study of a dipeptide.
HAMMERSLEY, J. M. and HANDSCOMB, D. C. *Monte Carlo Methods*, Methuen, London (1964)
Introduction to Monte Carlo methods.
HARRISON, S. W., SWAMINATHAN, S. and BEVERIDGE, D. L. *Int. Journal Quantum Chemistry*, **14**, 319 (1978)
Methane-water.
KRISTENMACHER, H., POPKIE, H. and CLEMENTI, E. *J. Chem. Phys.*, **59**, 5842 (1973)
Ion–water pair potentials.

MATSUOKA, O., CLEMENTI, E. and YOSHIMINE, M. *J. Chem. Phys.*, **64**, 1351 (1976)

OMIKI, J. C. and SCHERAGA, H. A. *J. Am. Chem. Soc.*, **99**, 7413 (1977)

PULLMAN, A. and PULLMAN, B. *Quart. Rev. Biophys.*, **7**, 505 (1975)
A review of applications of the supermolecule approach.

PULLMAN, B. (ed) 'Environmental effects on molecular structure and properties', *Proc. the 8th Jerusalem Symposium on Quantum Chemistry and Biochemistry*, D. Reidel, Dordrecht (1976)

ROSSKY, P. J. and KARPLUS, M. *J. Am. Chem. Soc.*, **101**, 1913 (1979)
Study of a dipeptide.

STILLINGER, F. H. and RAHMAN, A. *J. Chem. Phys.*, **60** (4), 1545 (1974)
Improved simulation of liquid water by molecular dynamics.

SWAMINATHAN, S., WHITEHEAD, R. J., GUTH, E. and BEVERIDGE, D. L. *J. Am. Chem. Soc.*, **99**, 7817 (1977)
Formaldehyde-water.

WEINSTEIN, H. and GREEN J. P. (eds) 'Quantum chemistry in biomolecular sciences', *Annals of the New York Academy of Sciences*, **367** (1981)
Pages 83–181 cover applications of Monte Carlo and molecular dynamics methods to solvation.

Chapter 18

Entropy effects

Far and away the most important entropy effect in the binding of pharmacologically active molecules to receptors involves the solvent. This has been discussed in the last chapter, but the importance bears repetition. Small molecules influence water structure for a considerable distance away from the solute molecule. Although in principle this may be studied by Monte Carlo or molecular dynamics methods, frequently the repeat distance allowed between solute molecules in published work has been insufficient to permit an accurate assessment to be made of solvation effects. Entropy differences due to solvent when a receptor site has bound water replaced by a previously solvated ligand are unknown quantities. They are, however, likely to be significant.

In addition there are other entropic contributions which may be of great importance.

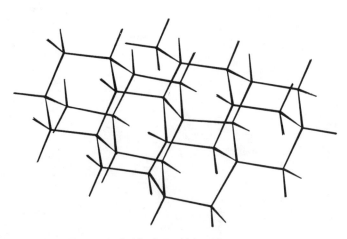

Figure 18.1. The tetrahedral lattice model

Flexible ligands

As a real and crucial example we may consider small peptides as examples of flexible binding partners. There is evidence that hormonal peptides of less than about thirty residues are very flexible in solution. Probably only a subset of the very large number of possible conformations is significantly populated, but there is no evidence for a single dominant shape. When bound to its specific receptor on the other hand, at least a section of the chain must adopt a unique conformation and the configurational entropy of the flexible molecule must contribute to the overall free energy of binding to the receptor.

It is possible that part of the chain binds while the rest forms a loop or a loose end. Larger peptides such as β-endorphin are believed to bind to their receptors in such a way as to form loops. The probability of loop formation will clearly depend on the shape of the binding site and particularly on the distances between individual binding subsites.

The tendency of the ligand to adopt a particular shape will effect kinetic behaviour in terms of whether the binding occurs by a multistep process or by an 'all-or-none' mechanism as discussed by Burgen and his colleagues. If the ligand binds sequentially there will be a much greater loss of entropy at the initial contact than in each of the subsequent attachments leading to cooperativity.

Thus, quite generally, the thermodynamics of binding for a long and flexible ligand may be influenced by factors such as the relative geometry of binding subsites or strong binding positions in the ligand, even if all other things are equal. Some of these influences can be revealed in model studies using the techniques of statistical thermodynamics.

Model calculations

A model suggested by Burgen and Roberts has been set up and exploited by Humphries to answer some of the thermodynamic questions about the binding of flexible ligands to receptors. In the absence of any real knowledge about intermolecular pair potentials appropriate to ligand–protein inter-

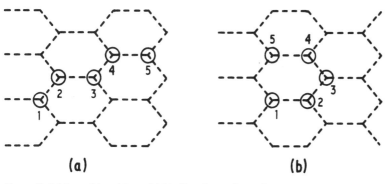

Figure 18.2. Linear (a) and bent (b) binding site configuration

actions a highly stylized model was taken. It consists of a Monte Carlo computer program aimed at studying flexible alkyl chains on a biological surface in a tetrahedral model (*Figure 18.1*).

The extended diamond lattice is the space above the binding surface which is the base of the lattice. On this base, specific points can be defined as binding sites. In its most general form, each lattice site on or above the plane is occupied either by a chain segment or a solvent molecule. Successive configurations of the chain are generated by random configuration changes in the conventional Monte Carlo fashion and normal boundary conditions are applied.

The model is capable of being made increasingly realistic in a step-wise manner. The simplest situation will ignore solvent and have no specificity between sites along the chain and the binding positions in the receptor. Next a variety of specificities can be incorporated as can competition with solvent molecules and perhaps restricted rotation within the ligand.

Even the simplest starting model can indicate some effects which may be biologically significant. Humphries first addressed the question as to whether, all other things being equal, it is beneficial to have the receptor binding subsites arranged in a linear or bent configuration. Specifically he chose a binding site with five subsites either linear or bent (*Figure 18.2*). These receptors were taken with flexible ligands with from three to twelve subunits.

The results may be presented in a variety of ways. *Figure 18.3* shows the average energy per bound configuration as a function of chain length for the two types of binding site. The ordinate is a measure of how tightly the chain is bound to the receptor, related to non-specific binding as measured perhaps by radio-chemical dialysis methods. The results in the figure indicate that the bent binding site is a more efficient receptor at all chain lengths up to twelve segments.

The explanation of this is the greater chance of multiple site occupancy

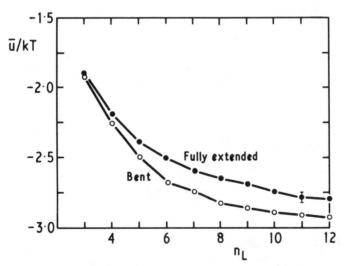

Figure 18.3. The average energy per bound configuration ($\bar{u}/kT$) as a function of chain length for bent and linear binding sites

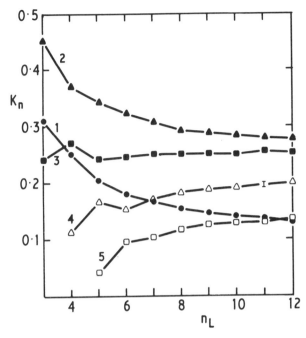

Figure 18.4. The relative 'time' spent in bound configuration with n subsites simultaneously occupied (K_n) as a function of chain length for a bent binding site

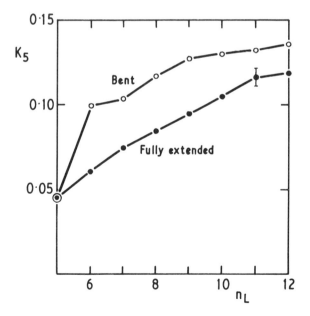

Figure 18.5. Comparison of the relative time spent with all binding subsites occupied (K_5) as a function of chain length for the two receptor configurations

for bent receptor configurations. Entropy of looping plays a more important role for bent receptors.

An alternative way of looking at the results from the simulation is to sample the relative times spent in states with the number sites $(1 \leqslant n \leqslant 5)$ simultaneously occupied. *Figure 18.4* shows these relative times for a bent receptor in the form of equilibrium binding constants as a function of chain length.

The figure demonstrates just how for a relatively simple and pure system the binding constants are a very complex function of energy, entropy and excluded volume.

Biochemically perhaps the most interesting constant in *Figure 18.4* is K_5 which corresponds to having all five receptor subsites occupied, possibly the requirement for triggering the subsequent biochemical event. *Figure 18.5* compares the alternative receptor shapes in the light of this measure. As chain length increases we see a rapid increase in K_5 for the bent receptor due to the possibility of entropy of looping.

A similar set of calculations explored the question of whether having one particularly strongly binding specific subsite (perhaps an ionic group) is more effective with this placed at the end or the middle of the ligand chain. Middle specificity was shown to be preferable with chains of up to about eight subunits. On the other hand with two strong binding specific interactions these are more helpful if at opposite ends of the chain.

Other questions

The model system studied has not yet been pushed to anything close to reality. It should be possible to extend the work just described to include solvent and ligand-bond rotational energy barriers without any serious complications. The potentials describing ligand–site interactions need also to be made more realistic with, in particular, repulsive forces being introduced as well as increasingly specific interactions. The reasonable limit for the model would be a receptor with sites $A, B, C, D \ldots$ and a ligand $a\ b\ c\ d \ldots$, with specific potentials for all ligand–receptor site–site interactions, $M–n$, as well as solvent interactions and rotational barriers.

A difficulty in this type of work is the sheer volume of data accumulated by computer simulations so that in this area an unsolved problem is just how to display results in a form which can be comprehended and lead to a more general understanding.

Summary

As well as solvent entropy effects there are contributions from conformational entropy for chain-like ligands such as peptides. These may be studied in model systems which even at an early stage reveal that entropy effects may confer an advantage on one shape of a binding site as opposed to another even if from enthalpy considerations they are identical. These statistical mechanical effects are normally ignored in quantum mechanical calculations. As with solvation studies, quantum mechanics can provide potentials to be used in statistical thermodynamical studies.

Further reading

BURGEN, A. S. V., ROBERTS, G. C. K. and FEENY, J. *Nature, Lond.*, **253**, 753 (1975)
HUMPHRIES, R. L. *J. theoret. Biol.*, **91**, 477 (1981)

Chapter 19

Activity correlations

Despite all the scientific effort expended in the pharmaceutical industry and academic laboratories, the finding of new useful drugs remains essentially an inspired hit-and-miss procedure. Typically only one in 15 000 compounds tested ever emerges as a commercial drug and it has been estimated that the investment required to develop a useful therapeutic agent to the point of US regulatory approval may be of the order of $50 million. Thus it is a small wonder that any rationalization of activity which will reduce the number of compounds to be tested is attractive, not only from the scientific point of view but also commercially.

Tremendous efforts have been made to produce useful quantitative structure–activity relationships and although these methods cannot yet claim to have been responsible for the development of one particularly successful drug, they have been shown capable of directing synthetic effort to improved variants.

It is also fair to point out that some successful structure–activity correlations have been discovered but not revealed for commercial reasons. Sensible commercial precautions are also behind recent International Union of Pure and Applied Chemistry (IUPAC) recommendations about structure–activity relations (SAR). The recommendation is that only *tested* predictions of activity be published because the publishing of untested predictions tends to preclude others from synthesizing pertinent structures because they will not be patentable.

Quantitative structure–activity relationships

Before discussing the role of theoretical calculations in activity correlations it is essential to have some idea of the status of correlations which use measured data.

The approach is statistical, establishing correlations between biological activity and measured properties associated with the chemical structure of the molecule,

$$\text{biological activity} = \text{constant} + \sum_{i=1}^{m} a_i x_i$$

with x_i being the structural properties and a_i the coefficients which emerge from the analysis. The number of compounds in the series must exceed m by, if possible, a factor of five or more. The a_i are normally found using a least-squares multiple regression program and the quality of fitting is judged by the usual statistical criteria.

The most popular and successful approach of this kind is associated with the name of Hansch. Although many measurable quantities may be related to the physico-chemical properties associated with binding, the vast majority of published correlations have been based on Hansch's π factor augmented by the classical Hammett σ.

The π value of a substituent is defined as $\log (P/P_0)$, where P is the partition coefficient between octanol and water for the substituted compound and P_0 the coefficient for the unsubstituted compound. The π values are additive so that the value for an unknown substituent can be approximated by summing the values for fragments of the substituent. The π values are essentially related to hydrophobic interactions, and in a given series of compounds may be proportional to molecular surface area.

This type of analysis is likely to lead to impressive correlations between activity and functions of parameters in cases where the relationship is dominated by physico-chemical properties. Such properties are frequently additive for the constituent parts of a molecule. Partition, like refractive index, is largely additive. On the other hand in instances where drug action is highly specific the biological activity may not be an additive reflection of the constituent parts of a molecule but rather dependent on the fine details of the manner in which the drug molecule is constituted.

For cases where the physico-chemical forces are dominant, Hansch analysis is both powerful and impressive. Quantum mechanics has little to offer in such cases save for the possibility of using calculations to compute some of the parameters involved. Quantum chemical methods will offer the possibility of rationalization in cases where activity is highly dependent on the details of molecular structures in series of compounds with almost identical physical properties but dramatic variations of potency. Instances of very successful Hansch correlations can be found in the references cited at the end of this chapter.

There is no doubt that the Hansch approach is successful and relatively simple to use. It is not a criticism of the method, however, to point out that it does not lead to a molecular picture of what is happening at the receptor. This is not its aim. If one does seek to understand drug action in a structural sense then it becomes attractive to try to produce activity correlations not with measured properties but with sub-molecular factors which might be involved in binding drugs to receptors and this is where the potential of theoretical calculation comes in.

The potential value of theoretical calculations

The logic behind many correlations of activity with sub-molecular factors is that the sub-molecular factors correlate with binding free energies and these in turn are directly related to activity, i.e.

Calculated sub-molecular properties $\propto$ binding $\propto$ activity.
(I)   (II)   (III)

The relationship between binding (II) and activity (III) follows from either of the alternative theories of drug action, so for correlations of I with III to be justified it is only necessary to show that I correlates with II.

Most of the work published has assumed this correlation exists. A simple attempt to verify whether the simple molecular orbital calculations being used would lead to a correlation with binding chose as a test case the binding free energies of haptens to antibodies. For a series of haptens which are phenyl trimethylammonium ions, free energies of binding are known and since the binding site is on the antibody protein it should serve as a reasonable model for drug–receptor interactions.

It seems likely in this case that the binding is largely electrostatic so that a correlation might follow the relation

$$\Delta G = \frac{ke_1 e_2}{r} + c$$

where for the series of haptens only e_1 varies, e_2 being the charge on the receptor, k an appropriate dielectric constant and r the separation of hapten and anti-body. Even using crude extended Hückel calculations and Mulliken population analyses for charge on the nitrogen atom of the quaternary ammonium hapten a reasonable correlation between charge and binding is produced as shown in *Figure 19.1.*

This correlation offers some encouragement to the calculation of sub-molecular parameters and correlation not with binding but with activity. However, it must be pointed out that the wave functions used are of poor quality; a multipole expansion for charge interaction would be preferable

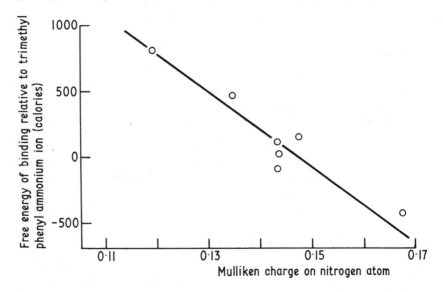

Figure 19.1. Correlation between nitrogen charge and free energy of interaction between trimethyl ammonium hapten groups on ovalbumin and antibody

and in any case Mulliken population analyses are suspect. Furthermore, the antibody is also heterogeneous.

It ought now to be possible to refine a study of this type just to see whether the calculation of sub-molecular properties can reveal anything about small molecule interaction with receptors. There now exist data from studies with homogeneous antibodies (for example MOPC 315) not only for binding free energies but also for rate constants of the hapten associating with and dissociating from the protein. These data coupled with good calculations of wave functions and charge or potential should precede application to more complicated biological interactions. On the other hand, so attractive is the idea of learning about binding factors in real situations that a lot of work has gone forward without prior physico-chemical justification.

The sub-molecular properties which are used in correlations with activity include charge on particular atoms, energies of filled and empty orbitals, bond orders and free valence indices. In principle all that is required is to have a set of chemically and physically similar compounds with varying biological activities. For each compound all the parameters which can possibly be computed are calculated. A multiple regression analysis program is then used to search for correlations.

The danger of this type of operation is that too much significance is placed on the statistical tests. It is all too easy to produce high correlation co-efficients if the regression involves say a dozen compounds and perhaps five disposable coefficients. There is nothing easier than producing correlations but with too many parameters very little is learned about what are the essential features of sub-molecular structure which must be optimized to produce effective binding. It is probably far more useful to produce statistically less impressive correlations but using at most three sub-molecular properties. In this way it might be possible to focus attention on say three points in the molecular framework which are involved in specific bonds.

Examples

The benzothiadiazine antihypertensive agents: From the many attempts to use indices computed by means of molecular orbital correlations to correlate with biological activity one of the more careful and thoughtful examples is the work of Wohl. This is an early study which uses the primitive extended Hückel molecular orbital method and is complicated by the possible tautomerism shown in *Figure 19.2*. In other ways the set of compounds and the biological data meet the requirements for a detailed study: all the compounds in the series of over 30 are thought to act at the same site as competitive antagonists of Ca^{2+} induced vasoconstriction and the biological

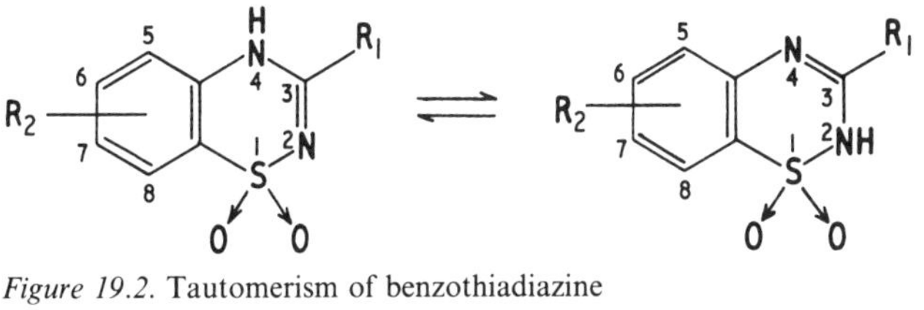

Figure 19.2. Tautomerism of benzothiadiazine

measurements were accurate and made *in vitro*. The pharmacological potency in the series of blocking agents, pA_2, is the negative logarithm of the molar concentration of antagonist which necessitates a doubling of agonist concentration for an equivalent effect when the antagonist is present. Mathematically pA_2 is related to the drug–receptor dissociation constants and the set of such values was treated as the dependent variable.

Independent variables were provided from the wave functions. Amongst those tried were net σ and π charges on nitrogen atoms, the energy of the highest occupied molecular orbital E_{HOMO}, nucleophilic superdelocalizabilities, S^N.

Of the various regressions tried the following proved most satisfactory

$$pA_2 = 64.12 - 15.6\ E_{HOMO} + 55.09\ S_3^N + 115.78\ S_6^N + 5.16\ q\ (3R)$$

where $q(3R)$ is the sum of the charges on atoms in the 3-R group. The statistics of the correlation are impressive with $R^2 = 0.96$ for 23 compounds and the probability that the relationship is a chance occurrence less than 0.0005.

Anti-allergy agents

An example which illustrates the best possible sort of correlation, that between activity and a single computed electronic factor, is provided by a structure–activity correlation for a series of anti-allergy agents—oxanilic,

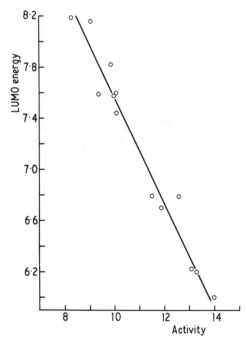

Figure 19.3.

quinaldic and benzopyran carboxylic acids. The correlation illustrated in *Figure 19.3* can be fitted by

$$-\ln ED_{50} = -64.4\,\varepsilon + 29.0$$

Here the ED_{50} is the dose required for 50 per cent inhibition of the anaphylactic response in rats and ε is the energy of the unoccupied pi molecular orbital. The correlation coefficient is -0.98 and the standard deviation 0.37.

The mechanistic conclusion which can be drawn from this study is that the molecules probably act by a charge transfer mechanism in stabilizing the drug–receptor complex. Particularly striking in this instance is the way in which compounds of very different structures can be accommodated in the same simple correlation.

β-Lactam compounds

Antibacterial activity of β-lactam compounds has been rationalized by Boyd and his co-workers in terms of the energetics of the hypothesized reaction of *Figure 19.4*. The stability of a model gas-phase transition intermediate with OH^- placed near the reactive carbon atom of the lactam ring is greater than that of the infinitely separated reactants. This energy increase (ΔE), as predicted by CNDO calculations permits a rational of reactivity to be produced. Qualitatively a small ΔE is believed to correspond to a less-reactive β-lactam ring. In such circumstances biological activity is expected to be low as the compound may be poor at acylating the bacterial cell-wall enzymes. Conversely, very large ΔE compounds may be unstable. As a result a parabolic relationship between ΔE and activity might be expected. With a variety of choices of compound, some twenty molecules can be fitted to a parabolic curve to a satisfactory statistical level.

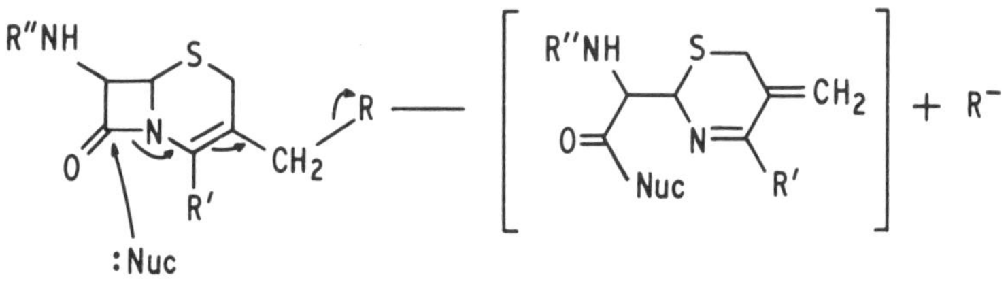

Figure 19.4. Hypothesized reaction of a β-lactam compound

Carcinogenicity of aromatic hydrocarbons

Perhaps of all examples of structure–activity relations based upon quantum mechanical calculations, the most studied is that of the carcinogenicity of aromatic hydrocarbons. The story dates back to the 1940s when the Pullmans, using simple pi-electron Hückel theory, produced a striking linear relationship between measured biological activity and theoretical indices of reactivity of a specific area of the molecules (*see Figure 19.5*).

The very encouraging beginning has been followed by years of elaboration

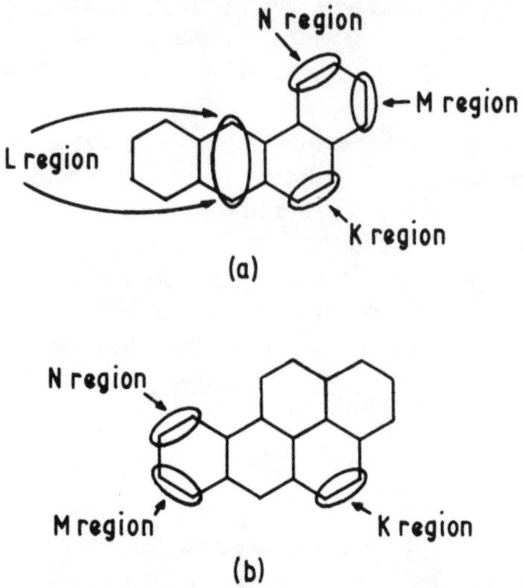

Figure 19.5. Molecular regions involved in carcinogenesis by polycyclic aromatic hydrocarbons. (a) Benz (α) anthracene. (b) Benzo (α) pyrene

and numerous articles which have served to show the complexity of using calculations on unperturbed molecules as the basis for activity correlations.

The carcinogenic activity relates to the presence in the molecule of particularly favourable regions (K) which are susceptible to the involvement in reactions leading to carcinogenic products and to the simultaneous absence or weakness of other potentially reactive regions (L). The latter, if too effective, involve the molecules in alternative reactions which lead to non-carcinogenic products.

The actual reagents which produce the carcinogenic step are metabolites or even second-order metabolites of the original hydrocarbon whose reactivity is computed in terms of static reactivity indices. Thus as well as K and L regions, areas marked M denote the metabolically more reactive parts of the molecule. The key step in chemical carcinogenesis is covalent bonding

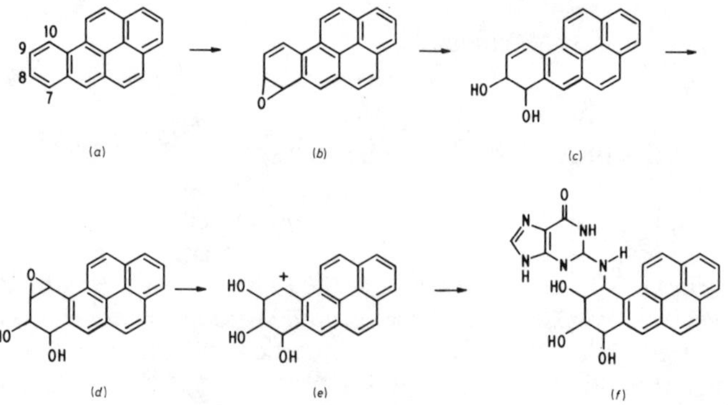

Figure 19.6. The metabolic fate of benz (α) pyrene

between the active metabolites and DNA, probably the amino group of guanine. The complexity of these metabolite transformations is illustrated in *Figure 19.6*. The probable importance of the diol epoxide has led to an alternative reformation of the K,L,M region rationalization in terms of a 'bay region' theory, a bay being a concave exterior region of a polycyclic aromatic hydrocarbon bordered by three phenyl rings at least one of which is a terminal ring (*Figure 19.7*). Diol epoxides can exist in alternative conformations whose ease of solvation and activity differ giving a further complication in an already tortuous story.

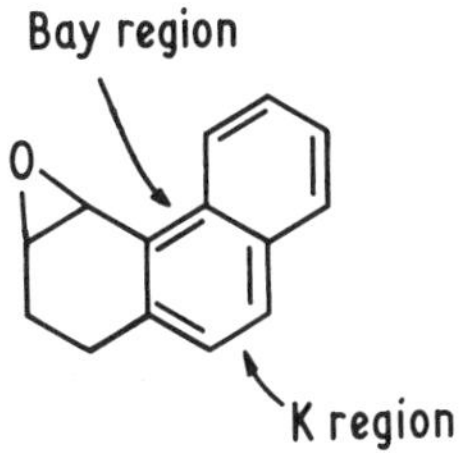

Figure 19.7. The 'bay region' of a polynuclear hydrocarbon

At the present time, despite the many years of work on this problem there are many loose ends: molecules which do not fit in with the theories. In a sense the work has not lived up to its early promise but, more reasonably, too much has been expected from a simple early statistical correlation.

Summary

Despite the apparent successes of activity correlations, it would be unwise to be too enthusiastic about this approach, even though it probably contains the basis of a useful procedure. The problems of knowing the conformation, ionic form and tautomeric form of molecules in the receptor environment remain, as does the problem of using isolated molecule calculations. Most of the parameters computed are very crude and again apply to the unperturbed rather than the bound molecule. The rewards for success in drug design are so inviting that no doubt more and more attempts will be made to use molecular orbital calculations, if only to provide extra parameters for Hansch analyses although theoretical calculations are not well suited to this task.

There have been many correlations published but few are totally convincing. In general too few compounds are considered for the results to be compelling.

Further reading

ARIENS, E. J. *Drug Design*, Academic Press, New York and London (1971)
  Vol. 1 p. 271 C. HANSCH: 'Quantitative structure activity relationships in drug design'
    p. 381 A. J. WOHL: 'An MO approach to quantitative drug design'
    p. 406 R. L. SCHNAARE: 'Electronic aspects of drug action'
  Vol. 2 (1972) J. J. KAUFMAN and W. SKORSKI
BOYD, D. B. *Annals New York Acad. Sci.*, **367**, 531 (1981)
  Theoretical studies of β-lactam antibiotics.

BURGER, A. *Medicinal Chemistry*, Part 1, Wiley-Interscience, New York (1970)
CHENEY, B. V., WRIGHT, J. B., HALL, C. M., JOHNSON, H. G. and CHRISTOF-
    FERSEN, R. E. *J. med. Chem.*, **21**, 936 (1978)
    Anti-allergy agents.
GOODFORD, P. J. *Adv. Pharmac. Chemother.*, **11**, 51 (1973)
HANSCH, C. *Acc. chem. Res.*, **3**, 232 (1969)
PULLMAN, B. *Int. J. Quantum Chem.*, **16**, 669 (1979)
    Carcinogenicity of aromatic hydrocarbons.
PURCELL, W. P., BASS, G. E. and CLAYTON, J. M. *Strategy of Drug Design*, John Wiley
    & Sons, New York (1973)
REDL, G., CRAMER, R. D. *tert* and BERKOFF, C. E. *Chem. Soc. Rev.*, **3**, 273 (1974)
WOHL, A. J. *Molec. Pharmac.*, **6**, 195 (1970)

Chapter 20

Enzymes as receptors

Apart from the neglect of solvation, the chief criticism of quantum pharmacology has been that it focuses attention on isolated molecules while in reality it is their interaction with receptors which is of importance. Generally this is both true and inevitable. Little is known about pharmacological receptors at the atomic level. On the other hand many enzymes have been crystallized and the binding sites are studied both by diffraction methods and by n.m.r. Furthermore enzymes are targets for medicinal chemists who may want to provide false substrates, or more usually block the active site. It may, for example, be useful to design inhibitors for enzymes which are vital to abnormal or invading cells while being inactive in the host.

From the point of view of quantum mechanical calculations, enzymes are very large molecules—too large to be incorporated in full atomic detail in any currently available computer program. Some approximations must be made and the obvious possibilities include considering just the substrate and studying the reaction pathway, limiting the enzyme to a model containing only those groups involved in the active site, or making approximations in the quantum mechanical method to permit the incorporation of dozens, even hundreds of enzyme atoms. Whichever approach is followed, entropy effects are normally ignored as is solvent so that as in so many other theoretical calculations of relevance to biology, differences between results for similar molecules are to be preferred to studies of single substrate–enzyme pairs.

Reaction pathways

The most significant part of a reaction pathway from the point of view of rate enhancement by an enzyme is the transition state. A comparison of transition state energies may indicate a preferred path or even suggest that one active site may be responsible for two reactions. An example of this latter state of affairs is provided by the work of Andrews and Heyde which suggests that there is a common active site for the two reactions catalysed by chorismate mutase–prephenate dehydrogenase. The two reactions are shown in *Figure 20.1*.

A geometry optimizing semi-empirical program (MINDO/3) permits a

229

(a)

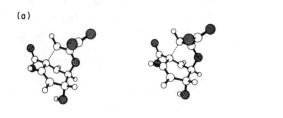

(b)

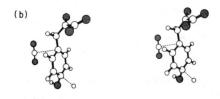

Figure 20.1. (a) The isomerization of chorismate to prephenate. (b) The dehydrogenation of prephenate to 4-hydroxyphenylpyruvate

(a)

(b)

Figure 20.2. Stereoscopic drawings of the transition states for (a) the isomerization of chorismate to prephenate, (b) the dehydrogenation of prephenate to 4-hydroxyphenylpyruvate. Oxygen atoms are shaded [reproduced with permission from P. R. Andrews and E. Heyde, *J. theoret. Biol.*, **78**, 393–403 (1979)]

reasonable prediction of the transition states for the two reactions to be made and compared (*Figure 20.2*). The similarities are strong enough for the hypothesis of a single active site to be made and therefore lead to suggestions of groups which are likely to be involved on the enzyme.

If the enzyme structure is already known then the reaction pathway can be followed much more realistically. More than any other case the famous protease charge–relay system involving serine, histidine and aspartate has been investigated (*Figure 20.3*). The debate has been between two similar but alternative mechanisms which lead to an enhanced reactivity of the O^{γ} atom in serine. One alternative has the aspartate pulling the $N^{\delta 1}$ proton from histidine followed by an $O^{\gamma} \ldots N^{\varepsilon 2}$ proton transfer to the imidazolium anion. A highly reactive hydroxylate anion is then formed and this readily attacks the carbon atom of the peptide bond cut by the enzyme. The other possibility involves no free hydroxylate anion being formed. The relative reactive profiles of the two alternatives are amenable to straightforward calculation, but just how many amino acids residue must be included remains problematic.

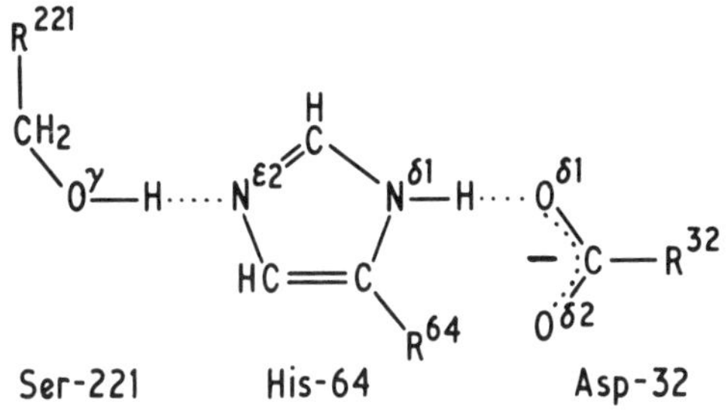

The charge–relay mechanism structure (Figure 20.3):

Ser-221   His-64   Asp-32

Figure 20.3. The charge–relay mechanism

Model enzyme studies

Model enzyme studies concentrate solely on the active site of the enzyme and replace the neighbouring amino acid residues by simple groups. For example models of the active sites of metalloenzymes have been studied by Lipscomb, Madame Pullman's French group and by Weinstein and his collaborators. The model enzyme is stark to say the least, being for carboxy-peptidase nothing more than $[M(OH)(NH_3)_2]^+$. In the crystal a central zinc atom in the active site is bound to three protein residues: histidine, glutamine and another histidine. The fourth position in a distorted tetrahedron is occupied by a water molecule (*Figure 20.4*). The substrate peptide or ester is believed to displace the water molecule and bind to the Zn through the carbonyl of the substrate.

In Lipscomb's work the metal M is taken to be Be^{2+} but other workers have used Zn^{2+} as in the native enzyme. Imidazoles are replaced by ammonia molecules since trial calculations suggest that the binding is similar.

Electrostatic potential computations show that the zinc complex generates a localized attractive field for ligands with high electron density such as the carbonyl of a substrate. The gradient of the field moreover hints at a directing effect of the complex towards the incoming ligands.

Using pseudopotential SCF methods the model has been pushed slightly closer to reality for the zinc-containing enzyme carbonic anhydrase (*Figure*

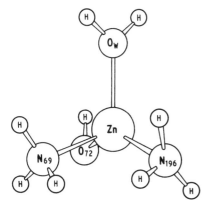

Figure 20.4. Model for the active site of carboxypeptidase

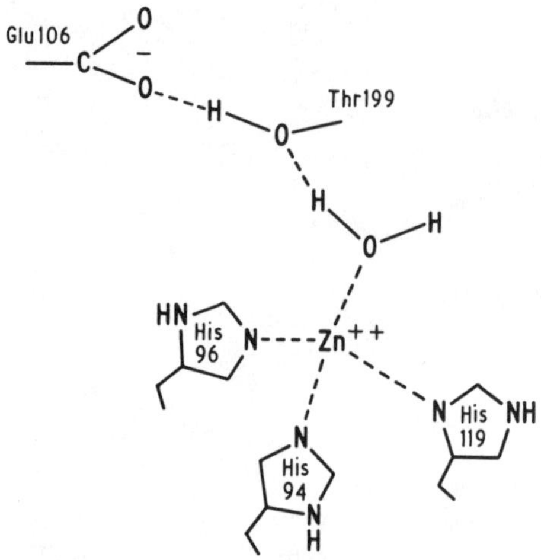

Figure 20.5. The active site of carbonic anhydrase

20.5). The hydrogen bonded chain glutamate–threonine–water is stable when unbound but prefers the form glu–thr–OH$^-$ when bound to the zinc and the proton relay to that form occurs with no barrier. The calculations also showed that the reaction

$$OH^- + CO_2 \rightleftharpoons HCO_3^-$$

proceeds readily on zinc at the active site with no activation energy and a small exothermicity.

These examples are impressive in their way and make a serious contribution to the understanding of enzyme mechanism. They do not, however, lead towards the design of new therapeutic compounds and two major criticisms can be levelled. In the first place the atoms of the active site incorporated are so few in number that the reality of the model is not convincing. Secondly no heed has been paid to solvation or other entropic factors.

Incorporation of many enzyme atoms

A method of incorporating a large number of atoms in the neighbourhood of the enzyme's active site stems from an important paper by Hayes and Kollman in 1976. In essence they showed that one can place atoms, perhaps a few hundred, in the known positions using crystal data. These atoms on the enzyme may, however, be replaced by dummy atoms which have a partial net positive or negative charge. The substrate or blocker on the other hand is treated in a normal full *ab initio* computation.

The time-consuming part of an *ab initio* calculation involves the integrals over electrons; one-centre terms such as nuclear attraction are by comparison trivial. Thus if we have a site consisting of perhaps a hundred point partial charges plus a small molecule we can solve the modified Hartree–Fock equations in a reasonable time and vary relative molecular orientations and distances. The actual partial charges to use on the amino acid residues are found from calculations on model side chains. The origin of this idea lies in the fact that electrostatic potentials generated from a point charge model agree with the picture which emerges from a full calculation, at least in regions removed from the atomic nuclei.

It must be emphasized that interaction energies computed in this way will be dominated by the electrostatic contribution. No account is taken of dispersion forces or entropic factors such as hydrophobic interactions, although polarization of substrate by the enzyme is included but not the counter effect of ligand on the binding site. Nonetheless, since many drug–receptor interactions involve ions of opposite charge then certainly for the long-range to mid-distance interaction, this is probably not a serious handicap. Repulsion is taken into account by not allowing the substrate to penetrate within the Van der Waals radii of the protein atoms.

The original paper was an application to carboxypeptidase A, its apo derivative and the complex between the enzyme with glycine–tyrosine. The authors predicted that an o–OH–Gly–Tyr analogue should bind more strongly to carboxypeptidase A than the natural substrate.

This type of study has tremendous possibilities particularly if combined with computer graphics. The binding site picture can be displayed using files of crystallographic data and the relative orientations of protein and small molecules varied on the screen as the energy calculations are made. Colour to distinguish site and substrate has obvious advantages.

The remaining drawback is the neglect of solvent and other unknown environmental influences. This can only be circumvented by studying the relative binding energies of a series of similar small molecules to the same enzyme active site.

The study of a series

This next step, the study of a series, is only being attempted now that graphics capabilities have become available. Robins in Oxford has considered the problem of the binding of n-alkyl boronic acid substrates, $B(OH)_2(CH_2)_nH$ to α-chymotrypsin (n being in the range 0 to 8).

The initial step is to fit the boronic acid conformation into the known active site pocket. This is only feasible using computer graphics; even a good geometrical model is insufficient. The stages in this fitting start qualitatively and are then made increasingly quantitative. The starting point is to fit the substrate into the cleft by eye, using as a guide the known crystal structure of bound ligands. Secondly the skeleton of the substrate with hydrogens removed can be fitted into the pocket represented by a surface on the van der Waals spheres of the enzyme atoms plus one carbon van der Waals radius. This will provide a more restricted, tightly fitting picture. Quantitative adjustments can then be added using the methods of molecular mechanics with Lennard–Jones potentials. These methods are rapid enough for an energy minimum to be sought. A final check that the optimum bound configuration has been found comes from the *ab initio* calculation with point charges on the enzymic atoms.

Energies, broken down into total electronic, nuclear–nuclear repulsion and point-charge-nuclear or point-charge-electron terms are calculated for the substrate in free space and optimally bound surrounded by over two hundred point charges. The point charges were derived directly from Mulliken population analysis of amino acid residues using coordinates from crystallographic data on α-chymotrypsin with modification of each of these sets of charges to ensure electrical neutrality. Tests have shown that the modified conformationally averaged charges must maintain electrical neutrality if the amino acid residue is uncharged, but the small variation of point charge with adjustment of conformation of the residue is unimportant: it affects only the absolute value of binding energy and not relative binding energies.

The binding energy is determined as the difference between the total energy of the separate site and ligand and the combination. It can be analysed in terms of its electrostatic and polarization contributions. In this instance the former predominates approximately in the ratio of two to one.

Binding to α-chymotrypsin depends both on the attraction to the charge relay system and upon a hydrophobic interaction. If we wish to compare the calculated binding energies with those determined experimentally as free energies we have to allow for the fact that experimentally the substrate goes from solution to the active site. The hydrophobic contribution to binding is related to entropic changes in the solvent so that it is necessary to correct the calculated binding energy by solvation terms. Estimates of ΔG solvation for an alkyl chain are known in terms of the number of $-(CH_2)-$

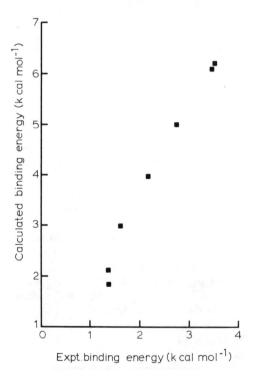

Figure 20.6. Calculated and experimental binding energies of alkyl boronic acids to chymotrypsin

groups in the substrate. They amount to 0.85 kcal/mole per methylene unit.

The corrected calculated binding energies of the series of substrates are plotted and compared with experimental values in *Figure 20.6*. In this work the larger substrate with $n = 7$ and $n = 8$ had to be divided into two fragments, $B(OH)_2(CH_2)_4H$ and $H(CH_2)_{n-4}H$. The consistency of the result indicates, encouragingly, that this is a safe procedure.

Thus from a knowledge of the active site it does seem possible to estimate relative binding energies of hypothetical substrates. Further, it may be possible to do the converse: to gain information about the nature of the receptor site from binding energy data on known substrates.

The drug-docking problem

Aided by computer graphics techniques it is clear that useful calculations on binding between an enzymic active site and a small ligand are possible. The next problem which comes ripe for solution is then that of the docking between a drug and its receptor; bringing the problem of recognition down to a molecular level. There are a number of extra features which will have to be incorporated over and above those involved in computations of relative binding energies. In the first place as a ligand approaches the appropriate binding site a process of desolvation will be involved, encompassing both partners. This may be circumvented yet again by doing difference studies. Much more important will be the flexibility not only of the approaching small molecule, but also of the protein itself. It should never be forgotten that oxygen will not bind to haemoglobin in the latter's crystal structure geometry. Even the incorporation of oxygen demands adjustment of atomic positions.

Ideally for a study of this problem one requires a fairly rigid ligand and details of the binding site. Then it is really necessary to compute the energy of the system as docking proceeds, allowing flexibility. A graphics system may allow the docking to be visualized but very rapid energy calculations are also a prerequisite. The method discussed above is one possibility as are molecular mechanics calculations which might allow the embrace of the ligand by the receptor to be studied in real time.

One heroic attempt to grapple with this important problem has been made by Dean and Wakelin. They took as a prototype model the intercalative attack of the rigid molecule ethidium and its carboxylated derivative on a fragment of DNA. Charge distributions were calculated for both the intercalative site and the drug molecules. From the charge distributions the molecular electrostatic potential was derived. The variation as relative separations and orientations are sampled indicates quite clearly that the receptor induces an orientation change in the incoming ligand. For this particular instance two types of interaction predominate: coulombic interactions and electron delocalization. Changes are also induced in the electronic distributions and orbital energy levels.

The molecular electrostatic potentials surrounding the receptor and binding drugs do seem to be complementary. Dean and Wakelin showed this by using stereoprojections. The electrostatic potential appears to play a major role in positioning the drug before molecular contact. This was highlighted by inspecting the vectors of the field generated by the receptor. Orientation of the drugs corresponded to the receptor's local field vector.

This particular study represents something of a milestone. It demonstrates just how much depends on electrostatic interactions and how crudely computed electrostatic fields may enable quite intimate details of the docking mechanism to be followed. What is lacking and must soon be incorporated are the essential flexibility of receptor and substrate together with some account of solvation and desolvation.

Summary

Both as model systems for drug–receptor interactions and as targets for medicinal chemists the enzyme–substrate and enzyme–blocker combinations deserve to be studied. Graphics systems may circumvent the problems of visual complexity and the adjustment of the position of a small molecule within a binding site on a protein. At present calculations are restricted. The *ab initio* variety reduce the protein to a model with very few atoms. A more realistic binding site involving hundreds of atoms necessitates an approximation such as replacing nuclei plus electrons by point partial charges. Nonetheless it does seem possible to compute relative binding enthalpies. Solvation and entropic effects have to be introduced empirically or assumed to be a constant feature for a series of similar ligands. Particularly between charged species the electrostatic potential can indicate orientational effects and complementarity prerequisites.

Further reading

ANDREWS, P. R. and HEYDE, E. *J. theoret. Biol.* **78**, 393 (1979)
   A common active site for catalysis by chorismate mutase-prephenate dehydrogenase.
DEAN, P. M. and WAKELIN, L. P. G. *Phil. Trans. R. Soc. London, B.*, **287**, 571 (1979)
   The docking manoeuvre at a drug receptor: a quantum mechanical study of intercalative attack of ethidium and its carboxylated derivative on a DNA fragment.
DEAN, P. M. and WAKELIN, L. P. G. *Proc. R. Soc. London, B.*, **209**, 472 (1980)
   Elecrostatic components of drug receptor recognition: 2, the DNA-binding antibiotic actinomycin.
DEMOULIN, D. and PULLMAN, A. in B. PULLMAN (ed), *Catalysis in Chemistry and Biochemistry. Theory and Experiment*, D. Reidel, Dordrecht (1979)
   Theoretical studies on models of the active site of carbonic anhydrase.
HAYES, D. M. and KOLLMAN, P. A. *J. Am. chem. Soc.*, **98**, 3335 (1976)
   Electrostatic potentials of proteins. 1. Carboxypeptidase A.
HAYES, D. M. and KOLLMAN, P. A. *J. Am. chem. Soc.*, **98**, 7811 (1976)
   Electrostatic potentials of proteins. 2. Role of electrostatics in a possible catalytic mechanism for carboxypeptidase A.
OSMAN, R. and WEINSTEIN, H. *Israel J. Chem.*, **19**, 149 (1980)
   Models for active sites of metalloenzymes: comparison of zinc and beryllium containing complexes.
WEINSTEIN, H. and GREEN, J. P. (eds) 'Quantum chemistry in biomedical sciences', *Annals of the New York Academy of Sciences*, **367** (1981)
   Pages 326–451 cover calculations on enzyme–substrate interactions.

Chapter 21

Conclusions

Every attempt has been made in this book to adopt an honest and critical attitude while trying to be constructive. Finally, it seems appropriate to ask some of the questions which ought to occur to open-minded readers concerning the value and status of work in the field of applying theory to pharmacological problems.

Can calculations be useful?

First it is possible to answer the obvious corollary in the affirmative: calculations can be useless. It is so very easy to run molecular orbital calculations of an approximate type for a small biologically active molecule, but the assumptions made in order to produce explanations of effects in living systems may be so gross that the work may be futile.

The theoretician should be very humble when approaching biology. In physics theoreticians have a highly productive role; in chemistry much has been illuminated as a result of theoretical work. In biology there have been few striking successes. On the other hand, provided the theoretician or experimentalist using theoretical tools is aware of the difficulties then his calculations can be useful.

In the opinion of the author it is essential to work with a series of compounds in order to highlight the variations in activity which are molecular in origin in order to rule out environmental effects. If care over such matters is taken, calculations should add to experimental structural data on conformation and electronic distribution. The calculations are not restricted to forms of molecules found in equilibrium experimental conditions. Molecules need not be synthesized before calculations are run.

Is the time ripe?

In principle the Schrödinger equation does contain all the answers and in time it will no doubt be possible to run calculations for huge systems which will include solvent, receptor, counter ions and all the particles involved in biological recognition and activity. That ideal world is not yet with us so is it too soon to start work in this area?

The question of ripe time is difficult since the best time to enter a research field is just too soon, just before the work becomes possible. Once it is obviously routine, bright minds want to move on. Estimating how far one is from a threshold is clearly impossible. It is perhaps salutary to consider the case of the crystallography of proteins. Its beginning in the 1930s was decades before the work was to become routine. Major scientific break-throughs were necessary before the work had any chance of the success which has since been achieved. Yet who would deny that the pioneers who went into this work in the early days made the correct decision?

The state of theoretical computation of meaningful biological systems is much nearer to fruition than was crystallography when the first workers entered that field. Furthermore it does not seem necessary for there to be any major breakthrough. All that is required are the obvious developments in both theory and experiment to continue as they are doing currently.

Two factors, one experimental and the other on the theory side, suggest that the time is ripe. Experimentally, pharmacology is becoming more molecular. Receptors are being isolated, labelled binding studies and cyclase activities are being measured. Enzymes are being studied in atomic detail. The activity figures with which a theoretician must grapple should become more like physico-chemical data and less prone to depend on complex biological mechanisms other than the one being studied.

The development of bigger and faster computers together with the falling price of minicomputers and microcomputers suggest that on the computation side it may no longer be necessary to use calculations which are intrinsic-ally untrustworthy. It is becoming possible to do better calculations on more reliable data.

The role of computer graphics

Theoretical approaches in drug design have until recently concentrated on energy calculations and descriptions of molecular shape in terms of nuclear positions. Computer graphics systems have been used to display and mani-pulate molecular structures in an increasingly sophisticated manner. Many pharmaceutical research laboratories now employ systems which can go from a hand-drawn, two-dimensional structural formula to a realistic picture using the data from a crystal structure data bank and optimizing energy calculations of the molecular mechanics type. Pictures may be produced in quasi-three-dimensional form. This is achieved by 'depth-cueing' where parts of the picture distant from the viewer are fainter. Alternatively pairs of images suitable for stereo-viewing are produced. With colour, molecules may be superimposed to seek out structural similarities which could have biological significance.

The increasing availability of graphics systems is now leading to the logical extension of such work from molecular pictures in terms of nuclear position to the far more important and potentially revealing electronic description. When molecules interact with each other, or indeed with receptors, it is the clouds of electronic density which mingle rather than the point positive nuclei.

Quantum mechanical calculations furnish not only the energy of a molecule for a prescribed nuclear conformation but also a wave function, whose square at any point in space gives an electron density. Since the earliest days of molecular quantum mechanics the use of Ψ^2 to give electron density has been used, but only for simple model systems. The advent of computer graphics systems has permitted the utility of these calculations to be realized for complex non-symmetrical structures.

The problem of visualization is only rendered feasible if colour and depth-cueing are employed. The 'shape' of a molecule can be presented as a net covering the exterior of a molecule at a prescribed electron density contour. The choice of the appropriate contour is arbitrary but a logical choice may be taken from consideration of separate quantum mechanical computations of molecular interaction energies. Molecules can be displayed on a graphics screen as a skeleton of the Dreiding model type with the electron density net superimposed. This is only comprehensible when two colours are employed or alternatively by using colour filters. The use of this system has been of real value in highlighting similarities in molecules which are not apparent with the use of structural formulae or indeed space-filling models.

The quantum mechanical wave function can alternatively be used to reveal the electrostatic potential field generated by a molecule and used pharmacologically as a means of defining what a molecule should 'look like' to a positive centre.

Computers with graphical output are perhaps for the first time being used to provide information which could not be obtained in any other way and the commercial results are already beginning to flow. Practitioners of quantum pharmacology used to be taunted by sceptics with the question of how many drugs they had discovered. Now at least there are several instances where the computational chemist has been included on commercial patents as a testimony to the practicality of the approach.

The role of colour graphics in this progress is quite crucial in enabling chemists to see things which would otherwise be lost in complexity. For this reason the bibliography includes a section on molecular computer graphics.

How should calculations be used?

Running calculations is very easy but sensible work is most likely to be produced if it is done in close collaboration with or directly by experimental groups, particularly those in the pharmaceutical industry. In such a context the use of calculations can be very helpful even though the work may not produce the material for a publication.

This, in the long term, may be the future of calculations. They may be used rather in the manner in which molecular models are now used—an invaluable aid to thought and discussion or rationalization but not a field in their own right. Used in this type of 'in-house' fashion, theoretical calculations should be more and more widely used. Calculations should stimulate the work of synthetic organic chemists by putting additional rationale into synthesis. Compounds should be synthesized for good scientific reasons rather than merely to be screened.

Moral questions

Moral questions may seem out of place in a scientific text although they should not. However of all areas of science few attract more reaction than the pharmaceutical industry despite its excellent record in almost every moral aspect.

There are two sources of moral indignation most often raised against the industry. One is the argument that pharmaceutical companies do most of their research in areas where the sale of products is likely to be highest, producing tremendous competition in areas such as tranquillizers, but much less effort is expended on diseases which involve only a small percentage of the population or people in underdeveloped countries. The second cause of hostile reaction is the large number of animals used in screening compounds for activity.

The two problems have at root the same cause. Finding new drugs requires the synthesis and testing of perhaps thousands of chemicals before a successful new compound is found.

The money spent on research by the pharmaceutical industry now runs into billions of dollars. Because of the investment required it only makes sense commercially to focus attention on areas where the research expenditure is likely to be recouped.

If theory can help to rationalize drug design then it would contribute towards alleviating both moral problems. If less compounds are screened then less populous markets can be investigated and for any given successful drug less animal experimentation may be required.

Sub-molecular biology

As a final comment on the role of calculations of molecular wave functions in pharmacology we should remember that the wave function tells us above all about the properties and positions of the electrons in the molecule.

Molecular biology has been both successful and fashionable in the last two decades. Now many research workers are looking beyond questions as to which molecule does what. One direction in which to move is obviously towards cell biology, moving one step up the hierarchy of biological complication. The alternative direction should also prove rewarding: stepping down to the sub-molecular level.

Once it is clear that particular molecules fulfil specific roles it then becomes interesting to ask why? What is it about a particular molecule which enables it to perform some function?

The answer to such questions must be in terms of the electrons in the molecule as it is they which are involved in interactions. Molecular wave functions can give far more detail about electronic distribution than any experimental technique.

Part IV

Bibliography

Bibliography

Molecules are grouped in a manner corresponding to the text in Part I. Entries are arranged chronologically and are intended to be complete up to the end of 1981.

Acetylcholine

GILL, E. W. *Prog. med. Chem.*, **4,** 39 (1965)
  Empirical calculation of conformation.
KIER, L. B. *Molec. Pharmac.*, **3,** 487 (1967)
  EHT conformation compared with X-ray structure.
KIER, L. B. *Molec. Pharmac.*, **4,** 70 (1968)
  EHT calculation; comparison with nicotine; charge densities.
LIQUORI, A. M., DAMIANI, A. and DeCOEN, J. L. *J. molec. Biol.*, **33,** 445 (1968)
  Empirical calculation.
FARKAS, M. and KRUGLYAK, J. A. *Nature, Lond.*, **223,** 523 (1969)
  EHT calculation.
KIER, L. B. and TRUITT, E. B. *Experientia*, **26,** 988 (1970)
  EHT calculation.
HEGYHATI, M. M. and FARKAS, M. *J. chem. Phys.*, **52,** 2778 (1970)
  EHT study of hydrolysis.
BEVERIDGE, D. L. and RADNA, R. J. *J. Am. chem. Soc.*, **93,** 3759 (1971)
  INDO conformational study.
PULLMAN, B., COURRIÈRE, P. and COUBEILS, J. L. *Molec. Pharmac.*, **7,** 397 (1971)
  PCILO calculation.
AJO, D., BOSSA, M., DAMIANI, A., FIDENZI, R., GIGLI, S., LANZI, L. and LAPICCIRELLA, A. *J. theoret. Biol.*, **34,** 15 (1972)
  Electrostatic stabilization of cholinergic compounds.
PULLMAN, B. and COURRIÈRE, P. *Molec. Pharmac.*, **8,** 612 (1972)
  PCILO calculation compared with other methods.
FROIMOWITZ, M. and GANS, P. J. *J. Am. chem. Soc.*, **94,** 8020 (1972)
  Semiclassical and INDO conformational study.
SARAN, A. and GOVIL, G. *J. theoret. Biol.*, **37,** 181 (1972)
  CNDO conformational study.
KIER, L. B. and GEORGE, J. M. *Experientia*, **29,** 501 (1973)
  EHT calculation.
PULLMAN, B. and COURRIÈRE, P. *Theoret. chim. Acta*, **31,** 19 (1973)
  PCILO calculation on acetylcholine and derivatives.
AJO, D., BOSSA, M., FIDENZI, R., GIGLI, S. and JEROMIDIZ, G. *Theoret. chim. Acta*, **30,** 275 (1973)
  EHT compared with other methods.

AJO, D., BOSSA, M., DAMIANI, A., FIDENZI, R., GIGLI, S. and RAMUNNI, G. in 'Conformation of biological molecules and polymers', E. D. Bergmann and B. Pullman (eds), *Proc. 5th Jerusalem Symposium on Quantum Chemistry and Biochemistry*, Academic Press, New York, p. 571 (1973)
EHT, CNDO and empirical calculations.

PULLMAN, B. and COURRIÈRE, P. in 'Conformation of biological molecules and polymers', E. D. Bergmann and B. Pullman (eds), *Proc. 5th Jerusalem Symposium on Quantum Chemistry and Biochemistry*, Academic Press, New York, p. 547 (1973)
PCILO conformational potential energy map.

BEVERIDGE, D. L., RADNA, R. J. and GUTH, E. in 'Conformation of biological molecules and polymers', E. D. Bergmann and B. Pullman (eds), *Proc. 5th Jerusalem Symposium on Quantum Chemistry and Biochemistry*, Academic Press, New York, p. 73 (1973)

PORT, G. N. J. and PULLMAN, A. *J. Am. chem. Soc.*, **95**, 4059 (1973)
Ab initio conformational study.

GRENSON, D. W. and CHRISTOFFERSEN, R. E. *J. Am. chem. Soc.*, **95**, 362 (1974)
Ab initio fragment study.

PULLMAN, B. in R. Daudel and B. Pullman (eds), *The World of Quantum Chemistry*, D. Reidel, Dordrecht, p. 61 (1974)
PCILO conformational study.

BEVERIDGE, D. L., KELLY, M. M. and RADNA, R. J. *J. Am. chem. Soc.*, **96**, 3769 (1974)
Contiuum model of solvation.

BEVERIDGE, D. L. in 'Molecular and quantum pharmacology', E. D. Bergmann and B. Pullman (eds), *Proc. 7th Jerusalem Symposium on Quantum Chemistry and Biochemistry*, D. Reidel, Dordrecht, p. 153 (1974)
INDO conformation and solvent effect.

PULLMAN, B. and COURRIÈRE, P. *C. r. hedb. Séanc. Acad. Sci., Paris*, **278**, 1785 (1974)
PCILO calculation. Includes other molecules, anticholinergics and atropine.

PULLMAN, A. and PORT, G. N. J. *Theoret. chim. Acta*, **32**, 77 (1975)
Ab initio conformational maps.

WEINSTEIN, H. *Int. J. Quantum Chem. Quantum Biol. Symp.*, **2**, 59 (1975)
Analysis of drug–receptor interaction.

GELIN, B. R. and KARPLUS, M. *J. Am. chem. Soc.*, **97**, 6996 (1975)
Role of structural flexibility in conformational calculations.

PULLMAN, B., BERTHOD, H. and GRESH, H. *C. r. hebd. Séanc. Acad. Sci., Paris*, **280**, 1741 (1975)
Conformation in solution.

HEGYHATI, M. M. *Prog. theoret. org. Chem.*, **2**, 319 (1977)
Enzyme-facilitated hydrolysis using interative extended Hückel method.

SMEYERS, Y. G., De BUEREN, A. and HERNANDEZ LAGUNA, A. *An. Quim. Farm.*, **75**, 102 (1979)
Charge distribution.

SUBBA, RAO, G., TYAGI, R. S. and MISHRA, R. K. *Int. J. Quantum Chem.*, **20**, 273 (1981)
Calculation of minimum conformational energy.

β Methyl acetylcholine

GELIN, B. R. and KARPLUS, M. *J. Am. chem. Soc.*, **97**, 6996 (1975)
Role of structural flexibility in conformational calculations.

Acetylthiocholine, carbamoylcholine and cetylcholine

PULLMAN, B. and COURRIÈRE, P. *Molec. Pharmac.*, **8**, 612 (1972)
PCILO conformational study.

PULLMAN, B. and COURRIÈRE, P. in 'Conformation of biological molecules and polymers', E. D. Bergmann and B. Pullman (eds), *Proc. 5th Jerusalem Symposium on Quantum Chemistry and Biochemistry*, Academic Press, New York, p. 547 (1973)
PCILO conformational potential energy map.

PULLMAN, B. in R. Daudel and B. Pullman (eds), *The World of Quantum Chemistry*, D. Reidel, Dordrecht, p. 61 (1974)
  PCILO conformational study.

Nicotine

KIER, L. B. *Molec. Pharmac.*, **4**, 70 (1968)
  EHT calculation.
PULLMAN, B., COURRIÈRE, P. and COUBEILS, J. L. *Molec. Pharmac.*, **7**, 317 (1971)
  PCILO conformation and charge distribution.
PULLMAN, B. and COURRIÈRE, P. in 'Conformation of biological molecules and polymers', E. D. Bergmann and B. Pullman (eds), *Proc. 5th Jerusalem Symposium on Quantum Chemistry and Biochemistry*, Academic Press, New York, p. 547 (1973)
  PCILO conformational potential energy map. Includes nicotinamide and 1,4 reduced nicotinamide.
RADNA, R. J., BEVERIDGE, D. L. and BENDER, A. L. *J. Am. chem. Soc.*, **95**, 3831 (1973)
  INDO calculation on nicotine.
KUTHUN, J. and MUSIL, L. *Colln. Czech. chem. Commun. Engl. Edn*, **40**, 3169 (1975)
  CNDO calculations in nicotinamide and dihydronicotinamide.
LEE, I. and PARK, D. H. *Taehan Hwatiak Hoechi*, **22**, 195 (1978)
  Molecular orbital study.

Muscarine

KIER, L. B. *Molec. Pharmac.*, **3**, 487 (1967)
  EHT calculation.
LIQUORI, A. M., DAMIANI, A. and ELEFANTA, G. *J. molec. Biol.*, **33**, 439 (1968)
  Empirical potential calculation.
KIER, L. B. *J. Pharm. Sci.*, **59**, 112 (1970)
  Oxtremorine compared with muscarine.
PULLMAN, B., COURRIÈRE, P. and COUBEILS, J. L. *Molec. Pharmac.*, **7**, 397 (1971)
  PCILO calculation of conformation and charge distribution.
RADNA, R. J., BEVERIDGE, D. L. and BENDER, A. L. *J. Am. chem. Soc.*, **95**, 3831 (1973)
  INDO calculation on muscarine and methyl compounds.
HÖLTJE, H. D. *Arch. Pharm.*, **307**, 969 (1974)
  Conformational study.
HOELTJE, H. D. *Arch Pharm.*, **311**, 311 (1978)
  Structure of muscarine-like piperidinium and thioniacyclohexane compounds.

Pilocarpine

KANG, S. *Int. J. Quantum Chem. Quantum Biology Symposium*, **1**, 109 (1974)
  INDO and empirical potential calculation on this muscarinic agonist.

Substituted ammonium ions

PORT, G. N. J. and PULLMAN, A. *Theoret. chim. Acta*, **31**, 231 (1973)
  Study of hydration.
CROW, J. W. *J. med. Chem.*, **16**, 728 (1973)
  EHT calculation on furfuryl trimethyl ammonium.
KIER, L. B. and ALDRICH, H. S. *J. theoret. Biol.*, **46**, 529 (1974)
  Trimethylammonium; receptor site model.
WEINSTEIN, H., APFELDORFER, B. Z., COHEN, S., MAAYANI, S. and SOKOLOVSKY, M. in 'Conformation of biological molecules and polymers', E. D. Bergmann and B. Pullman (eds), *Proc. 5th Jerusalem Symposium on Quantum Chemistry and Biochemistry*, Academic Press, New York, p. 531 (1973)
  Calculations on 3-acetoxyquinuclidine.

NELSON, S. D., KOLLMAN, P. A., TRAGER, W. F. and ROTHENBERG, S. *J. med. Chem.*, **16**, 1034 (1973)
Calculation on intermediates of amine metabolism.
KIMURA, I., MORISHIMA, I., YONEZAWA, T. and KIMURA, M. *Chem. pharm. Bull.*, *Tokyo*, **22**, 429 (1974)
MO interpretation for cholinergic activities.
WEINSTEIN, H., MAAYANI, S., SREBRENIK, S., COHEN, S. and SOKOLOVSKY, M. *Molec. Pharmac.*, **11**, 671 (1975)
Receptor interaction electrostatic potential for 3-acetoxyquinuclidine.

Anticholinergics cholinesterase inhibitors and related compounds

PULLMAN, B. and VALDERMO, C. *Biochim. Biophys. Acta*, **43**, 548 (1960)
Hückel calculations.
NEELY, W. B. *Molec. Pharmac.*, **1**, 137 (1965)
Structure–activity relationships for inhibitors.
PURCELL, W. P. *J. med. Chem.*, **9**, 294 (1966)
Activity of N-alkyl substituted amides as function of charge density.
MILLNER, O. E. and PURCELL, W. P. *J. med. Chem.*, **14**, 1134 (1971)
Inhibitory potencies of decyl piperidines as function of charge density.
CROW, J. W. and HOLLAND, W. C. *J. med. Chem.*, **15**, 429 (1972)
Neostigmine studied by EHT.
WEINSTEIN, H., MAAYANI, S., SREBRENIK, S., COHEN, S. and SOKOLOVSKY, M. *Molec. Pharmac.*, **9**, 820 (1973)
Interaction potentials of 1-cyclohexylpiperidine with receptor.
PULLMAN, B. and COURRIÈRE, P. *C. r. hebd. Séanc. Acad. Sci., Paris*, **278D**, 1785 (1974)
PCILO calculation on atropine.
HÖLTJE, H. D. and KIER, L. B. *J. pharm. Sci.*, **64**, 418 (1975)
Nature of anionic site of cholinesterase.
WEINSTEIN, H. SREBRENIK, S., MAAYANI, S. and SOKOLOVSKY, M. *J. theoret. Biol.*, **64**, 295 (1977)
Anti-muscarinics, atropine and scopolamine.
BARONE, V., LILJ, F. and RUSSO, N. *Molec. Pharmac.*, **18**, 331 (1980)
Conformation of N-(βacetoxyethyl) pyridinium ion and comparison with acetylcholine.
REED, K. W., MURRAY, W. J., ROCHE, E. B. and DOMMELSMITH, L. N. *Gen. Pharmac.*, **12**, 177 (1981)
Conformation of reverse ester of acetylcholine.
BARONE, V., LELJ, F., RUSSO, N. and GEMELLI, M. L. *Gazz. chim. ital.*, **111**, 75 (1981)
Conformational analysis of phosphonium and arsonium acetylcholine.

Noradrenaline

KIER, L. B. *J. Pharm. Pharmac.*, **21**, 93 (1969)
EHT calculation.
PEDERSEN, L. HOSKINS, R. E. and CABLE, H. *J. Pharm. Pharmac.*, **23**, 216 (1971)
INDO calculation of conformation.
PULLMAN, B., COUBEILS, J. L., COURRIÈRE, P. and GEROIS, J. P. *J. med. Chem.*, **15**, 17 (1972)
PCILO conformation study.
KATZ, R., HELLER, S. R. and JACOBSON, A. E. *Molec. Pharmacol.*, **9**, 486 (1973)
CNDO study of conformation of protonated species. Structure-activity relationships.
PULLMAN, B. and COURRIÈRE, P. in 'Conformation of biological molecules and polymers', E. D. Bergmann and B. Pullman (eds), *Proc. 5th Jerusalem Symposium on Quantum Chemistry and Biochemistry*, Academic Press, New York, p. 547 (1973)
PCILO conformational potential energy map.
KATZ, R., HELLER, S. R. and JACOBSON, A. E. *Molec. Pharmac.*, **9**, 486 (1973)
Structure–activity study using CNDO and INDO.

PULLMAN, B., BERTHOD, H. and COURRIÈRE, P. *Int. J. Quantum Chem. Quantum Biology Symp.*, **1**, 93 (1974)
  PCILO and *ab initio* calculations including solvation.
RICHARDS, W. G., ASCHMAN, D. G. and HAMMOND, J. *J. theoret. Biol.*, **52**, 223 (1975)
  EHT study of conformational flexibility, including methylated compounds.

Related compounds

KANG, S., OLSEN, J. F. and HAMONN, J. R. *J. theoret. Biol.*, **28**, 195 (1970)
  Phenylalanine studied by CNDO.
GEORGE, J. M., KIER, L. B. and HOYLAND, J. R. *Molec. Pharmac.*, **7**, 328 (1971)
  EHT study of isoprenaline.
COUBEILS, J. L., COURRIÈRE, P. and PULLMAN, B. *J. med. Chem.*, **15**, 453 (1972)
  PCILO conformational study of sympatholytics.
PULLMAN, B., COUBEILS, J. L., COURRIÈRE, P. and GERVOIS, J. P. *J. med. Chem.*, **15**, 17 (1972)
  PCILO study of isoprenaline.
PULLMAN, B. and COURRIÈRE, P. in 'Conformation of biological molecules and polymers', E. D. Bergmann and B. Pullman (eds), *Proc. 5th Jerusalem Symposium on Quantum Chemistry and Biochemistry*, Academic Press, New York, p. 547 (1973)
  PCILO conformational potential energy map for Iproniazid—an MAO inhibitor.
NEBON, S. D., KOLLMAN, P. A. and TRAGER, W. F. *J. med. Chem.*, **16**, 1034 (1973)
  CNDO study of amine oxidase intermediates.
PULLMAN, B., BERTHOD, H. and COURRIÈRE, P. *Int. J. Quantum Chem. Quantum Biology Symp.*, **1**, 93 (1974)
  PCILO and *ab initio* calculations, including solvation, on isoprenaline.
GERMER, H. A. *J. Pharm. Pharmac.*, **26**, 799 (1974)
  MO study of tissue selectivity in β-blockers.
RICHARDS, W. G., CLARKSON, R. and GANELLIN, C. R. *Phil. Trans. R. Soc. B*, **272**, 75 (1975)
  Phenoxypropanolamine β-agonism related to conformation.
HÖLTJE, H. D. *Arch. Pharm.*, **308**, 438 (1975)
  Theoretical structure–activity relationship for monoamineoxidase inhibitors.

Adrenaline

GEORGE, J. M., KIER, L. B. and HOYLAND, J. R. *Molec. Pharmac.*, **7**, 328 (1971)
  EHT calculation.
PULLMAN, B., COUBEILS, J. L., COURRIÈRE, P. and GERVOIS, J. P. *J. med. Chem.*, **15**, 17 (1972)
  PCILO conformational study.
PULLMAN, B., BERTHOD, H. and COURRIÈRE, P. *Int. J. Quantum Chem. Quantum Biology Symp.*, **1**, 93 (1974)
  PCILO and *ab initio* calculations including solvation.
RICHARDS, W. G., ASCHMAN, D. G. and HAMMOND, J. *J. theoret. Biol.*, **52**, 223 (1975)
  EHT study of flexibility including methylated compounds.
SHINAGAWA, Y. and SHINAGAWA, Y. *J. Am. chem. Soc.*, **100**, 67 (1978)
  INDO calculation.
SOLMAJAR, T., KOCJAN, D. and HADZI, D. *Int. J. Quantum. Chem.*, **20**, 1225 (1981)
  Interaction of catecholamine with an anion.

Related compounds

PATIL, P. N., MILLER, D. D. and TRINDELE, U. *Pharm. Rev.*, **26**, 323 (1974)
  Extensive bibliography on adrenergic drug activity.
PETRONGOLO, C. and TOMASI, J. *J. med. Chem.*, **17**, 501 (1974)
  Conformation and reactivity of isoproterenol; electrostatic molecular potential.

Norephedrine, ephedrine and pseudo-ephedrine

KIER, L. B. *J. Pharmac. exp. Ther.*, **164**, 75 (1968)
EHT conformational study.
PULLMAN, B., COUBEILS, J. L., COURRIÈRE, P. and GERVOIS, J. P. *J. med. Chem.*,
15, 17 (1972)
PCILO conformational map.
PULLMAN, B. and COURRIÈRE, P. in 'Conformation of biological molecules and polymers',
E. D. Bergmann and B. Pullman (eds), *Proc. 5th Jerusalem Symposium on Quantum Chemistry
and Biochemistry*, Academic Press, New York, p. 547 (1973)
PCILO conformational potential energy map.
PULLMAN, B., BERTHOD, H. and COURRIÈRE, P. *Int. J. Quantum Chem. Quantum
Biology Symp.*, **1**, 93 (1974)
PCILO and *ab initio* calculations including solvation.

Phenylethylamine

KIER, L. B. *J. Pharmac. exp. Ther.*, **164**, 75 (1968)
EHT conformational study.
PULLMAN, B., COUBEILS, J. L., COURRIÈRE, P. and GERVOIS, J. P. *J. med. Chem.*,
15, 17 (1972)
PCILO conformational map.
KATZ, R. and JACOBSON, A. E. *Molec. Pharmac.*, **9**, 495 (1973)
Polyhydroxyphenylethylamines studied by CNDO.
WEINTRAUB, H. J. R. and HOPFINGER, A. J. *J. theoret. Biol.*, **41**, 53 (1973)
Empirical potential calculation including solvent.
PULLMAN, B. and COURRIÈRE, P. in 'Conformation of biological molecules and polymers',
E. D. Bergmann and B. Pullman (eds), *Proc. 5th Jerusalem Symposium on Quantum Chemistry
and Biochemistry*, Academic Press, New York, p. 547 (1973)
PCILO conformational potential energy map; includes amphetamine.
PULLMAN, B., BERTHOD, H. and COURRIÈRE, P. *Int. J. Quantum Chem. Quantum Biology
Symp.*, **1**, 93 (1974)
PCILO and *ab initio* calculations including solvation; includes amphetamine.
HALL, G. G., MILLAR, C. J. and SCHNUELLE, G. W. *J. theoret. Biol.*, **53**, 475 (1975)
Ab initio conformational energies.
MARTIN, M., CARBO, R., PETRONGOLO, C. and TOMASI, J. *J. Am. chem. Soc.*, **97**,
1338 (1975)
Structure–activity relationships; comparison of *ab initio* and semi-empirical calculations.
DOMELSMITH, L. N., MUNCHAUSEN, L. L. and HOUK, K. N. *J. Am. chem. Soc.*, **99**,
4311 (1977)
Photoelectron spectrum of phenylethylamine.
LAI, A., MONDUZZI, M. and SABA, G. *J. chem. Soc. Faraday Trans. II.*, **77**, 227 (1981)
CNDO studies and n.m.r. on biogenic amines.

Adrenergic compounds

PETRONGOLO, C., MACCHIA, B., MACCHIA, F. and MARTINELLI, A. *Chim. Ind.
(Milan)*, **58**, 520 (1976)
Conformation of 1-isopropylamino-3-(2-hydroxy)-2-propranol.
PETRONGOLO, C., MACCHIA, B., MACCHIA, F. and MARTINELLI, A. *J. med. Chem.*,
20, 1645 (1977)
Study of β-adrenergic compounds.
PETRONGOLO, C., MACCHIA, B., MACCHIA, F. and MARTINELLI, A. *J. med. Chem.*,
20, 1645 (1977)
Explanation of the aromatic moity in β-adrenergics.
MARTIN, M. L. and HERNANDEZ, J. A. *Afinidad*, **35**, 187 (1978)
Hypothesis on nature of β-adrenergic receptor.

GADRET, M., LEGAR, J. M., CARPY, A. and BERTHOD, H. *Eur. J. med. Chem.*, **13**, 367 (1978)
Conformation of aryloxypropanolamines.
ANDERSON, G. M., CASTAGNOLI, N. and KOLLMAN, P. A. *Natn. Inst. Drug Abuse Res. Monogr. Ser.*, **23**, 199 (1978)
2,4,5-ring substituted phenylisopropylamines.
KULKARNI, V. M., VASANTHKUMAR, N., SARAN, A. and GOVIL, G. *Int. J. Quantum Chem. Quantum Biol. Symp.*, **6**, 153 (1977)
Conformation of propranolol.
MACCHIA, B., MACCHIA, F. and MARTINELLI, A. *Eur. J. med. Chem.*, **15**, 515 (1980)
Adrenergic reactivity of Fazolol.
de JONG, A. P. and van DAM, H. *J. med. Chem.*, **23**, 889 (1980)
Electronic structure of clonidine and related molecules.
SCHARFENBERG, P. and SAUER, J. *Int. J. Quantum Chem.*, **18**, 1309 (1980)
Biological response as a function of conformation for adrenergic compounds.
DAVIES, R. H. and SMITH, L. H. *Int. J. Quantum Chem. Quantum Biol. Symp.*, **7**, 331 (1980)
β-blockers and competitive conformer–receptor occupancy.
DE, A. U. and GHOSE, A. K. *Indian J. Chem.*, **20B**, 58 (1981)
Exploration of adrenergic receptor through potentials.
MOTOHASHI, M. and NISHIKAWA, N. *Molec. Pharmac.*, **20**, 22 (1981)
Conformation of β-2 adrenergic agents.

Histamine

GREEN, J. P. *Histamine Club Symp. Federation Proc.*, **26**, 211 (1967)
Hückel parameters for imidazoles.
KIER, L. B. *J. med. Chem.*, **11**, 441 (1968)
EHT calculation.
PERITI , P. F. *Pharmac. Res. Commun.*, **2**, 309 (1970)
Empirical potential.
COUBEILS, J. L., COURRIÈRE, P. and PULLMAN, B. *C. r. hebd. Séanc. Acad. Sci., Paris*, **272**, 1813 (1971)
PCILO calculation.
MARGOLIS, S., KANG, S. and GREEN, J. P. *Int. J. clin. Pharmacol. ther. Tox.*, **5**, 279 (1971)
INDO calculation.
GANELLIN, C. R., PEPPER, E. S., PORT, G. N. J. and RICHARDS, W. G. *J. med. Chem.*, **16**, 610 (1973)
EHT results compared with NMR.
GANELLIN, C. R., PORT, G. N. J. and RICHARDS, W. G. *J. med. Chem.*, **16**, 616 (1973)
Conformational preferences of methyl substituted compounds.
GANELLIN, C. R. *J. med. Chem.*, **16**, 620 (1973)
Model conformational study.
GANELLIN, C. R., PORT, G. N. J. and RICHARDS, W. G. in 'Conformation of biological molecules and polymers', E. D. Bergmann and B. Pullman (eds), *Proc. 5th Jerusalem Symposium on Quantum Chemistry and Biochemistry*, Academic Press, New York, p. 579 (1973)
Conformer population of substituted compounds.
PULLMAN, B. and PORT, G. N. J. *Molec. Pharmac.*, **10**, 360 (1974)
Effect of solvent on conformation.
FARNELL, L., RICHARDS, W. G. and GANELLIN, C. R. *J. theoret. Biol.*, **43**, 389 (1974)
Conformational free energies.
PULLMAN, A. in R. Daudel and B. Pullman (eds), *The World of Quantum Chemistry*, D. Reidel, Dordrecht, p. 239 (1974)
Effect of hydration.
PULLMAN, B. in 'Molecular and quantum pharmacology', E. D. Bergmann and B. Pullman (eds), *Proc. 7th Jerusalem Symposium on Quantum Chemistry and Biochemistry*, D. Reidel, Dordrecht, p. 9 (1974)
Effect of solvent.
KUMBAR, M. *J. theoret. Biol.*, **53**, 333 (1975)
Empirical potential study of conformation.

ABRAHAM, R. J. and BIRCH, D. *Molec. Pharmac.*, **11**, 663 (1975)
Use of a counter ion in CNDO conformational calculation.
RICHARDS, W. G., CLARKSON, R. and GANELLIN, C. R. *Phil. Trans. R. Soc. B*, **272**, 75 (1975)
Conformational requirements to bind to receptor.
FARNELL, L., RICHARDS, W. G. and GANELLIN, C. R. *J. med. Chem.*, **18**, 662 (1975)
Definition of essential conformation for activity by comparative study.
RICHARDS, W. G., HAMMOND, J. and ASCHMAN, D. G. *J. theoret. Biol.*, **51**, 237 (1975)
Barriers to rotation in histamine and 4-methylhistamine by *ab initio* calculation.
RICHARDS, W. G., ASCHMAN, D. G. and HAMMOND, J. *J. theoret. Biol.*, **52**, 223 (1975)
Conformational flexibility of methyl substituted compounds.
KANG, S. and CHOU, D. *Chem. Phys. Letters*, **34**, 537 (1975)
Tautomerism studied by INDO and *ab initio* calculations.
ABRAHAM, R. J. in 'Environmental effects on molecular structure and properties', B. Pullman (ed.), *Proc. 9th Jerusalem Symposium on Quantum Chemistry and Biochemistry*, D. Reidel, Dordrecht, p. 41 (1976)
Solvent effect on conformation.
WEINSTEIN, H., CHOU, D., JOHNSON, C. L., KANG, S. and GREEN, J. P. *Molec. Pharmac.*, **12**, 738 (1976)
Tautomerism and receptor action: molecular potential fields given.
RICHARDS, W. G. and WALLIS, J. *J. med. Chem.*, **19**, 1250 (1976)
Charge distribution of essential conformation for H1 activity.

Related compounds

MURPHEY, M. F., HAARSTAD, V. B. and HAHN, F. B. *Int. J. Quantum Chem. Quantum Biology Symp.*, **1**, 149 (1974)
Mast cell zinc–histamine complex studied by IEHT.
PULLMAN, B., COURRIÈRE, P. and BERTHOD, H. *Molec. Pharmac.*, **11**, 268 (1975)
Conformational properties of antihistamine drugs; ethylene diamine and pheniramine derivatives.
DEFINA, J. A. and VAUGHAN, G. N. *Aust. J. pharm. Sci.*, **6**, 15 (1977)
Study of histamine isosteres.
RICHARDS, W. G., WALLIS, J. and GANELLIN, C. R. *Eur. J. med. Chem.*, **14**, 9 (1979)
Tautomer preference for histamine.
AKHREM, A. A., GOLUHOVICH, V. P. and GALAKTIONOV, S. G. *Dokl. Akad. Nauk. USSR*, **23**, 753 (1979)
Calculation of stable conformations.
XIAO-YUAN, F. and SHU-JUN, S. *Int. J. Quantum Chem. Quantum Biol. Symp.*, **8**, 197 (1981)
Correlation of energy of tautomerization with activity.

Dopamine

KIER, L. B. and TRUITT, E. B. *J. Pharmacol. exp. Ther.*, **174**, 94 (1970)
EHT calculation.
BUSTARD, T. M. and EGAN, R. S. *Tetrahedron*, **27**, 4457 (1971)
Conformation derived from EHT and NMR compared.
PULLMAN, B., COUBEILS, J. L., COURRIÈRE, P. and GERVOIS, J. P. *J. med. Chem.*, **15**, 17 (1972)
REKKER, R. F., ENGEL, D. J. C. and NYS, G. G. *J. Pharm. Pharmac.*, **24**, 589 (1972)
Dopamine–apomorphine comparison.
KIER, L. B. *J. theoret. Biol.*, **40**, 211 (1973)
EHT conformational study.
PULLMAN, B. and COURRIÈRE, P. in 'Conformation of biological molecules and polymers', E. D. Bergmann and B. Pullman (eds), *Proc. 5th Jerusalem Symposium on Quantum Chemistry and Biochemistry*, Academic Press, New York, p. 547 (1973)
PCILO conformational potential energy map.

PULLMAN, B., BERTHOD, H. and COURRIÈRE, P. *Int. J. Quantum Chem. Quantum Biol. Symp.*, **1**, 93 (1974)
  PCILO and *ab initio* calculations including solvation.
RICHARDS, W. G., ASCHMAN, D. G. and HAMMOND, J. *J. theoret. Biol.*, **52**, 223 (1975)
  Conformational flexibility of methyl substituted compounds.
GROL, C. J. and ROLLEMA, H. *J. Pharm. Pharmac.*, **29**, 153 (1977)
  INDO conformational study.
GUHA, S. *J. Indian chem. Soc.*, **54**, 551 (1977)

Related compounds

KUMBAR, M. and SANKAR, D. V. *Res. Commun. Chem. Pathol. Pharmac.*, **4**, 707 (1972)
  Quantum chemical study of inhibition of synoptosome dopamine uptake by antihistaminic pheniramines.
KATZ, R. and JACOBSON, A. E. *Molec. Pharmac.*, **9**, 495 (1973)
  CNDO calculation on 6-hydroxydopamine.

Serotonin

KIER, L. B. *J. pharm. Sci.*, **57**, 1188 (1968)
  EHT calculation.
COURRIÈRE, P., COUBEILS, J. L. and PULLMAN, B. *C. r. hebd. Séanc. Acad. Sci., Paris*, **272**, 1697 (1971)
  PCILO calculation.
KANG, S. and CHO, M. H. *Theoret. chim. Acta*, **22**, 176 (1971)
  INDO calculation.
KANG, S., JOHNSON, C. L. and GREEN, J. P. *J. molec. Struct.*, **15**, 453 (1973)
  EHT and empirical conformational map.
KIER, L. B. *J. theoret. Biol.*, **40**, 24 (1973)
  EHT conformational study.
JOHNSON, C. L., KANG, S. and GREEN, J. P. in 'Conformation of biological molecules and polymers', E. D. Bergmann and B. Pullman (eds), *Proc. 5th Jerusalem Symposium on Quantum Chemistry and Biochemistry*, Academic Press, New York, p. 547 (1973)
  Conformational analysis by combined classical and MO methods.
PULLMAN, B. and COURRIÈRE, P. in 'Conformation of biological molecules and polymers', E. D. Bergmann and B. Pullman (eds), *Proc. 5th Jerusalem Symposium on Quantum Chemistry and Biochemistry*, Academic Press, New York, p. 547 (1973)
  PCILO conformational potential energy map.
PULLMAN, B. in 'Molecular and quantum pharmacology', E. D. Bergmann and B. Pullman (eds), *Proc. 7th Jerusalem Symposium on Quantum Chemistry and Biochemistry*, D. Reidel, Dordrecht, p. 9 (1974)
  Effect of solvent.
PORT, G. N. J. and PULLMAN, B. *Theoret. chim. Acta*, **33**, 275 (1974)
  Ab initio calculation.
PULLMAN, B., COURRIÈRE, P. and BERTHOD, H. *J. med. Chem.*, **17**, 439 (1974)
  Isolated and solvated molecule by PCILO.
RICHARDS, W. G., ASCHMAN, D. G. and HAMMOND, J. *J. theoret. Biol.*, **52**, 223 (1975)
  Conformational preferences of methyl substituted compounds.
KUMBAR, M. and SANKAR, D. V. *Res. Commun. Chemotherap.*, **10**, 433 (1975)
  Preferred conformations in relation to receptor sites.

Related compounds

KANG, S. and GREEN, J. P. *Nature, Lond.*, **222**, 794 (1969)
  Indolealkylamines; resonance constants correlate with activity.
GREEN, J. P. and KANG. S. in L. B. Kier (ed), *Molecular Orbital Studies in Chemical Pharmacology*, Springer, New York (1970)
  Study of activity.

KUMBAR, M. and SANKAR, D. V. *Res. Commun. chem. Pathol. Pharmac.*, **6**, 65 (1973)
  Correlation of hallucinogenic and anti-serotonin activity of lysergic acid derivatives.
SANKAR, D. V. and KUMBAR, M. *Res. Commun. chem. Pathol. Pharmac.*, **7**, 259 (1974)
  Correlation of substituent structures and anti-serotonin activity.
PULLMAN, B., COURRIÈRE, P. and BERTHOD, H. *J. med. Chem.*, **17**, 439 (1974)
  Indolealkylamines studied by PCILO isolated and solvated.
JOHNSON, C. L. and GREEN, J. P. *Int. J. Quantum Chem. Quantum Biol. Symp.*, **1**, 159 (1974)
  MO studies of tryptamine activities on LSD receptors.
PORT, G. N. J. and PULLMAN, B. *Theoret. chim. Acta*, **33**, 275 (1974)
  Ab initio study of bufotenine cation.
GLENNON, R. A. and GESSNER, P. K. *Pharmacology*, **17**, 259 (1975)
  Correlation of activity of antagonists with quantum mechanical parameters.
KUMBAR, M., CUSIMANO, V. and SANKAR, D. V. S. *J. Pharm. Sci*, **65**, 1014 (1976)
  Uptake inhibition correlated with total energy.
WEINSTEIN, H., CHOU, D., KANG, S., JOHNSON, C. L. and GREEN, J. P. *Int. J. Quantum Chem. Quantum Biol. Symp.*, **3**, 135 (1976)
CAILLET, J., CLAVERIE, P. and PULLMAN, B. *Acta crystallogr.*, **A33**, 885 (1977)
  Conformation of serotonin in crystal.
WEINSTEIN, H. and OSMAN, R. *Int. J. Quantum Chem. Quantum Biol. Symp.*, **4**, 253 (1977)
  Serotonin complex with imidazolium cation.
DOMELSMITH, L. N., MUNCHAUSEN, L. L. and HOUK, K. N. *J. Am. chem. Soc.*, **99**, 4311 (1977)
  Photoelectron spectrum of serotonin.
OSMAN, R. and WEINSTEIN, H. *Chem. Phys. Lett.*, **49**, 69 (1977)
  Comparison of *ab initio* and pseudopotential results.
CAILLET, J., CLAVERIE, P. and PULLMAN, B. *Acta. crystallogr.*, **A33**, 885 (1977)
  Conformation of 5-methoxy, N-N dimethyltryptamine.
WEINSTEIN, H., OSMAN, R., EDWARDS, W. D. and GREEN, J. P. *Int. J. Quantum Chem. Quantum Biol. Symp.*, **5**, 449 (1978)
  Tryptamine congeners acting on LSD-serotonin receptor.
WEINSTEIN, H., GREEN, J. P., OSMAN, R. and EDWARDS, W. D. in G. Barnett, M. Trsic, and R. Willette (eds), *QuaSAR Research Monograph*, **22**, National Institute on Drug Abuse (1978)
  Mechanism on LSD/serotonin receptor.
KANG, S., ERNST, L., WEINSTEIN, H. and OSMAN, R. *Molec. Pharmac.*, **16**, 1031 (1979)
  Relation of electronic structure to activity of serotonin congeners.
BALDWIN, S., KIER, L. B. and SHILLADY, D. *Molec. Pharmac.*, **18**, 455 (1980)
  Molecular potential of mescalin and serotonin.
REGGIO, P. H., WEINSTEIN, H., OSMAN, R. and TOPIOL, S. *Int. J. Quantum Chem. Quantum Biol. Symp.*, **8**, 373 (1981)
  Molecular determinants for binding methylenedioxytryptamines at the serotonin–LSD receptor.

GABA (γ amino butyric acid)

KIER, L. B. and TRUITT, E. B. *Experientia*, **26**, 988 (1970)
  EHT conformational study.
KIER, L. B. and GEORGE, J. M. *Experientia*, **29**, 501 (1973)
  EHT calculations.
PARTHASAN, S., DHINGRA, M. M. and GOVIL, G. *Ind. J. Chem.*, **12**, 805 (1974)
  Conformations of amino acids.
KIER, L. B., GEORGE, J. M. and HÖLTJE, H. D. *J. Pharm. Sci.*, **63**, 1435 (1974)
  Structure–activity relationships for GABA-like agents.
PULLMAN, B. and BERTHOD, H. *C. r. hebd. Séanc. Acad. Sci., Paris*, **278**, 1433 (1974)
  PCILO conformational study.

PULLMAN, B. and BERTHOD, H. *Theoret. chim. Acta*, **36**, 317 (1975)
Conformations of isolated and solvated molecules.
WARNER, D., BORTHWICK, P. W. and STEWARD, E. G. *J. molec. Struct.*, **25**, 397 (1975)
CNDO study of electronic structure, conformation and dipole moment.
WARNER, D. and STEWARD, E. G. *J. molec. Struct.*, **25**, 403 (1975)
CNDO conformational study; net atomic populations.
PULLMAN, B. in 'Environmental effects on molecular structure and properties', B. Pullman
(ed), *Proc. 9th Jerusalem Symposium on Quantum Chemistry and Biochemistry*, D. Reidel,
Dordrecht, p. 55 (1976)
Solvent effect.
BORTHWICK, P. W. and STEWARD, E. G. *J. molec. Struct.*, **41**, 253 (1977)
CNDO calculations.
LAMBORELLE, C. and TAPIA, O. *Chem. Phys.*, **42**, 25 (1979)
Solvent effect by virtual charge model.
BLAKO, I. and ORTEGA, L. A. *Int. J. Quantum Chem.*, **19**, 463 (1981)
Mg^{2+} and Ca^{2+} interaction with GABA.

Related compounds

KIER, L. B., GEORGE, J. M. and HÖLTJE, H. D. *J. Pharm. Sci.*, **63**, 1435 (1974)
EHT on GABA-like agents.
WARNER, D., BORTHWICK, P. W. and STEWARD, E. G. *J. molec. Struct.*, **25**, 397
(1975)
4-amino tetrolic acid studied with CNDO.
ANDREWS, P. R. and JOHNSTON, G. A. R. *Biochem. Pharmac.*, **28**, 2697 (1979)
Discussion of agonists and antagonists.
ANDREWS, P. R. and JOHNSTON, G. A. R. *J. theoret. Biol.*, **79**, 263 (1979)
MINDO study of conformation of muscimol.

Central nervous system drugs

Anti-anxiety drugs

ANDREWS, P. R. *J. med. Chem.*, **12**, 761 (1969)
Charge distribution and energy by EHT of barbiturates.
PULLMAN, B. in L. B. Kier (ed), *Molecular Orbital Studies in Chemical Pharmacology*, Springer
Verlag, Berlin, p. 1 (1970)
PCILO calculation on barbiturates.
PULLMAN, B., COUBEILS, J. L. and COURRIÈRE, P. *J. theoret. Biol.*, **35**, 375 (1972)
PCILO conformational study of barbiturates.
ANDREWS, P. R. and JONES, G. P. *Int. J. Quantum Chem. Quantum Biol. Symp.*, **6**, 439
(1979)
Conformational analysis of barbiturates.
JONES, G. P. and ANDREWS, P. R. *J. med. Chem.*, **23**, 444 (1980)
Conformation of convulsant and anticonvulsant barbiturates.

Antipsychotic and anti-anxiety drugs

MALRIEU, J. P. and PULLMAN, B. *Theoret. chim. Acta*, **2**, 293 (1964)
Hückel calculations and spin densities of phenothiazines.
COUBEILS, J. L. and PULLMAN, B. *Theoret. chim. Acta*, **24**, 35 (1972)
Side chain conformations of phenothiazines by PCILO; comparison with X-ray structures.
KAUFMAN, J. J. and KERMAN, E. *Int. J. Quantum Chem.*, **6**, 319 (1972)
CNDO and INDO calculations on chlorpromazine.
PULLMAN, B. and COURRIÈRE, P. in 'Conformation of biological molecules and polymers',
E. D. Bergmann and B. Pullman (eds), *Proc. 5th Jerusalem Symposium on Quantum
Chemistry and Biochemistry*, Academic Press, New York, p. 547 (1973)
PCILO conformational potential energy map.

KIER, L. B. *J. theoret. Biol.*, **40,** 211 (1973)
    EHT conformational study of chlorpromazine.
KAUFMAN, J. J. and KERMAN, E. *Adv. Biochem. Psychopharmac.*, **9,** 55 (1974)
    Calculations on phenothiazines.
KAUFMAN, J. J. and KERMAN, E. in I. S. Forrest, C. J. Karr and E. Usdin (eds),
    Phenothiazines and Structurally Related Drugs, Raven Press, New York (1974)
KAUFMAN, J. J. and KERMAN, E. *Int. J. Quantum Chem. Quantum Biol. Symp.*, **3,** 187 (1976)
    Thioridazine.
KAUFMAN, J. J. and KERMAN, E. *Int. J. Quantum Chem.*, **10,** 559 (1976)
    Conformation using CNDO.
POPKIE, H. E. and KAUFMAN, J. J. *Int. J. Quantum Chem.*, **10,** 569 (1976)
    Ab initio calculation of chlorpromazine and promazine.
DOMELSMITH, L. N., MUNCHAUSEN, L. L. and HOUK, K. N. *J. Am. Chem. Soc.*,
    99, 6506 (1977)
    Photoelectron spectra of phenothiazine and related tranquillizers.
BLAIR, T. and WEBB, G. A. *J. med. Chem.*, **20,** 1206 (1977)
    Structure–activity study of 1,4, benzodiazepin-2-ones.
RIGA, J., VERBIST, J. J., DEGELAEN, J., TOLLENAERE, J. P. and KOCH, M. H. J.
    Molec. Pharmac., **13,** 892 (1977)
    Electron densities of neuroleptic compounds using CNDO.
PETRONGOLO, C., PRESTON, H. J. T. and KAUFMAN, J. J. *Int. J. Quantum Chem.*, **13,**
    457 (1978)
    Electrostatic potentials for chlorpromazine and promazine.
DOMELSMITH, L. N. and HOUK, K. N. *Int. J. Quantum Chem. Quantum Biol. Symp.*, **5,**
    257 (1978)
    Photoelectron spectra and partition coefficients.
VANE, F. M., and BENZ, W. *Org. Mass Spectrom.*, **14,** 233 (1979)
    Rearrangements of ions of benzodiazepin in mass spectrum.
MAHAJAN, S. and SUNDARAM, K. *Physiol. Chem. Phys.*, **13,** 183 (1981)
    Molecular orbitals of tricyclic nuclei and of biogenic amines.

Amphetamine

DOMELSMITH, L. N. and HOUK, K. N. *Int. J. Quantum Chem. Quantum Biol. Symp.*, **5,**
    257 (1978)
    Ionization potentials of substituted amphetamines.
DIPAOLO, T., HALL, L. H. and KIER, L. B. *J. theoret. Biol.*, **71,** 295 (1978)
    Model interaction calculations.
WEINTRAUB, H. J. R. and NICHOLS, D. E. *Int. J. Quantum Chem. Quantum Biol. Symp.*,
    5, 321 (1978)
    Conformational calculation including solvent.
GRUNEWALD, G. L., CRESSE, M. W. and WALTER, D. E. *ACS Symposium* (*Computer-
    assisted drug design*), **112,** 439 (1979)
    Conformationally defined amphetamine analogues.
DOMELSMITH, L. N., EATON, T. A., HOUK, K. N., ANDERSON, G. M., GLENNON,
    R. A., SHULGIN, A. T., CASTAGNOLI, N. and KOLLMAN, P. A. *J. med. Chem.*, **24,**
    1484 (1981)
    Photoelectron spectra and relationship to pharmacological properties.

Psychotropic drugs

KAUFMAN, J. J. and KERMAN, E. *Int. J. Quantum Chem.*, **6,** 319 (1972)
KAUFMAN, J. J. in *Psychopharmacology, Sexual Disorders and Drug Abuse*, North-Holland,
    Amsterdam, London (1973)
KAUFMAN, J. J. and KERMAN, E. in 'Chemical and biochemical reactivity', E. D. Berg-
    mann and B. Pullman (eds), *Proc. 6th Jerusalem Symposium on Quantum Chemistry and
    Biochemistry*, Academic Press, New York, p. 523 (1974)
KAUFMAN, J. J. and KERMAN, E. *Int. J. Quantum Chem. Quantum Biology Symp.*, **1,** 259
    (1974)
    CNDO and INDO prediction of a new class of neuroleptics.

KAUFMAN, J. J. and KOSKI, W. S. *J. Pharmac.*, **5**, 49 (1974)
KAUFMAN, J. J. *Cancer Chemother. Rep. Suppl.*, **4**, 49 (1974)
KAUFMAN, J. J. *Psychopharmac. Bull.*, **11**, 64 (1975)
GREEN, J. P. *Psychopharmac. Bull.*, **11**, 44 (1975)
KAUFMAN, J. J. and KOSKI, W. S. *Int. J. Quantum Chem. Quantum Biol. Symp.*, **2**, 35 (1975)
    CNS agents, narcotics and psychotropic drugs; electron densities; lengthy discussion of
    mechanisms and comparison with experiment.
SNYDER, S. H. and MERRIL, C. R. *Proc. Nat. Acad. Sci. U.S.A.*, **54**, 285 (1965)
    Hückel calculation leads to activity correlation.
KANG, S. and GREEN, J. P. *Proc. Nat. Acad. Sci. U.S.A.*, **67**, 62 (1970)
    INDO calculation of steric and electronic relationships.
KANG, S. and GREEN, J. P. *Nature, Lond.*, **226**, 645 (1970)
    Correlation of activity with orbital energy.
ARCHER, R. A., BOYD, D. B., DEMARCO, P. V., TYMINSKI, I. J. and ALLINGER, N. L.
    J. Am. chem. Soc., **92**, 5200 (1970)
    EHT on marijuana constituents.
GREEN, J. P. and KANG, S. in L. B. Kier (ed), *Molecular Orbital Studies in Chemical
    Pharmacology*, Springer, New York (1970)
COURRIÈRE, P., COUBEILS, J. L. and PULLMAN, B. *C. r. hebd. Séanc. Acad. Sci., Paris*,
    272D, 1697 (1971)
    PCILO calculation.
GREEN, J. P., DRESSLER, K. P. and KHAZAN, N. *Life Sciences*, **12**, 475 (1973)
    Mescalin-like activity.
JOHNSON, C. L., KANG, S. and GREEN, J. P. in 'Conformation of biological molecules and
    polymers', E. D. Bergmann and B. Pullman (eds), *Proc. 5th Jerusalem Symposium on Quantum
    Chemistry and Biochemistry*, Academic Press, New York, p. 517 (1973)
    Mescalin and psilocin; comparison with serotonin.
KANG, S., JOHNSON, C. L. and GREEN, J. P. *Molec. Pharmac.*, **9**, 640 (1973)
    INDO and empirical potential study of mescalin and psilocin showing possible congruence
    with LSD.
JOHNSON, C. L. and GREEN, J. P. *Int. J. Quantum Chem. Quantum Biol. Symp.*, **1**, 159 (1974)
    CNDO calculation.
PULLMAN, B., BERTHOD, H. and PULLMAN, A., *An Quím. Farm.*, **70**, 1204 (1974)
    Mescalin and related compounds studied by PCILO.
PULLMAN, B., COURRIÈRE, P. and BERTHOD, H. *J. med. Chem.*, **17**, 439 (1974)
    PCILO study of conformation and solvent effects.
KANG, S., JOHNSON, C. L. and GREEN, J. P. *J. molec. Struct.*, **15**, 453 (1977)
    INDO calculation.
LARA, O. F., OMANA, P. F. V. and CETINA, R. *Revta Soc. quim. Méx.*, **23**, 77 (1979)
    Indole hallucinogens.

Anti-epileptic compounds

ANDREWS, P. R. *J. med. Chem.*, **12**, 761 (1969)
    EHT and CNDO energy and charge distribution of anti-convulsants.
ALDRICH, H. S. and KIER, L. B. in 'Molecular and quantum pharmacology', E. D.
    Bergmann and B. Pullman (eds), *Proc. 7th Jerusalem Symposium on Quantum Chemistry and
    Biochemistry*, D. Reidel, Dordrecht, p. 229 (1974)
    CNDO calculations show anti-epileptic agents can mimic conformations of GABA.
WEINTRAUB, H. J. R. *Int. J. Quantum Chem. Quantum Biol. Symp.*, **4**, 111 (1977)
    Solvent-dependent energy calculations on succinimides.
ANDREWS, P. R. and DEFINA, J. A. *Int. J. Quantum Chem. Quantum Biol. Symp.*, **7**, 297
    (1980)
    Stereochemistry and electronic structure.
TAMIR, I., MECHOULAM, R. and MEYER, A. Y. *J. med. Chem.*, **23**, 220 (1980)
    Structural comparison of cannabidiol and phenytoin.

Analgesics

KAUFMAN, J. J. and KERMAN, E. *Int. J. Quantum Chem.*, **6**, 319 (1972)

KAUFMAN, J. J. and KERMAN, E. *Int. J. Quantum Chem. Symp.*, **6,** 319 (1973)
CNDO, INDO and PCILO on morphine activity.
UMEGAMA, H. *Chem. pharm. Bull. Tokyo.*, **22,** 2518 (1974)
KAUFMAN, J. J., KERMAN, E. and KOSKI, W. S. *Int. J. Quantum Chem. Quantum Biol. Symp.*, **1,** 289 (1974)
CNDO, INDO and empirical potential computations.
CAPPOREL, A. L., MARANON, J., SORARRAL, O. M. and FILGUEIR, R. R. *J. molec. Struct.*, **23,** 145 (1974)
Morpholine: CNDO and INDO studies.
LOEW, G. H., BERKOWITZ, D., WEINSTEIN, H. and SREBRENIK, S. in 'Molecular and quantum pharmacology', E. D. Bergmann and B. Pullman (eds), *Proc. 7th Jerusalem Symposium on Quantum Chemistry and Biochemistry*, D. Reidel, Dordrecht, p. 355 (1974)
Morphine compounds including interaction potentials.
LOEW, G. H. and BERKOWITZ, D. S. *J. med. Chem.*, **18,** 656 (1975)
Effects of N substituent variations in morphine opiates.
LOEW, G. H., JESTER, J. R., BERKOWITZ, D. S. and NEWTH, R. C. *Int. J. Quantum Chem. Symp.*, **2,** 25 (1975)
PCILO conformation and charge density on methadone, meperidine and prodines.
LOEW, G. H. and JESTER, J. R. *J. med. Chem.*, **18,** 1051 (1975)
Electronic distribution and conformational energy of meperidine and prodine.
LOEW, G. H., BERKOWITZ, D. S. and NEWTH, R. C. *J. med. Chem.*, **19,** 863 (1976)
Methadone using PCILO.
LOEW, G. H., WEINSTEIN, H. and BERKOWITZ, D. S. in B. Pullman (ed), *Environmental Effects on Molecular Structure and Properties*, D. Reidel, Dordrecht (1976)
POPKIE, H. E., KOSKI, W. S. and KAUFMAN, J. J. *J. Am. chem. Soc.*, **98,** 1342 (1976)
Morphine and nalorpine including photoelectron spectra.
KAUFMAN, J. J. and KERMAN, E. *Int. J. Quantum Chem.*, **11,** 181 (1977)
PCILO conformational study of nalorpine.
BARNETT, G., TRSIC, M. and WILLETTE, R. (eds) *QuaSAR Research Monograph*, **22,** National Institute on Drug Abuse (1978)
Several papers both on methodology and specific compounds.
CHENEY, B. V., DUCHAMP, D. J. and CHRISTOFFERSEN, R. E. in G. Barnett, M. Trsic and R. Willette (eds), *QuaSAR Research Monograph*, **22,** 218, National Institute on Drug Abuse (1978)
Assessment of quantum mechanical calculations.
KAUFMAN, J. J. in G. Barnett, M. Trsic and R. Willette (eds), *QuaSAR Research Monograph*, **22,** 250, National Institute on Drug Abuse (1978)
LOEW, G. H., BERKOWITZ, D. S. and BURT, S. K. in G. Barnett, M. Trsic and R. Willette (eds), *QuaSAR Research Monograph*, **22,** 278, National Institute on Drug Abuse (1978)
Structure–activity studies of narcotic agonists and antagonists.
LOEW, G. H. and BERKOWITZ, D. S. *J. med. Chem.*, **21,** 101 (1978)
N-substituent variation in the oxymorphone series.
De GRAW, J. I., LAWSON, J. A., CRASE, J. L., JOHNSON, H. L., ELLIS, M., UYENO, E. T., LOEW, G. H. and BERKOWITZ, D. S. *J. med. Chem.*, **21,** 415 (1978)
N-alkyl normorphines; conformation.
BREON, T. L., PETERSEN, H., PARUTA, A. N. *J. Pharm. Sci.*, **67,** 73 (1978)
Isoelectrostatic potentials.
LOEW, G. H., BURT, S., NOMURA, P. and MACELROY, R. in E. C. Olson and R. E. Christoffersen (eds), *Computer Assisted Drug Design*, American Chem. Soc., Washington (1979)
Interaction of model receptor with opiates.
KLASNIC, L., RUSCIC, B., SABLJIC, A. and TRINAJSTIC, N. *J. Am. chem. Soc.*, **101,** 7477 (1979)
Photoelectron spectra of narcotics.
RANDIC, M. and WILKINS, C. L. *Int. J. Quantum Chem. Quantum Biol. Symp.*, **6,** 55 (1979)
Graph theory study of benzomorphans.
LOEW, G. H. and BERKOWITZ, D. S. *J. med. Chem.*, **21,** (1978)
Conformation of N-derivatives of oxymorphone.
LOEW, G. H. and BERKOWITZ, D. S. *J. med. Chem.*, **22,** 603 (1979)
Intramolecular hydrogen bonding and conformation of thebaine and oripavine opiate narcotic agonists and antagonists.

AGRESTI, A., BUFFONI, F., KAUFMAN, J. J. and PETRONGOLO, C. *Molec. Pharmac.*, **18,** 461 (1980)
Electrostatic potentials of eseroline and morphine and interaction with water.
RAZZAK, K. S. A. and HAMID, K. A. *J. Pharm. Sci.*, **69,** 769 (1980)
The analgesic aryl moity: prodine analogues.
BURT, S. K., LOEW, G. H. and HASHIMOTO, G. M. *Ann. N. Y. Acad. Sci.*, **367,** 219 (1981)
LOWREY, A. H., HARIHARAN, P. C. and KAUFMAN, J. J. *Int. J. Quantum Chem. Quantum Biol. Symp.*, **8,** 149 (1981)
Conformation and isopotential maps.
CHENEY, B. V. and ZICHI, D. A. *Int. J. Quantum Chem. Quantum Biol. Symp.*, **8,** 201 (1981)
Effects of N-protonation on morphine and naloxone.

Anaesthetics

COUBEILS, J. L. and PULLMAN, B. *Molec. Pharmac.*, **8,** 278 (1972)
Conformational properties of esters and lidocaine by PCILO.
PULLMAN, B. and COURRIÈRE, P. *Theoret. chim. Acta*, **31,** 19 (1973)
Structure–activity relationships on choline derivatives.
LOEW, G. H., TRUDELL, J. and MOTULSKY, H. *Molec. Pharmac.*, **9,** 152 (1973)
General anaesthetics; IEHT conformational study.
LOEW, G. H., MOTULSKY, H., TRUDELL, J., COHEN, E. and HJELMELAND, L. *Molec. Pharmac.*, **10,** 406 (1974)
EHT and PCILO study of metabolism of inhalation anaesthetics.
LIN, T. K. *J. med. Chem.*, **17,** 151 (1974)
Quantum statistical calculation of structure activity.
DAVIES, R. H., MASON, R. C., SMITH, D. A., McNEILLIE, D. J. and JAMES, R. *Int. J. Quantum Chem. Quantum Biol. Symp.*, **5,** 221 (1978)
Hydrogen bond, proton acceptor properties of anaesthetics.
REMKO, M. and CIZMARIK, J. *Eur. J. med. Chem.*, **15,** 556 (1980)
PCILO study of model of heptacaine.

Prostaglandins

HOYLAND, J. R. and KIER, L. B. *J. med. Chem.*, **15,** 84 (1972)
Empirical EHT calculation.
RYAN, J. A., HOVIS, F., SPANGLER, D., HYLTON, J. and CHRISTOFFERSEN, R. E. in 'Molecular and quantum pharmacology', E. D. Bergmann and B. Pullman (eds), *Proc. 7th Jerusalem Symposium on Quantum Chemistry and Biochemistry*, D. Reidel, Dordrecht, p. 319 (1974)
Ab initio fragment calculation.
GUND, P. and SHEN, T. Y. *J. med. Chem.*, **20,** 1146 (1977)
RUSU, I., MEDESAN, A., GRIGORAS, S., MOLDOVEAUNU, S. and PAUSESCU, E. *Rev. Roum. Biochem.*, **16,** 321 (1979)
Theoretical structure–activity study of some prostaglandin molecules.
KOTHEKA, V. and DUTTA, S. *Int. J. Quantum Chem.*, **15,** 481 (1979)
Conformation of PGF2. alpha.
KUTHAN, J., BOHM, S. and MOSTECKY, J. *Colln Czech, chem. Commun Engl. Edn*, **45,** 2199 (1980)
Prediction of relative stabilities of intermediates.
GRIGORAS, S., RUSU, I., PAUSESCU, E., MEDESAN, A. and MOLDOVEANU, S. *Int. J. Quantum Chem.*, **18,** 501 (1980)
Hydrophile–hydrophobe interaction of some prostaglandins by CNDO.
KOTHEKAR, V. and DUTTA, S. *Int. J. Quantum Chem.*, **18,** 891 (1980)
Conformation of PGA1 and role of Ca^{2+} in abortifacient action.
KOTHEKAR, V. *Int. J. Quantum Chem.*, **20,** 167 (1981)
Charge distribution in prostaglandins.

Hormones

KIER, L. B. *J. med. Chem.*, **11**, 915 (1968)
Oxopregnane, preferred conformation of model compound.
HERMANN, R. B., CULP, H. W., McMAHON, R. G. and MARSH, M. M. *J. med. Chem.*, **12**, 749 (1969)
Acetophenones; EHT on substrates for rabbit kidney reductase.
KIER, L. B. and HOYLAND, J. R. *J. med. Chem.*, **13**, 1182 (1970)
Conformational influence of halogens on trihalothyronine.
CAILLET, J. and PULLMAN, B. *Theoret. chim. Acta*, **17**, 377 (1970)
PCILO on sterane.
GALE, M. N. and SAUNDERS, L. *Biochim. biophys. Acta*, **248**, 466 (1971)
Steroid polarities by CNDO.
CAMERMAN, N. and CAMERMAN, A. *Science, N.Y.*, **175**, 764 (1972)
Triiodothyronine; EHT and crystal structure.
KIER, L. B. and GEORGE, J. M. *J. med. Chem.*, **15**, 384 (1972)
Gastrin tetrapeptide.
KOLLMAN, P. A., GIANNINI, D. D., DUAX, W. L., ROTHENBERG, S. and WOLFF, M. E. *J. Am. chem. Soc.*, **95**, 2869 (1973)
CNDO on cortisol.
KOLLMAN, P., MURRAY, W. J., NUSS, M. E., JORGENSEN, E. C. and ROTHENBERG, S. *J. Am. chem. Soc.*, **95**, 8518 (1973)
Thyroxine analogues; CNDO extended for halogen atoms.
GOUDARD, L. and OZIAS, Y. *C. r. hebd. Séanc. Acad. Sci., Paris*, **276**, 2085 (1973)
Anti-thyroid drugs.
GEORGE, J. M. and KIER, L. B. *J. theoret. Biol.*, **46**, 111 (1974)
Angiotensin conformational study using EHT.
MOMANY, F. *J. Am. chem. Soc.*, **98**, 2990 (1976)
Empirical calculation on decapeptide (LHRH).
MOMANY, F. *J. Am. chem. Soc.*, **98**, 2996 (1976)
Empirical calculation on peptides.
DIETRICH, S. W., BOLGER, M. B., KOLLMAN, P. and JORGENSEN, E. C. *J. med. Chem.*, **20**, 863 (1977)
Structure activity of thyromimetic agents.
LEE, D. L., KOLLMAN, P. A., MARSH, F. J. and WOLFF, M. E. *J. med. Chem.*, **20**, 1139 (1977)
Steroid bonding to progesterone receptors.
MOMANY, F. A. *J. med. Chem.*, **21**, 63 (1978)
Conformation of luteinizing hormone-releasing hormone.
ANDREA, T. A., DIETRICH, S. W., MURRAY, W. J., KOLLMAN, P. and JORGENSEN, E. C. *J. med. Chem.*, **22**, 221 (1979)
Model for thyroid hormone-receptor interactions.

Vitamins

PULLMAN, B., LANGLET, J. and BERTHOD, H. *J. theoret. Biol.*, **23**, 492 (1969)
Vitamin A; cis-trans isomerism.
LANGLET, J., PULLMAN, B. and BERTHOD, H. *J. Chim. phys.*, **67**, 480 (1970)
COURRIÈRE, P. and PULLMAN, B. *C. r. hebd. Séanc. Acad. Sci., Paris*, **273D**, 2674 (1971)
COUBIELS, J., PULLMAN, B. and COURRIÈRE, P. *Biochem. biophys. Res. Commun.*, **44**, 1131 (1971)
LONG, K. R. and GOLDSTEIN, J. H. *Theoret. chim. Acta*, **27**, 75 (1972)
EHT study of conformation of nicotinamide.
MAGGIORA, G. M. *J. theoret. Biol.*, **41**, 523 (1973)
Electronic structure of biotin by CNDO.

JORDAN, F. *J. Am. chem. Soc.*, **96**, 3623 (1974)
    Conformation study of thiamine by EHT and CNDO.
JORDAN, F. *J. Am. chem. Soc.*, **98**, 808 (1976)
    EHT and *ab initio* study of thiamine.
THOMSON, C. *J. molec. Struct.*, **67**, 133 (1980)
    Electronic structures of radicals derived from ascorbic acid and α-hydroxytetronic acid.

Sulphonamides

YONEZAWA, T., MURO, I., KATO, H. and KIMURA, M. *Molec. Pharmac.*, **5**, 446 (1969)
    Sulphonamides by EHT.
GERSON, S. H., WORLEY, S. D., BODOR, N. and KAMINSKI, J. J. *J. med. Chem.*, **21**, 686 (1978)
    Hydrogen-bonding in N-chloramines.
CAVELLIER, J. F. and PERADEJORDI, F. *Eur. J. med. Chem.*, **16**, 241 (1981)
    Conformation of unionized N1-phenylsulfanilamide.
PERADEJORDI, F. and CAVELLIER, J. F. *Eur. J. med. Chem.*, **16**, 247 (1981)
    Conformation of ionized N-phenylsulfanilamides.

Antibiotics

PERADEJORDI, F., MARTIN, A. and CAMMERATA, A. *J. pharm. Sci.*, **60**, 576 (1971)
    Study of tetracycline activity.
PERADEJORDI, F. in *Aspects de la Chimie quantique contemporaine*, CNRS, Paris, p. 261 (1971)
    Tetracycline structure–activity correlation.
BOYD, D. B. *J. Am. chem. Soc.*, **94**, 6513 (1972)
    Cephalosporin and penicillin moieties by EHT.
BOYD, D. B. *J. med. Chem.*, **16**, 1195 (1973)
    EHT structure–activity relationship for penicillin and cephalosporin.
TOPP, W. C. and CHRISTIANSEN, B. G. *J. med. Chem.*, **17**, 342 (1974)
    CNDO study of antibacterial activity.
BOYD, D. B. *J. phys. Chem.*, **78**, 2604 (1974)
    Cephalosporin structure and charge density; EHT and CNDO.
PULLMAN, B. in R. Daudel and B. Pullman (eds), *The World of Quantum Chemistry*, D. Reidel, Dordrecht, p. 61 (1974)
    PCILO conformation study. Penicillin G.
CAESAR, G. P. and GREEN, J. J. *J. med. Chem.*, **17**, 1122 (1974)
    Amino-immino tautomerism in formycin by CNDO.
SHIPMAN, L. L., CHRISTOFFERSEN, R. E. and CHENEY, B. V. *J. med. Chem.*, **17**, 583 (1974)
    Ab initio molecular fragment study of effects of chemical modification in lincomycin.
CHENEY, B. V. *J. med. Chem.*, **17**, 590 (1974)
    Ab initio fragment study of lincomycin, chloramphenicol and erythromycin.
HÖLTJE, H. D. and KIER, L. B. *J. med. Chem.*, **17**, 814 (1974)
    EHT and CNDO study; suggestion of binding site.
CAVELLIER, J. F. and PERADEJORDI, F. *C. r. hebd. Séanc. Acad. Sci., Paris*, **278D**, 1289 (1974)
    EHT and CNDO study.
BOYD, D. B., YEH, C. Y. and RICHARDSON, F. S. *J. Am. chem. Soc.*, **98**, 6100 (1976)
    Optical activity of penicillin nucleus chromophores.
GIESSNER-PRETTRE, C. and PULLMAN, B. *C. r. hebd. Séanc. Acad. Sci., Paris*, **283**, 675 (1976)
    Electrostatic potential of actinomycin.

UGHETTO, G. and WARING, M. J. *Molec. Pharmac.*, **13,** 579 (1977)
  Conformation of echinomycin.
SARAN, A., MITRA, C. K. and PULLMAN, B. *Int. J. Quantum Chem. Quantum Biol. Symp.*, **4,** 43 (1977)
  Conformation of Formycin and showdomycin.
BROWN, R. E., SIMAS, A. M. and BURNS, R. E. *Int. J. Quantum Chem. Quantum Biol. Symp.*, **4,** 357 (1977)
  CNDO calculation on chloramphenicols.
BOYD, D. B. *Int. J. Quantum Chem. Quantum Biol. Symp.*, **4,** 161 (1977)
  MINDO study of β-lactams.
SAMUNI, A. and MEYER, A. Y. *Molec. Pharmac.*, **14,** 704 (1978)
  Conformation of penicillins.
PACK, G. R., LOEW, G. H., YAMABE, S. and MOROKUMA, K. *Int. J. Quantum Chem. Quantum Biol. Symp.*, **5,** 417 (1978)
  The actinomycin–guanine complex.
SUNDARAM, K. and TYAGI, R. S. *Int. J. Quantum Chem.*, **15,** 491 (1979)
  Analogues of valinomycin.
BOYD, D. B. and LUNN, W. H. W. *J. med. Chem.*, **22,** 778 (1979)
  Departure of a leaving group in cephalosporins.
NUSS, M. and KOLLMAN, P. *J. med. Chem.*, **22,** 1517 (1979)
  Electostatic potentials of nucleotides and actinomycin.
SARAN, A. and CHATTERJEE, C. L. *Int. J. Quantum Chem. Quantum Biol. Symp.*, **7,** 123 (1980)
  Conformation of toyocamycin and sangivamycin.
BOYD, D. B., HERRON, D. K., LUNN, W. H. W. and SPITZER, W. A. *J. Am. chem. Soc.*, **102,** 1812 (1980)
  Prediction of β-lactam activities.
DEAN, P. M. and WAKELIN, L. P. G. *Proc. R. Soc. B*, **209,** 472 (1980)
  Actinomycin binding to DNA.
SARAN, A. and PATNAIK, L. N. *Int. J. Quantum Chem.*, **20,** 357 (1981)
  Conformation of cordycepin.
SARAN, A. *Int. J. Quantum Chem.*, **20,** 439 (1981)
  Conformation of nucleoside antibiotics.
CHATTERJEE, C. L. and SARAN, A. *Int. J. Quantum Chem. Quantum Biol. Symp.*, **8,** 129 (1981)
  Conformation of pyrazofurans.
BOYD, D. B. *Ann. N.Y. Acad. Sci.*, **367,** 531 (1981)
  Studies of β-lactam antibiotics.

Antimalarials

SINGER, J. A. and PURCELL, W. P. *J. med. Chem.*, **10,** 754 (1967)
  Hückel calculations.
MARTIN, Y. C., BUSTARD, T. M. and LYNN, K. R. *J. med. Chem.*, **16,** 1089 (1973)
  Activity correlation of antimalarials.
LOEW, G. H. and SAHAKIAN, R. *J. med. Chem.*, **20,** 103 (1977)
  Conformational study of phenanthrene amino alcohols.

Anti-cancer drugs and carcinogens

PULLMAN, B. and PULLMAN, A. *Biochem. biophys. Res. Commun.*, **2,** 239 (1960)
  Anti-tumour activity of pyrazines related to basicity.
COLLIN, R. and PULLMAN, B. *Biochim. biophys. Acta*, **89,** 232 (1964)
  Folic acid reductase inhibitors studied by the Hückel method.

LePÉCQ, J. B., LeBRET, M., GOSSE, C., PAOLETTI, C., CHALVET O. and DAT-XUONG, N. in 'Molecular and quantum pharmacology', E. D. Bergmann and B. Pullman (eds), *Proc. 7th Jerusalem Symposium on Quantum Chemistry and Biochemistry*, D. Reidel, Dordrecht, p. 515 (1974)

CHRISTOFFERSEN, R. E. *Cancer Chemother. Rep. Suppl.*, **4**, 47 (1974)
Ab initio molecular fragment study.

BERGES, J. and PERADEJORDI, F. in 'Molecular and quantum pharmacology', E. D. Bergmann and B. Pullman (eds), *Proc. 7th Jerusalem Symposium on Quantum Chemistry and Biochemistry*, D. Reidel, Dordrecht, p. 549 (1974)
Activity correlation for nitrogen mustards.

SCRIBNER, J. D. *J. Nat. Cancer*, **55**, 1038 (1975)
MO theory in carcinogenesis.

MIYAJI, M., ICHIKAWA, H. and OGATA, M. *Chem. Pharm.*, **23**, 1256 (1975)
MO study of tautomerism of carcinogenic 4-hydroxyamino quinoline-1-oxide.

HALL, G. G. and RODWELL, W. R., *J. theoret. Biol.*, **50**, 107 (1975)
Correlation of electronic structure with carcinogenic activity.

THOMSON, C., PROVAN, D. and CLARK, S. *Int. J. Quantum Chem. Quantum Biol. Symp.*, **4**, 205 (1977)
Intermedials from N-alkylnitrosamines.

POLITZER, P. and DAIKER, K. C. *Int. J. Quantum Chem. Quantum Biol. Symp.*, **4**, 317 (1977)
Comparison of electrostatic potentials of carcinogens.

MARSH, M. M. and JERINA, D. M. *J. med. Chem.*, **21**, 1298 (1978)
Arene oxides as models of carcinogens.

LOEW, G. H., WONG, J., PHILLIPS, J., HJELMELAND, L. and PACK, G. *Cancer Biochem. Biophys.*, **2**, 123 (1978)
Metabolism of benzo(α)pyrene.

DE, A. U. and GHOSHE, A. K. *Indian. J. Chem.*, **16B**, 1104 (1978)
Binding of nitrogen and sulphur mustards to DNA.

KAUFMAN, J. J., POPKIE, H. E., PALOLIKIT, S. and HARIHARAN, P. C. *Int. J. Quantum Chem.*, **14**, 793 (1978)
Benzopyrene and its metabolites.

LAVERY, R., PULLMAN, A. and PULLMAN, B. *Int. J. Quantum Chem. Quantum Biol. Symp.*, **5**, 21 (1978)
Reaction between benzopyrene diol epoxide and guanine.

KAUFMAN, J. J., POPKIE, H. E. and PRESTON, H. J. T. *Int. J. Quantum Chem. Quantum Biol. Symp.*, **5**, 201 (1978)
Ab initio and pseudopotential calculations.

SMITH, I. A. and SEYBOLD, P. G. *Int. J. Quantum Chem. Quantum Biol. Symp.*, **5**, 311 (1978)
Methylbenz[α]anthracenes.

KLOPMAN, G., GRINBERG, H. and HOPFINGER, A. J. *J. theoret. Biol.*, **79**, 355 (1979)
Conformation and carcinogenicity of metabolites of aromatic hydrocarbons.

KAUFMAN, J. J., POPKIE, H. E. and HARIHARAN, P. C. in E. C. Olson and R. I. Christoffersen (eds), *Computer Assisted Drug Design*, American Chem. Soc., Washington (1979)
Ab initio calculations.

LAVERY, R. and PULLMAN, B. *Int. J. Quantum Chem.*, **15**, 271 (1979)
Reactivity of diol epoxides and aromatic hydrocarbons.

MEMORY, J. D. *Int. J. Quantum Chem.*, **15**, 363 (1979)
Polynuclear hydrocarbons.

LAVERY, R. and PULLMAN, B. *Int. J. Quantum Chem.*, **16**, 175 (1979)
Reactivity of benzopyrene diol epoxide with nucleic acid bases.

KAUFMAN, J. J. *Int. J. Quantum Chem.*, **16**, 221 (1979)
Ab initio calculations.

POLITZER, P., DAIKER, K. C. and ESTER, V. M. *Int. J. Quantum Chem. Quantum Biol. Symp.*, **6**, 47 (1979)
Role of hydrogen bonds in some diol epoxides.

HARIHARAN, P. C., KAUFMAN, J. J. and PETRONGOLO, C. *Int. J. Quantum Chem. Quantum Biol. Symp.*, **6**, 223 (1979)
Electrostatic potential of benzopyrene and its metabolites.

LOEW, G. H., SUDHINDRA, B. S., BURT, S., PACK, G. R. and MACELROY, R. *Int. J. Quantum Chem. Quantum Biol. Symp.*, **6**, 259 (1979)
Aromatic amines.

BERGER, G. D. and SEYBOLD, P. G. *Int. J. Quantum Chem. Quantum Biol. Symp.*, **6**, 305 (1979)
Chrysene and its methyl derivatives.

KAUFMAN, J. J. *Int. J. Quantum Chem. Quantum Biol. Symp.*, **6**, 503 (1979)
Ab initio calculations.

HUNT, W. E., SCHWALBE, C. H., BIRD, K. and MALLINSON, P. D. *Biochem. J.*, **187**, 533 (1980)
Geometry of antifolate drugs.

THOMSON, C. *Int. J. Quantum Chem. Quantum Biol. Symp.*, **7**, 163 (1980)
Equilibrium geometry of β-propiolactone.

LOEW, G. H., PUDZIANOWSKI, A. T., CZERWINSKI, A. and FERRELL, J. E. *Int. J. Quantum Chem. Quantum Biol. Symp.*, **7**, 223 (1980)
Arene oxides and diol epoxides.

SEYBOLD, P. and GRÄSLUND, A. *Int. J. Quantum Chem. Quantum Biol. Symp.*, **7**, 261 (1980)
Phenols of benzo[α]pyrene.

BOUDREAUX, E. and CARSEY, T. P. *Int. J. Quantum Chem.*, **18**, 469 (1980)
Quasi-relativistic calculations on platinum complexes and interactions with DNA.

ALIEV, Z. G., KARTSEV, V. G., ATOVMYAN, L. O. and BOGDANOV, G. N. *Khim. Farm. Zh.* **14**, 84 (1980)
Structures of antineoplastic drug diazan.

SAIRAM, R., BHARGAVA, S. and RAY, N. K. *Natn. Acad. Sci. Lett.* (*India*), **3**, 31 (1980)
Molecular orbital study of biologically active coumarins.

ULMER, W. *Int. J. Quantum Chem.*, **19**, 337 (1981)
Electronic structure of metabolites of cyclophophamide.

LOEW, G. H. and POULSEN, M. T. *Int. J. Quantum Chem. Quantum Biol. Symp.*, **8**, 95 (1981)
Aflatoxins: metabolism and carcinogenic activity.

SEYBOLD, P. G., VESTEWIG, R. and SCRIBNER, J. D. *Int. J. Quantum Chem. Quantum Biol. Symp.*, **8**, 385 (1981)
Reactivity indices and carcinogenicity.

Anti-hypertensives

WOHL, A. J. *Molec. Pharmac.*, **6**, 189 (1970)
Tautomerism of benzothiadiazines.

WOHL, A. J. *Molec. Pharmac.*, **6**, 195 (1970)
Correlation of anti-hypertensive properties of benzothiadiazines with EHT parameters.

WOHL, A. J. in L. B. Kier (ed), *Molecular Orbital Studies in Chemical Pharmacology*, Springer, New York, p. 282 (1970)

KULKARMI, V. M. *J. Biochem. B.*, **12**, 367 (1975)
Structure–activity relationship for anti-hypertensives.

TIMMERMANS, P. B. M. W. M. and Van ZWIETEN, P. A. *J. med. Chem.*, **20**, 1636 (1977)
Structure–activity relationships in clonidine related molecules.

Carbohydrates

NEELY, W. B. *J. med. Chem.*, **12**, 16 (1969)
EHT on a D glucopyranose.

GIACOMINI, M., PULLMAN, B. and MAIGRET, B. *Theoret. chim. Acta*, **19**, 347 (1970)
PCILO on disaccharides.

KIER, L. B. *J. Pharm. Sci.*, **61**, 1394 (1972)
Molecular theory of sweet taste.

Peptides

HÖLTJE, H.-D. *Int. J. Quantum Chem. Quantum Biol. Symp.*, **4**, 245 (1977)
Interaction of model systems with amino acids.
MOMANY, F. A., DRAKE, L. G. and AUBUCHON, J. R. *Int. J. Quantum Chem. Quantum Biol. Symp.*, **5**, 381 (1978)
Conformation of somatostatin.
Del CONDE, G., ESTRADA, M. and CARDENAS, A. *Int. J. Quantum Chem. Quantum Biol. Symp.*, **5**, 393 (1978)
Interaction of glyoxal with glycine and N-methylacetamide.
URRY, D. W., KHALED, M. A., RENUGOPALAKRISHNAN, V. and RAPAKA, R. S. *J. Am. chem. Soc.*, **100**, 696 (1978)
Conformation of tropoelastin.
LOEW, G. H. and BURT, S. K. *Proc. natn. Acad. Sci. U.S.A.*, **75**, 7 (1978)
Conformation of enkephalin and resemblance to opiates.
LAMBURELLE, C. and TAPIA, O. *Chem. Phys.*, **42**, 25 (1979)
Solvation of β-alanine and glycine by virtual charge model.
CABROL, D., BROCK, H. and VASILESCU, D. *Int. J. Quantum Chem. Quantum Biol. Symp.*, **6**, 365 (1979)
Study of gly-pro-pro repetitive unit.
BEVERIDGE, D. L., MEZEI, M., MEHROTRA, P. K., MARCHESE, F. T., THIRUMALAI, V. and RAVI-SHANKAR, G. *Ann. N. Y. Acad. Sci.*, **367**, 108 (1981)
Solvation.
PATERSON, Y., NEMETHY, G. and SCHERAGA, H. A. *Ann. N. Y. Acad. Sci.*, **367**, 132 (1981)
Solvation.
KARPLUS, M. *Ann. N. Y. Acad. Sci.*, **367**, 151 (1981)
Solvation.

Enzymes

GUND, P., POE, M. and HOOGSTEEN, K. H. *Molec. Pharmac.*, **13**, 1111 (1977)
Action of dihydrofolate reductase.
MILES, D. L., MILES, D. W., REDINGTON, P. and EYRING, H. *J. theoret. Biol.*, **67**, 499 (1977)
Conformational basis for selection of apo-adenine.
ANDREWS, P. R. and HEYDE, E. *J. theoret. Biol.*, **78**, 393 (1978)
Model for chorismate mutase-prephenate dehydrogenase.
DEMOULIN, D. and PULLMAN, B. *Theoret. chim. Acta*, **49**, 161 (1978)
Binding of zinc in catalytic sites.
ANDREWS, P. R. in E. C. Olson and R. E. Christoffersen (eds), *Computer Assisted Drug Design*, American Chem. Soc. Symposium Series, **112**, p. 149 (1979)
Design of transition state analogues.
DEMOULIN, D. and PULLMAN, A. in B. Pullman (ed), *Catalysis in Chemistry and Biochemistry. Theory and Experiment*, D. Reidel, Dordrecht, p. 51 (1979)
ANDREWS, P. R. and HADDON, R. C. *Aust. J. Chem.*, **32**, 1921 (1979)
Rearrangement of chorismate to prephenate.
CASE, D. A., HUYNTH, B. H. and KARPLUS, M. *J. Am. chem. Soc.*, **101**, 4433 (1979)
Binding of O_2 and CO to haemoglobin.
NAGATA, C. and YAMAGUCHI, T. *J. med. Chem.*, **22**, 13 (1979)
Mechanism of irreversible inhibitors.
OTTO, P., SEEL, M., LADIK, J. and MÜLLER, R. *J. theoret. Biol.*, **78**, 197 (1979)
Correlation of N-methyl transferase inhibitors.
ANDREWS, P. R. and HEYDE, E. *J. theoret. Biol.*, **78**, 393 (1979)
Common site model for chorismate mutase-prephenate dehydrogenase.
SAWARYN, A. and SOKALSKI, W. A. *Int. J. Quantum Chem.*, **16**, 293 (1979)
Carbonic anhydrase.

PULLMAN, A. and DEMOULIN, D. *Int. J. Quantum Chem.*, **16**, 641 (1979)
Active site of carbonic anhydrase.
ROHMER, M.-M. and LOEW, G. H. *Int. J. Quantum Chem. Quantum Biol. Symp.*, **6**, 93 (1979)
Model of cytochrome P450.
PACK, G. R., and LOEW, G. H. *Int. J. Quantum Chem. Quantum Biol. Symp.*, **6**, 381 (1979)
Model for cytochrome P450.
LAVERY, R. and PULLMAN, B. *Int. J. Quantum Chem. Quantum Biol. Symp.*, **6**, 467 (1979)
Action of glyoxalase I.
PULLMAN, A. and DEMOULIN, D. in B. Pullman and K. Yagi (eds), *Water and Metal Cations in Biological Systems*, Japan. Sci. Soc. Press, Tokyo (1980)
Active site of carbonic anhydrase.
OSMAN, R. and WEINSTEIN, H. *Israel. J. Chem.*, **19**, 149 (1980)
Models for carboxypeptidase.
HERMAN, Z. S., LOEW, G. H. and ROHMER, M.-M. *Int. J. Quantum Chem. Quantum Biol. Symp.*, **7**, 137 (1980)
Model of carbonlyheme complexes.
NÁRAY-SZABÓ, G. and POLGÁR, L. *Int. J. Quantum Chem. Quantum Biol. Symp.*, **7**, 397 (1980)
Environmental effects on proton transfer in subtilisin.
Van DUIJNEN, P. T., THOLE, B. T., BROER, R. and NIEUWPOORT, W. C. *Int. J. Quantum Chem.*, **17**, 651 (1980)
Active site of papain.
ABDUL-AHAD, P. G., BLAIR, T. and WEBB, G. A. *Int. J. Quantum Chem.*, **17**, 821 (1980)
Enzyme-inhibitory quinazolines.
LOEW, G. H., HERMAN, Z. S. and ZERNER, M. C. *Int. J. Quantum Chem.*, **18**, 481 (1980)
Model oxylene complex.
PUDZIANOWSKI, A. T. and LOEW, G. H. *J. Am. Chem. Soc.*, **102**, 5443 (1980)
Model of cytochrome P450.
LOEW, G. H., HERMAN, Z. S., ROHMER, M.-M., GOLDBLUM, A. and PUDZIANOWSKI, A. *Ann. N. Y. Acad. Sci.*, **367**, 151 (1981)
Model cytochrome P450.
PULLMAN, A. *Ann. N. Y. Acad. Sci.*, **367**, 340 (1981)
Carbonic anhydrase model.
OSMAN, R., WEINSTEIN, H. and TOPIOL, S. *Ann. N. Y. Acad. Sci.*, **367**, 356 (1981)
Model of metalloenzymes.
WARSHEL, A. and WEISS, R. M. *Ann. N. Y. Acad. Sci.*, **367**, 370 (1981)
Empirical valence bond calculations.
ALLEN, L. C. *Ann. N. Y. Acad. Sci.*, **367**, 383 (1981)
Catalytic function of active amino acid side chains.
GODDARD, W. A. and OLAFSON, B. D. *Ann. N. Y. Acad. Sci.*, **367**, 419 (1981)
Study of oxygen binding.
KARPLUS, M. *Ann. N. Y. Acad. Sci.*, **367**, 407 (1981)
Aspects of protein dynamics.
GUND, P. and SCHLEGEL, H. B. *Ann. N. Y. Acad. Sci.*, **367**, 510 (1981)
Dihydrocolate reductase inhibitors.
KOLLMAN, P. A. and HAYES, D. M. *J. Am. chem. Soc.*, **103**, 2955 (1981)
Proton transfer mechanism in serine and cysteine proteases.
SHIBATA, M., KIEBER-EMMONS, T., DUTTA, S. and REIN, R. *Int. J. Quantum. Chem. Quantum Biol. Symp.*, **8**, 409 (1981)
Stability of chymotrypsin charge relay triad.

Nucleic acids

PACK, G. R. and LOEW, G. H. *Int. J. Quantum Chem. Quantum Biol. Symp.*, **4**, 87 (1977)
Ethidium nucleic acid intercalation.
SARAN, A., MITRA, C. and PULLMAN, B. *Biochim. biophys. Acta*, **517**, 255 (1978)
Conformation of 8-azapurine nucleosides.
POHORILLE, A., PERAHIA, D. and PULLMAN, B. *Biochim. biophys. Acta*, **517**, 511 (1978)
Conformation of amino and methyl adenosine monophosphate.

PERAHIA, D. and PULLMAN, A. *Theoret. chim. Acta*, **48**, 263 (1978)
Electrostatic potential of complementary bases.
LAVERY, R., PULLMAN, A. and PULLMAN, B. *Theoret. chim. Acta*, **50**, 67 (1978)
Acidity and basicity of amino groups.
DEMOULIN, D., ARMBRUSTER, A.-M. and PULLMAN, B. *Theoret. chim. Acta*, **50**, 75 (1978)
Interaction of methyl glyoxal with guanine.
NUSS, M. E. and KOLLMAN, P. *J. med. Chem.*, **22**, 1517 (1979)
Electrostatic potential of deoxynucleoside monophosphates.
PULLMAN, A., ZAKRZEWSKA, C. and PERAHIA, D. *Int. J. Quantum Chem.*, **16**, 395 (1979)
Electrostatic potential of B-DNA.
PERAHIA, D., PULLMAN, A. and PULLMAN, B. *Int. J. Quantum Chem. Quantum Biol. Symp.*, **6**, 353 (1979)
Electrostatic potential of B-DNA.
ZIELINSKI, T. J., SHIHATA, M. and REIN, R. *Int. J. Quantum Chem. Quantum Biol. Symp.*, **6**, 475 (1979)
Tautomerism of uracil.
PULLMAN, B., PERAHIA, D. and CAUCHY, D. *Nucleic Acids Res.*, **6**, 3821 (1979)
Electrostatic potential.
PULLMAN, B., MIERTUS, S. and PERAHIA, D. *Theoret. chim. Acta*, **50**, 317 (1979)
Hydration of bases and base pairs.
PERAHIA, D., PULLMAN, A. and PULLMAN, B. *Theoret. chim. Acta*, **51**, 349 (1979)
Electrostatic potential of B-DNA due to sugar–phosphate backbone.
PERAHIA, D. and PULLMAN, A. *Theoret. chim. Acta*, **50**, 351 (1979)
Electrostatic potential of B-DNA.
LAVERY, R. and PULLMAN, B. *Theoret. chim. Acta*, **53**, 175 (1979)
Electrostatic potential of B-DNA.
GRESH, N. and PULLMAN, B. *Biochim. biophys. Acta*, **608**, 47 (1980)
Interaction of guanine and cytosine with amino acids.
LANGLET, J., GIESSNER-PRETTRE, C., PULLMAN, B., CLAVERIE, P. and PIAZZOLA, D. *Int. J. Quantum Chem.*, **18**, 421 (1980)
Purine–water interactions in base stacking.
MILLER, K. J., LAUER, M. and ARCHER, S. *Int. J. Quantum Chem. Quantum Biol. Symp.*, **7**, 11 (1980)
Intercalation of thioxanthenones into DNA.
PULLMAN, A. and PULLMAN, B. *Int. J. Quantum Chem. Quantum Biol. Symp.*, **7**, 245 (1980)
Reactivity and chemical carcinogenesis.
LAVERY, R., PULLMAN, A. and PULLMAN, B. *Nucleic Acids Res.*, **8**, 1061 (1980)
Electrostatic potential of yeast tRNA.
ZAKRZEWSKA, K., LAVERY, R., PULLMAN, A. and PULLMAN, B. *Nucleic Acids Res.*, **8**, 3917 (1980)
Electrostatic potential and accessibility in Z-DNA.
LAVERY, R., PULLMAN, A., PULLMAN, B. and de OLIVEIRA, M. *Nucleic Acids Res.*, **8**, 5095 (1980)
Electrostatic molecular potential of tRNA.
DEAN, P. M. and WAKELIN, L. P. G. *Proc. R. Soc. B*, **209**, 453 (1980)
Electrostatic potential of polynucleotides.
LAVERY, R., PULLMAN, A. and PULLMAN, B. *Theoret. chim. Acta*, **57**, 233 (1980)
Molecular potential and steric accessibility of yeast tRNA.
CLEMENTI, E. and CORONGIU, G. *Ann. N. Y. Acad. Sci.*, **367**, 83 (1981)
Simulation of solvation.
PULLMAN, B. *Ann. N. Y. Acad. Sci.*, **367**, 182 (1981)
Electrostatic potentials.
PACK, G. R., HASHIMOTO, G. M. and LOEW, G. A. *Ann. N. Y. Acad. Sci.*, **367**, 240 (1981)
Mechanism of proflavin binding.
LAVERY, R., PULLMAN, A. and PULLMAN, B. *Int. J. Quantum Chem.*, **20**, 49 (1981)
Steric accessibility of reactive centre in RNA.
LONGLET, J., CLAVERIE, P., CARON, F. and BOEUVE, J. C. *Int. J. Quantum Chem.*, **20**, 299 (1981)
Role of charge distribution in interactions.

CHOJNACKI, H., LIPINSKI, J. and SOKALSKI, W. A. *Int. J. Quantum Chem.*, **20**, 339 (1981)
    Base pairs in model systems.
LAVERY, R., CORBIN, S. and PULLMAN, A. *Int. J. Quantum Chem. Quantum Biol. Symp.*, **8**, 171 (1981)
    Influence of counter ion on electrostatic potential.

Molecular graphics

BARRY, C. D. and NORTH, A. C. T. *Cold Spring Harb. Symp. quant. Biol.*, **36**, 577 (1971)
    Classic introduction.
MEYER, E. F. *Nature, Lond.*, **232**, 255 (1971)
    Description of the Brookhaven system.
FELDMAN, R. J., HELLER, S. R. and BACON, C. R. T. *J. chem. Documn*, **12**, 234 (1974)
    Accessing the Cambridge data base.
FELDMAN, R. J. *Ann. Rev. Biophys. and Bioeng.*, **5**, 477 (1976)
    Review of available systems.
EATON, D. F. and PENSAK, D. A. *J. Am. chem. Soc.*, **100**, 7428 (1978)
    Description of the Dupont system.
SMITH, G. M. and GUND, P. *J. chem. Inf. Comput. Sci.*, **18**, 207 (1978)
    Description of Merck system.
COLE, G. M., MEYER, E. F., SWANSON, S. M. and WHITE, W. G. in E. C. Olson and R. E. Christoffersen (eds), *Computer Assisted Drug Design*, Symp., **112**, 190, American Chem. Soc., New York (1979)
    Modelling active sites.
MARSHALL, G. R., BARRY, C. D., BOSSHARD, H. E., DAMMKOCHLER, R. A. and DUNN, D. A. in E. C. Olson and R. E. Christoffersen (eds), *Computer Assisted Drug Design*, Symp., **112**, 205, American Chem. Soc., New York (1979)
    The MMS-X system.
GUND, P., GRABOWSKI, E. J., SMITH, G. M., ANDOSE, J. D., RHODES, J. B. and WIPKE, W. T. in E. C. Olson and R. E. Christoffersen (eds), *Computer Assisted Drug Design*, Symp., **112**, 527, American Chem. Soc., New York, (1979)
    Merck system.
FULLERTON, D. S., YOSHIOKA, K., ROHRER, D. C., FROM, A. H. and AHMED, K. *Science, N.Y.*, **205**, 917 (1979)
    Description of NIH prophet system.
FERRIN, T. E. and LANGRIDGE, R. *Comput. Graphics*, **13**, 320 (1980)
    Description of UCSF system.
DYOTT, T. M., STUPER, A. J. and ZANDER, J. S. *J. chem. Inf. Comput. Sci.*, **20**, 28 (1980)
    Description of the Moly system at Rohm and Haas.
GUND, P., ANDOSE, J. D., RHODES, J. B. and SMITH, G. M. *Science, N.Y.*, **208**, 1425 (1980)
    Use of molecular graphics in drug design.
HUMBLET, C. and MARSHALL, G. R. *Drug Dev. Res.*, **1**, 409 (1981)
    Applications to drug design.
LANGRIDGE, R., FERRIN, T. E., KUNTZ, I. D. and CONNOLLY, M. L. *Science, N.Y.*, **211**, 661 (1981)
    The UCSF system including surfaces.

Miscellaneous

TINLAND, B., *Res. Commun. Chem. Pathol. Pharmac.*, **6**, 769 (1967)
    Phenols.
CROW, R., WASSERMAN, O. and HOLLAND, W. C. *J. med. Chem.*, **12**, 764 (1969)
    Phenylcholine ethers; Hückel study of charge densities.
WALD, R. W. and FEUER, G. *J. med. Chem.*, **14**, 1081 (1971)
    Structure–activity relationships for coumarin derivatives by EHT.

PERADEJORDI, F., MARTIN, A., CHALVET, O. and DAUDEL, R. *J. Pharm. Sci.*, **61,** 909 (1972)
Base strengths of benzacridines.
BUSTARD, T. M. and MARTIN, Y. C. *J. med. Chem.*, **15,** 1101 (1972)
Antisecretory agents: EHT on anti-peptic ulcer compounds.
SHINAGAWA, Y. *Jap. J. Pharmac.*, **23,** 615 (1973)
Diuretics; xanthine thiazide and triazine.
COURRIÈRE, P., PAUBEL, J. C. and NIVIÈRE, P. *C. r. hebd. Séanc. Acad. Sci.*, *Paris*, **279,** 1495 (1974)
Anti-fibrillation compounds.
CLONEY, R. D., KING, I. J., SCHERR, V. M. and FORGASH, A. J. in 'Molecular and quantum pharmacology', E. D. Bergmann and B. Pullman (eds), *Proc. 7th Jerusalem Symposium on Quantum Chemistry and Biochemistry*, D. Reidel, Dordrecht, p. 333 (1974)
Benzyl propynyl ethers.
IMAMURA, A. and NAGATA, C. *Gann*, **65,** 417 (1974)
MO study of activity of nitrosoguanidines.
UMEYAMA, H. *Chem. Pharm.*, **22,** 2518 (1974)
MO study of aspirin derivatives and acyl alpha chymotrypsin.
HOLEM, G. and SPURLING, T. H. *Experientia*, **30,** 480 (1974)
DDT analogues.
PULLMAN, B. and BERTHOD, H. *FEBS Letters*, **44,** 266 (1974)
Phospholipids; conformation of polar headgroups.
PULLMAN, B., PULLMAN, A., BERTHOD, H. and GRESH, N. *Theoret. chim. Acta*, **40,** 93 (1975)
Phosphate group hydration.
TINLAND, B. *Farmaco. Sci.*, **30,** 418 (1975)
Salicylaldehydes; activity relationship using CNDO and EHT.
WELLER, T. and FRISCHLEDER, H. *Chem. Phys. Lipids*, **15,** 5 (1975)
Quantum mechanics and empirical calculations on model headgroups.
ALDRICH, H. S. and CLAGETT, D. C. *J. Pharm. Sci.*, **65,** 1704 (1976)
CNDO conformational study of anti-schistomal agents.
ALEXANDER, K. S., PETERSON, H., TURCOTTE, J. G. and PARUTA, A. N. *J. Pharm. Sci.*, **65,** 851 (1976)
Structure–activity relationship of preservatives using IEHT.
KAUFMAN, J. J. *Int. J. Quantum Chem. Quantum Biol. Symp.*, **3,** 187 (1976)
Comprehensive discussion of molecular neuro-transmitter disorders.
SHINAGAWA, Y. *Int. J. Quantum Chem. Quantum Biol. Symp.*, **1,** 169 (1976)
Hückel MO studies on diuretics and carbonic anhydrase inhibitors.
GIESSNER-PRETTRE, C. and PULLMAN, B. *C. r. hebd. Séanc. Acad. Sci., Paris*, **283,** 675 (1976)
Electrostatic molecular potentials for ethidium guanacrine and proflavine.
PERAHIA, D., PULLMAN, A. and PULLMAN, B. *Theoret. chim. Acta*, **43,** 207 (1977)
Interaction of Na^+ with bases.
GUND, P. and SHEN, T. Y. *J. med. Chem.*, **20,** 1146 (1977)
Conformational analysis of indomethacin model for protaglandin synthetase site.
HALL, W. R. *J. med. Chem.*, **20,** 275 (1977)
Electronic structures of alloxan and its tautomers.
CHENEY, B. V., WRIGHT, J. B., HALL, C. L., JOHNSON, H. G. and CHRISTOFFERSEN, R. E. *J. med. Chem.*, **21,** 936 (1978)
Structure–activity relationship. Oxanilic quinaldic, and benzopyran-Z-carboxylic acids, anti-allergy agents.
WEBB, N. E. and THOMPSON, C. C. *J. Pharm. Sci.*, **67,** 165 (1978)
Complexing ability of quinoline and its simple derivatives.
CHRISTOFFERSEN, R. E. in E. C. Olson and R. E. Christoffersen (eds), *Computer Assisted Drug Design*, Symp., **112,** 3, American Chem. Soc., New York (1979)
Quantum pharmacology recent progress and current status.
DEMOULIN, D., ARMBRUSTER, A.-M., and PULLMAN, B. *Int. J. Quantum Chem.*, **16,** 631 (1979)
Interaction of glyoxal with arginine.

FULLERTON, D. S., YOSHIOKA, K., ROHRER, D. C., FROM, A. H. L. and AHMED, K. *Molec. Pharmac.*, **17**, 43 (1979)
Conformation of digitalis.
DENISOFF, O., Van DAMME, M., HANOCQ, M., MOLLE, L., GEERLINGS, P. and FIGEYS, H. P. *Nouv. J. Chim.*, **3**, 561 (1979)
Intramolecular hydrogen bonds in procainamide drugs.
KOROLKOVAS, A. and NICODEMO, S. A. *Quím. Nova.*, **2**, 2 (1979)
Mode of action of lucanthone and hycanthone at electronic and molecular levels.
KOCJAN, D. and HADZI, D. *Vest. slov. kem. Društ.*, **26**, 229 (1979)
Conformation of 2-phenylpropionic acid, anti-inflammatory.
OIKAWA, S., TSUDA, M., OHNOGI, S. and KURITA, N. *Chem. pharm. Bull., Tokyo*, **28**, 1946 (1980)
Application of molecular orbital theory for screening antifungal drugs.
FAWZI, M. B., DAVISON, E. and TUTE, M. S. *J. Pharm. Sci.*, **69**, 104 (1980)
Rationalization of complexation in solution using Hückel frontier orbitals.
FARRIMOND, J. A., ELLIOT, M. C. and CLACK, D. W. *Phytochemistry*, **20**, 1185 (1981)
Structure–activity relationship for aryloxyacetic acids.

Index